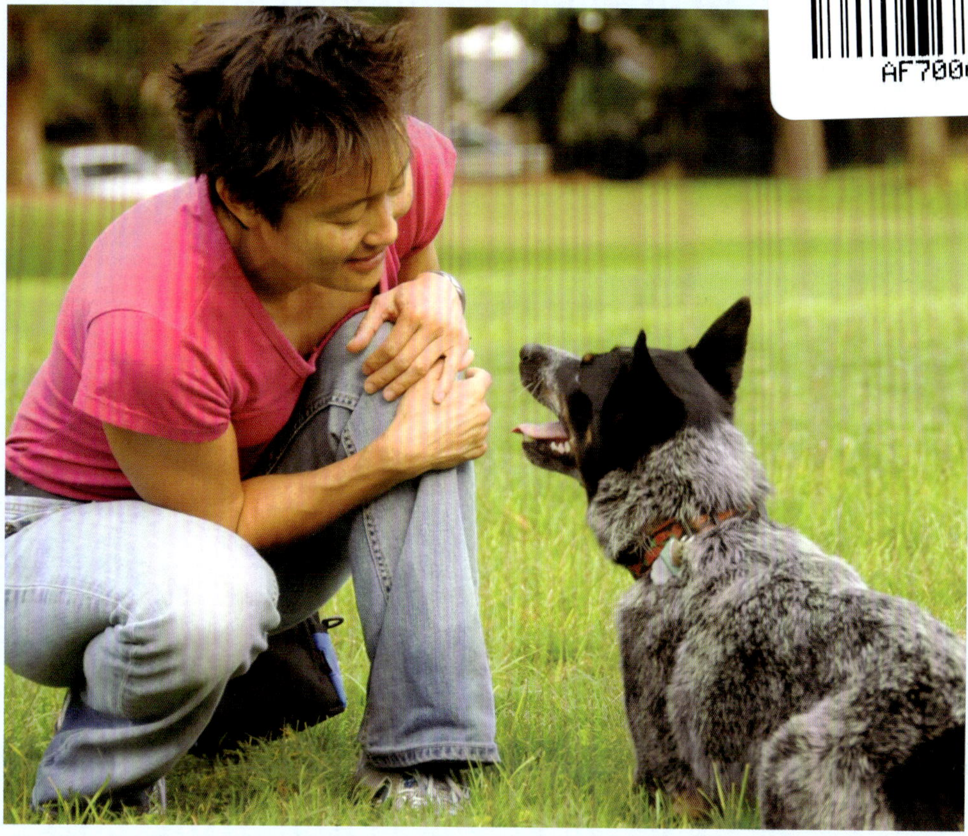

February 5, 1966 – September 28, 2014

In Memory of
Dr. Sophia Yin, DVM, CAAB, MS

Veterinarian, animal behaviorist, author, and
the creator of Low Stress Handling®.

Through scientific methods, rigorous research, and testing, she created the foundations of Low Stress Handling®, the origins for many modern animal behavior and training programs. Her methods are taught and applied in veterinary schools and clinics around the world. Her work reshaped the behavior, handling, and training standard of care for veterinary professionals, pet professionals, shelter workers, and pet owners. Dr. Yin passed away in September of 2014, but through CattleDog Publishing® and Veterinary Information Network®, Inc., her work and legacy lives on.

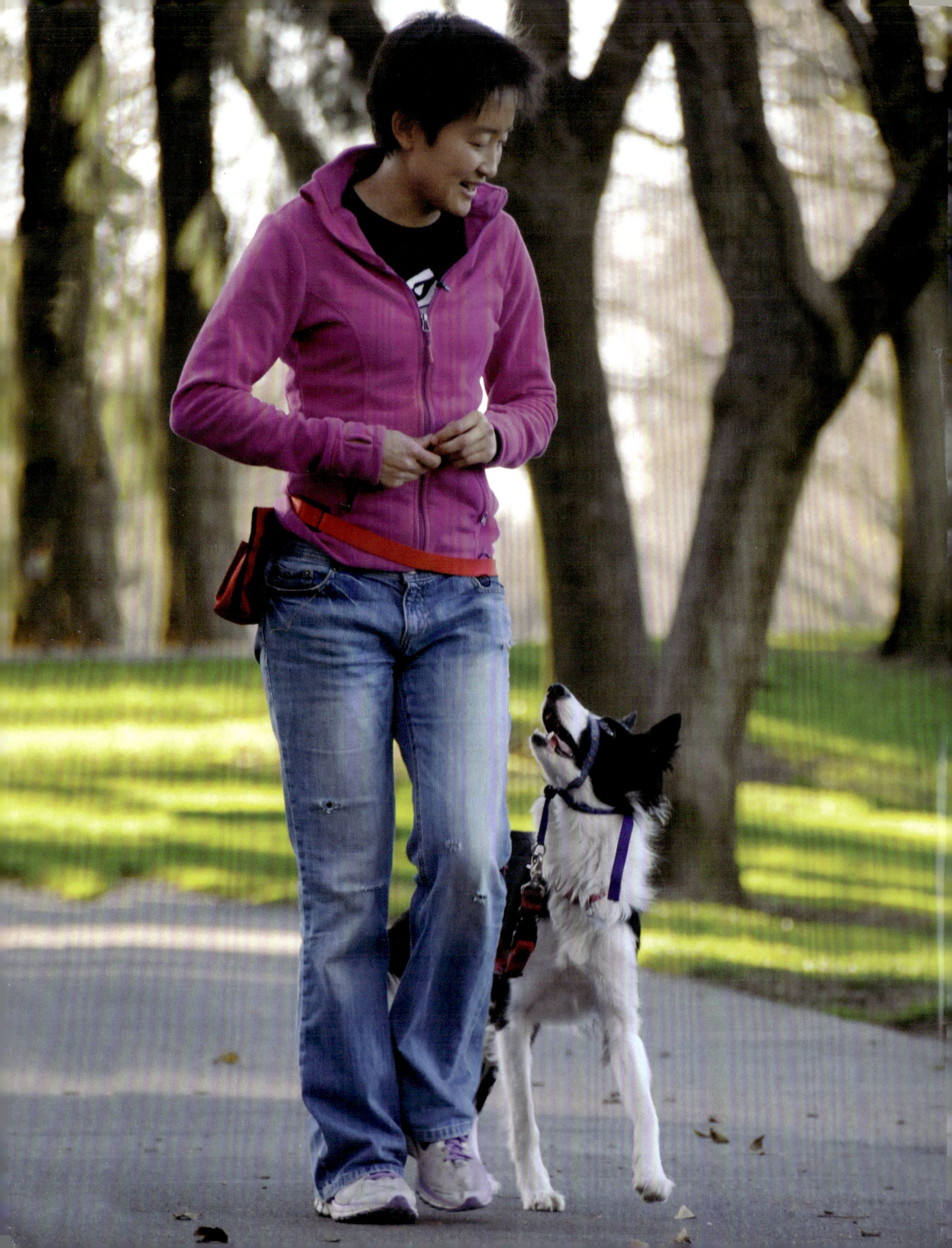

Second Edition

Dr. Sophia Yin's Low Stress Handling® and Behavior Modification of Dogs and Cats

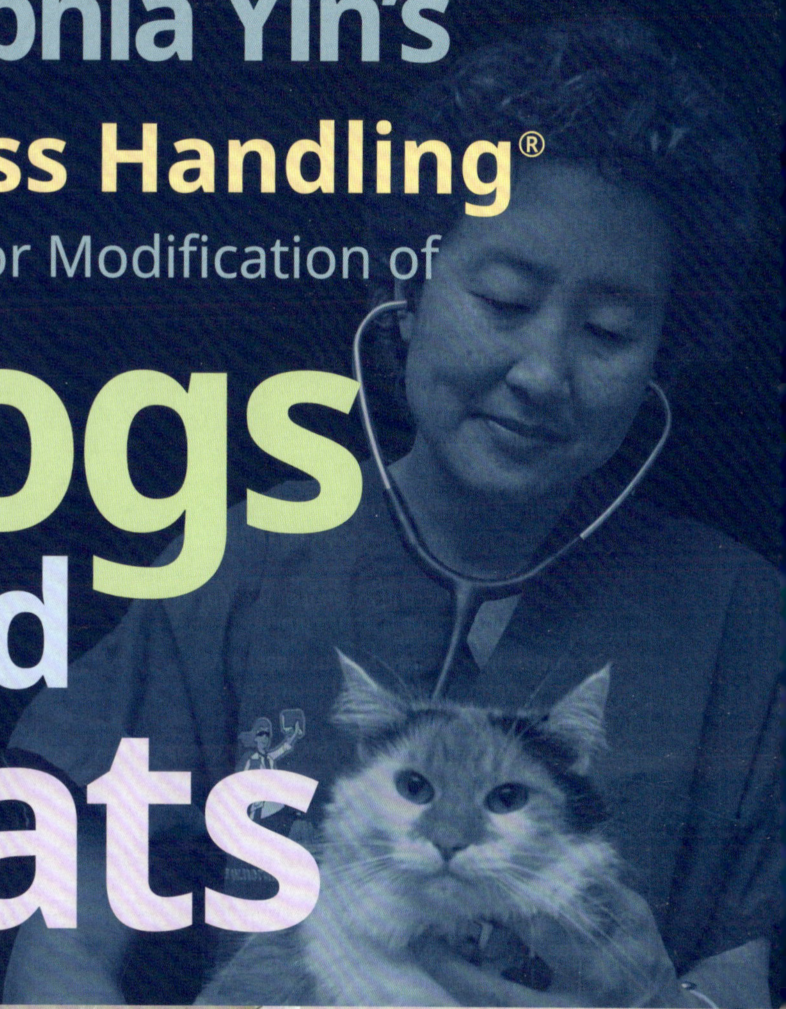

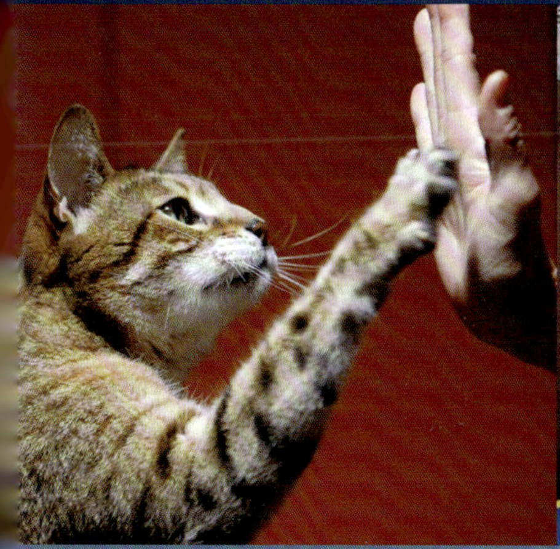

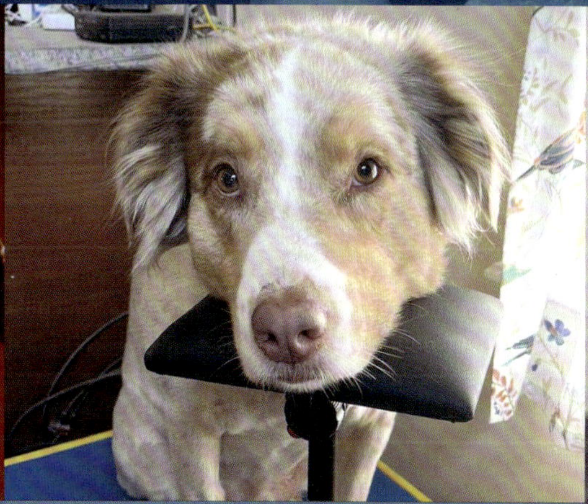

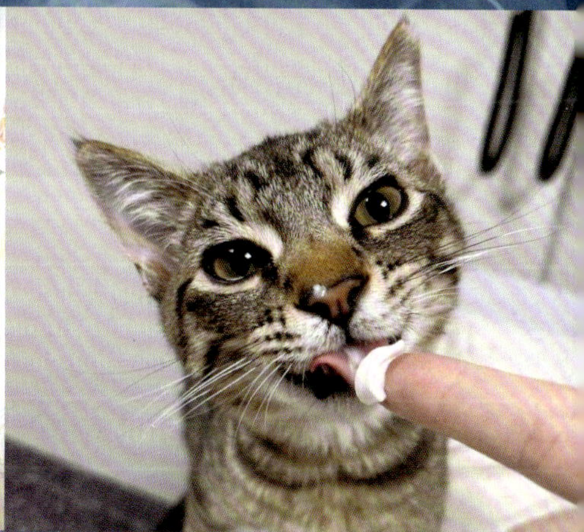

EDITED BY CHRISTINE D. CALDER AND PAT KOVEN

CattleDog Publishing®

Low Stress Handling® and Behavior Modification of Dogs and Cats
Second Edition
Edited by
Christine D. Calder DVM, DACVB
Pat Koven BA in Journalism, LVT, KPA-CTP

Published by Veterinary Information Network, Inc., Davis, California

Library of Congress Cataloging

ISBN: 978-0-9914953-9-9

Book Design by Michael Rohani, DesignforBooks.com
Cover Images: CattleDog Publishing

Limitation of Liability/Disclaimer of Warranty:

For general information on our other products and services or for technical support, please contact our Customer Care Department within the United States at (530)757-2383.

The Veterinary Information Network, Inc. also publishes its books in a variety of electronic formats. Some content that appears in print may not be available in electronic formats. For more information about CattleDog Publishing's products and additional copies of this work, visit our website at www.cattledogpublishing.com

Thank You

Heartfelt thanks to Jackie Brister, Heather Howell, and Pegi Webster for their exceptional editing wisdom and grammar expertise—they truly went above and beyond. Special thanks to all the reviewers, including Ilona Rodan, Kelly St. Denis, Nancy Welborn, Ali Gottlieb, Shannon Emmons, Ginny Price, Carla Pion, the CattleDog Publishing ®Team, and especially Christine Calder's mother, Dianne LeSage, whose fresh perspectives and invaluable feedback were instrumental in shaping this book. Sincere gratitude to Paul Pion and Raphael Moore for bringing this book to life. Lastly, a profound thank you to Jackie, Sophia's mother, for entrusting the Veterinary Information Network®, Inc. with Sophia's life's work, ensuring that her legacy continues to inspire future generations.

About the Editors

Dr. Christine Calder has practiced veterinary medicine in New Jersey, Maine, Louisiana, Alabama, and Mississippi for many years. She has worked in general practice, as part of the behavior service at the San Francisco SPCA, and held positions as a Clinical Instructor and Assistant Clinical Professor in community practice at several veterinary school teaching hospitals. With a deep interest in animal behavior, Dr. Calder completed a residency with the American College of Veterinary Behaviorists in 2016, becoming a Diplomate (DACVB) in 2017. She is currently the Chief Behavior Officer for CattleDog Publishing® and a Consultant with the Veterinary Information Network®, Inc. Dr. Calder is particularly passionate about education, with a focus on preparing veterinary students to be "Day One" ready for practice.

Pat Koven has been a Licensed Veterinary Technician (LVT) since 1993 and holds a BA in Journalism. In 2019, she became a Certified Training Partner from the Karen Pryor Academy and coauthored the Therapy Dog Team Training Course for the academy in 2023. With over 35 years of experience, Pat has trained and supervised team members in both clinical and behavioral skills. Since 2018, she has led the Maine chapter of Love on a Leash, supervising over 40 teams visiting schools, libraries, hospitals, nursing homes, and hospice facilities. She enjoys working with caregivers, teaching them how to develop and change animal behaviors using positive reinforcement methodologies and training techniques. Currently, Pat is the Customer Engagement Specialist at CattleDog Publishing® and owns her training and behavior modification business, Haulin' Aus Training, Inc.

List of Contributors

Jessica Benoit RVT, VTS (Behavior), KPA-CTP, CPDT-KA
Co-owner and Veterinary Technician Specialist in Behavior
Companion Veterinary Clinic
Edmonton, Ab, Canada

Stephanie Borns-Weil, DVM, DACVB
Assistant Clinical Professor, Department of Clinical Sciences
Cummings School of Veterinary Medicine
Tufts University
North Grafton, MA, USA

Desireé Broach, DVM, MS, DACVB
Deputy Director & Chief of Behavior
LTC Daniel E Holland MWD Hospital
JBSA-Lackland, TX, USA

Monique Feyrecilde BA, LVT, VTS(Behavior)
Teaching Animals
Auburn, WA, USA

Anneliese Heinrich MSc, DVM
Rockyview Veterinary Behaviour Consulting
Cochrane, AB, Canada

Colleen S. Koch, DVM. DACVB
Co-Owner Lincoln Land Animal Clinic, LTD.
Jacksonville, IL, USA

M. Leanne Lilly, DVM, DACVB
Assistant Professor-Clinical, Service Head-Behavioral Medicine
The Ohio State University
Veterinary Medical Center at Dublin
Dublin, OH, USA

Sandra Robbins CVT, VTS (anesthesia & analgesia), CPDT-KSA, KPA CTP
Behavior Technician Cummings School of Veterinary Medicine
Tufts University
North Grafton, MA, USA

Katharine Schwarz RVT, KPA-CTP
Owner Kat, Behaviour Tech
Ottawa, Ontario, Canada

Laura Ward Ansel, DVM
Owner and Veterinarian
Louisiana Veterinary Behavior Services
Mandeville, LA, USA

Sherrie Yuschak, RVT, VTS (Behavior), KPA-CTP
Faculty Karen Pryor Academy for Animal Training and Behavior
Lillington, NC, USA

Dedication to Dr. Sophia Yin

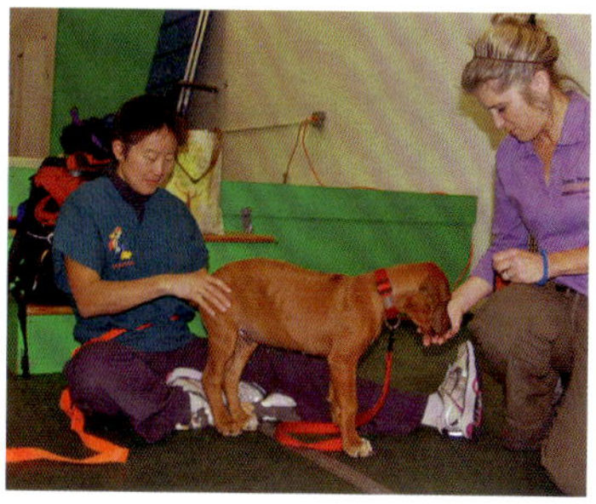

In the Summer of 2010, a two-day seminar, taught by Dr. Sophia Yin and Sarah Kalnajs, opened for registration in the Chicagoland area. I registered immediately, and couldn't wait to learn more about the Low Stress Handling® techniques featured in Dr. Yin's new book.

With the seminar date fast approaching, what I didn't predict upon signing up, was a new canine family member that would join our family that October. Santino was only nine weeks of age, and couldn't be left alone for that long.

I recall the heavy weight felt on my shoulders as I emailed Dr. Yin to share the need to withdraw attendance in order to care for our new puppy, due to arrive one week before the workshop.

Dr. Yin's enthusiastic response, one coupled with congratulations and an inclusive proposal, lifted that weight yet set the tone for an ongoing professional and personal friendship. She suggested that Santino join us for their workshop so he could remain close to me for puppy care, and perhaps participate in a few short hands-on demonstrations for their seminar guests to learn from.

So, with my new canine family member along for the ride, we drove to the two-day workshop to learn together with colleagues. I'm truly grateful that this treasured photograph was taken, for it epitomizing two treasured mentors working as a team. As I offered my sweet puppy his food, Dr. Yin and he demonstrated Low Stress Handling techniques.

Our communication between then and 2014 includes additional special memories; those I hold close to my heart. The constant theme within them are Dr. Yin's tremendous contributions to our community that educate canine and feline caregivers through continuing education. The excellent resources and content authored by her that promote ethical animal care. Collaboration within the veterinary and training community. The ongoing positive impact that others still speak of with admiration and appreciation.

Dr. Sophia Yin's memory continues to thrive as a direct reflection on the amazing person she is.

With gratitude to Sophia and her family,
Laura Monaco Torelli

Contents

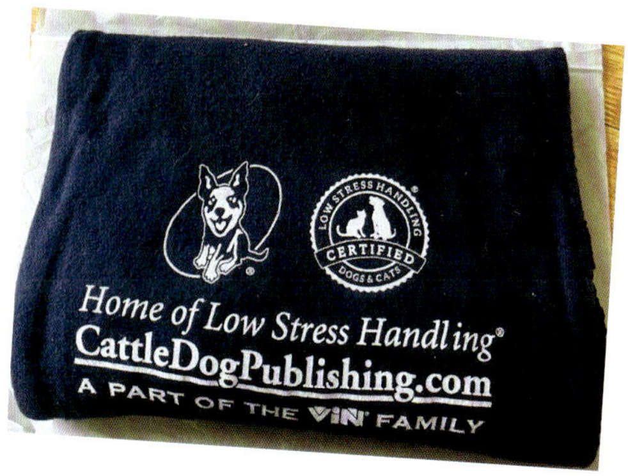

LOW STRESS HANDLING
CERTIFIED
DOGS & CATS
Home of Low Stress Handling®
CattleDogPublishing.com
A PART OF THE VIN® FAMILY

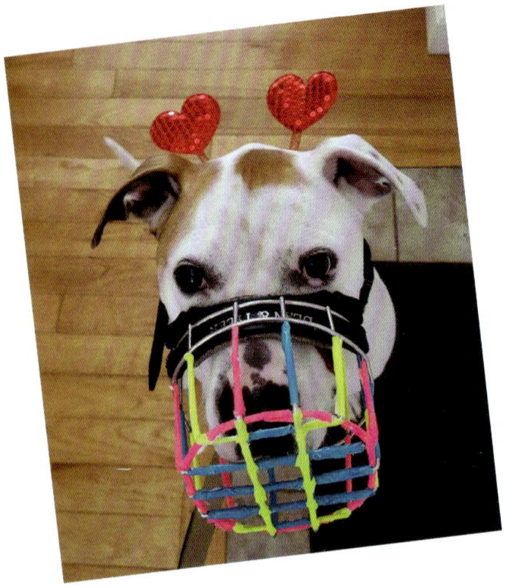

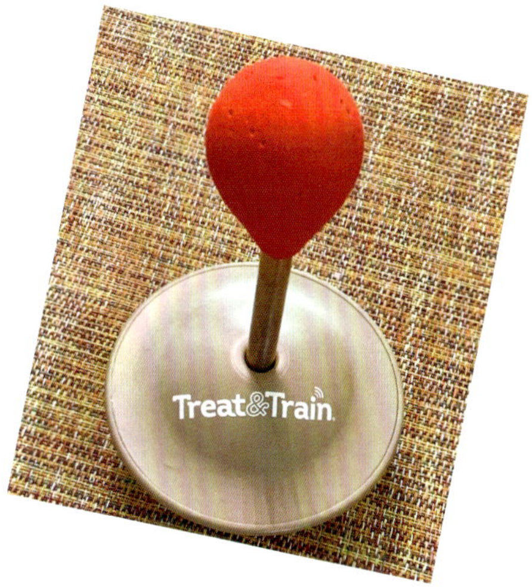
Treat&Train

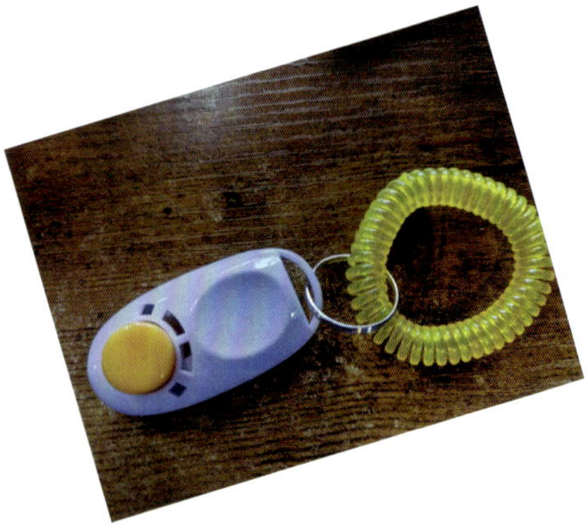

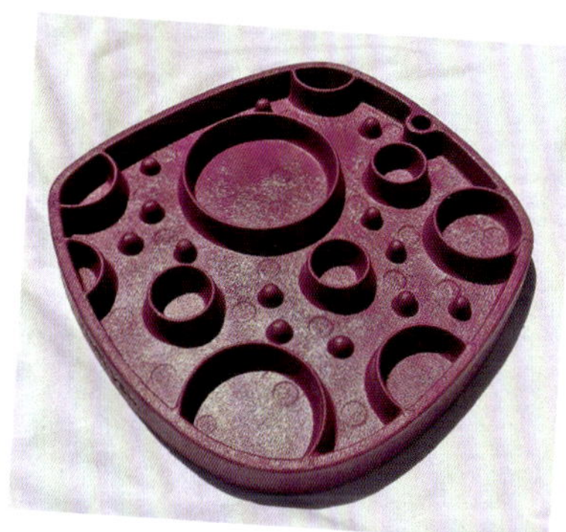

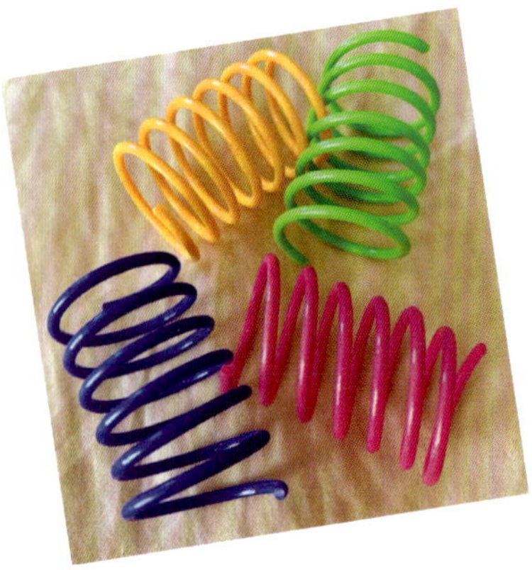

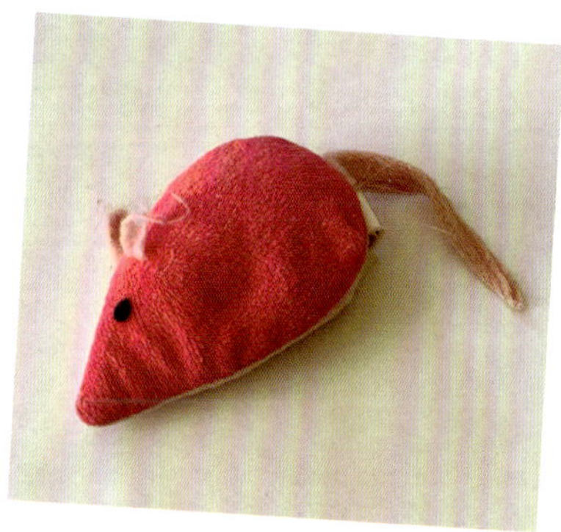

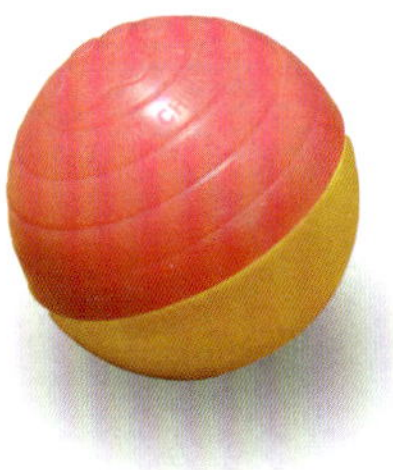

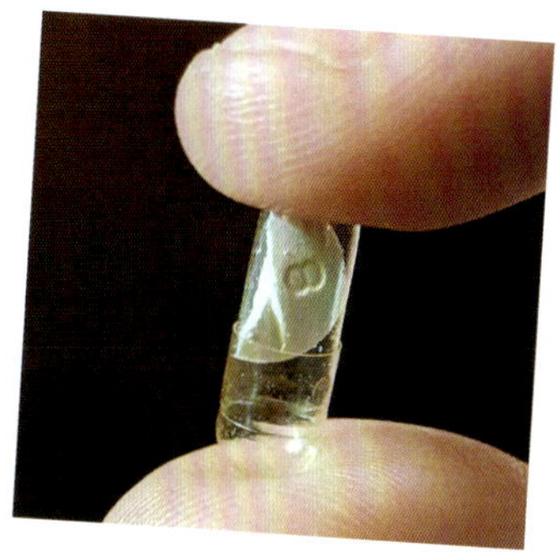

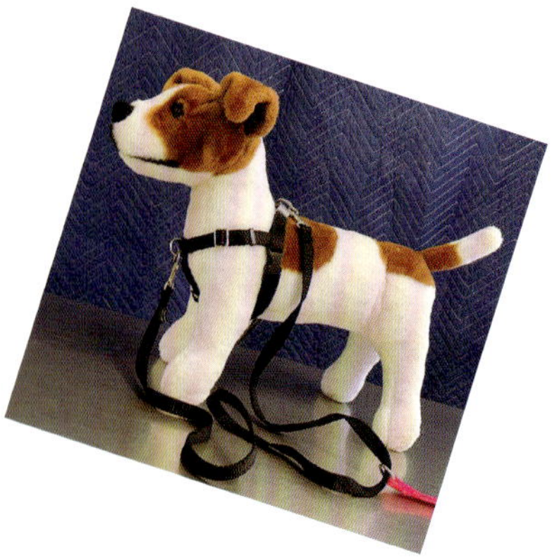

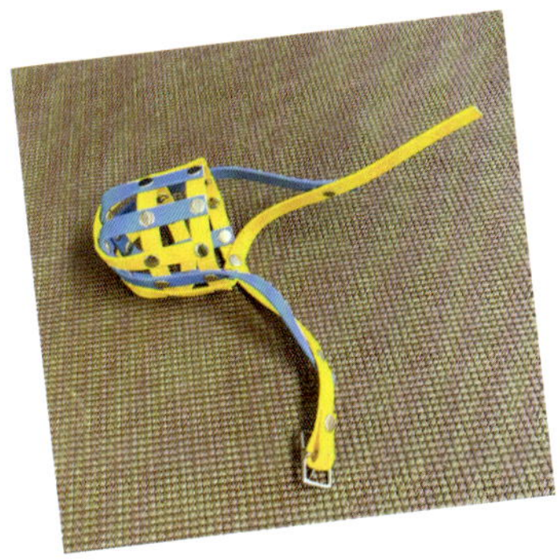

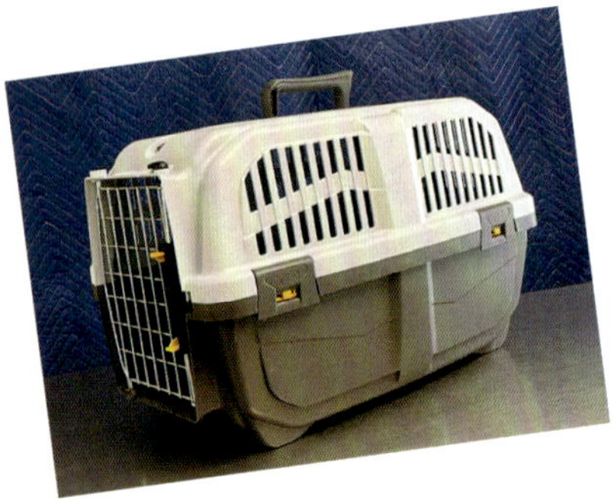

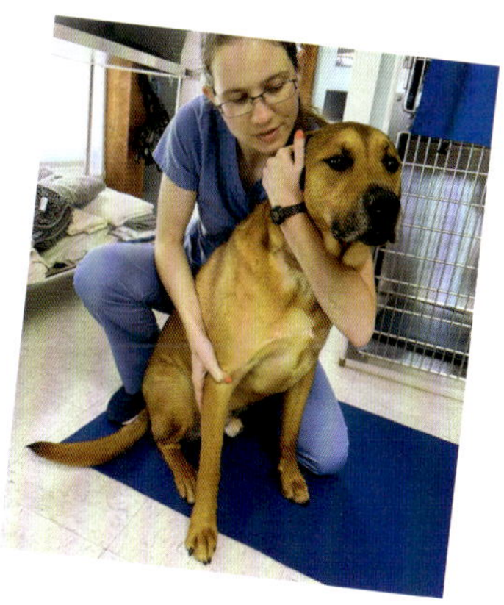

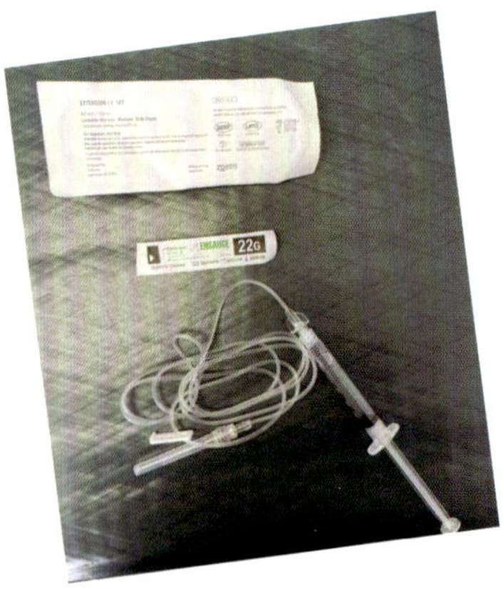

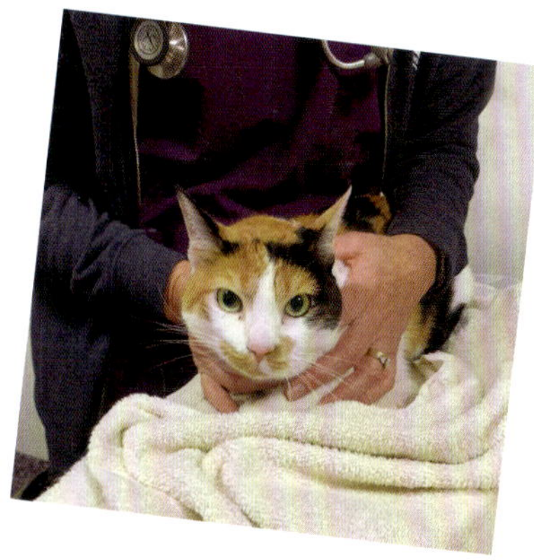

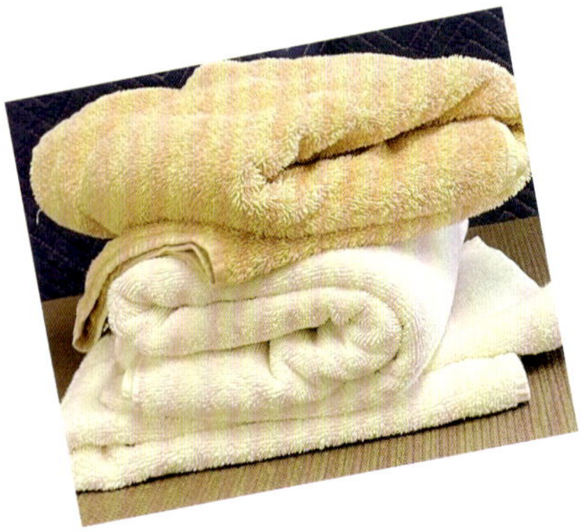

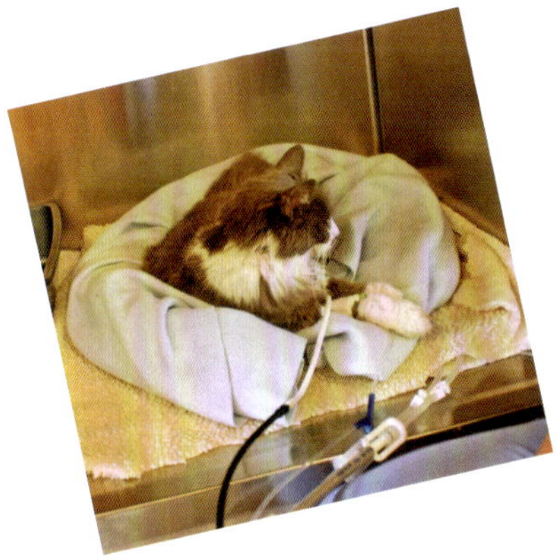

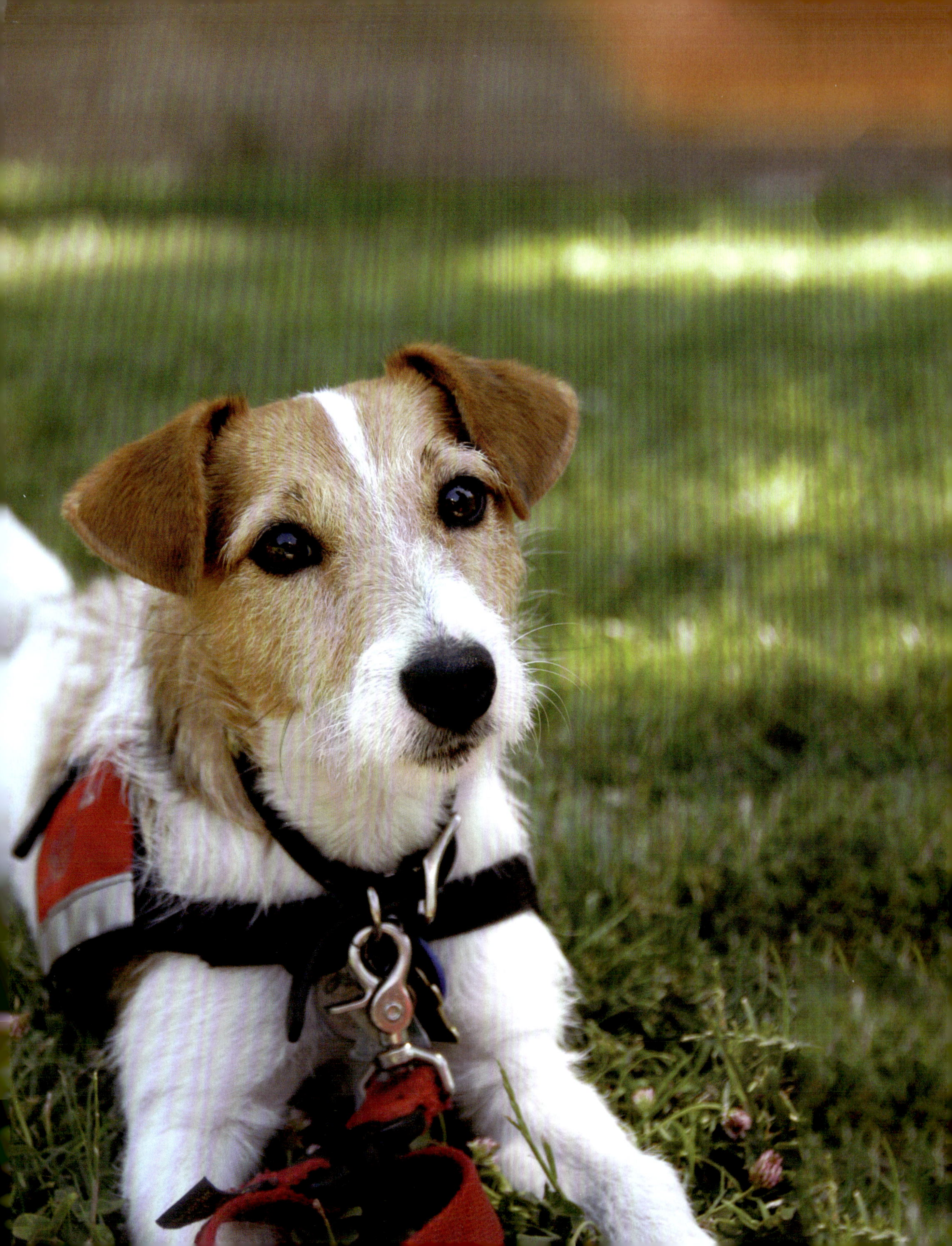

Low Stress Handling®

"Blessed is the match, consumed in kindling flame."

—Hannah Szenes

Introduction

With the publication of her ground-breaking work, *Low Stress Handling®, Restraint, and Behavior Modification of Dogs and Cats (2009),* Dr. Sophia Yin quietly sparked a revolution. With this book, she presented the radical notion that how we handle our patients matters. She demonstrated, point by point, how handling techniques designed to reduce an animal's stress work better than the use of force. Like all breakthroughs in medicine, Low Stress Handling® techniques have grown and evolved since they were first introduced by Dr. Yin.

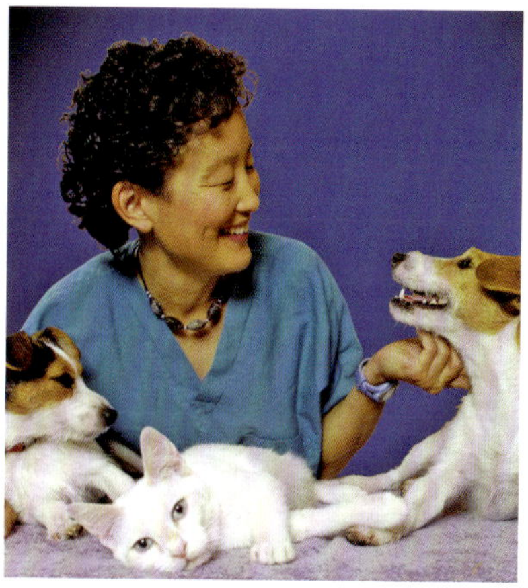

Low Stress Handling®, Restraint, and Behavior Modification of Dogs & Cats, 1st edition.

One aim of this second edition is to carry on Dr. Sophia Yin's groundbreaking approach. While some techniques have been modified and others added based on what has been learned since the first edition was published in 2009; the fundamental principles and spirit of her work remain unchanged.

Another aim of this book is to honor Dr. Sophia Yin's legacy and highlight her significant contributions to animal behavior. The roots of change, like those of the mightiest tree, are unseen and frequently unheralded. The very magnificence of the trunk and branches overshadows the strength of what they rest on. Dr. Yin's message of Low Stress Handling® continues to spread through CattleDog Publishing®, which she founded and which is now part of the Veterinary Information Network®, Inc. In this second edition of Dr. Sophia Yin's *Low Stress Handling® and Behavior Modification,* we, the contributors, wish to remember and honor Dr. Yin for the enduring flame she kindled, and for the lives, both human and animal, that are better for the light she shed.

General Principles of Low Stress Handling® and Care

Minimizing fear and anxiety in our patients is critical to successful veterinary care. Studies have shown that stress, fear, and anxiety compromise the emotional wellbeing of animals, interfere with physical examination and laboratory findings, and delay healing by 27%.[1] However, a visit to the veterinarian does not necessarily have to be a source of fear. As animal caregivers and handlers, we do not need to rely on force to get the job done. Our hearts need not be hardened to distress in order to treat our patients effectively and efficiently.

This book outlines ways that we can actively attend to our patients' emotional and medical needs throughout each stage of the animal's healthcare journey. The recommendations detailed in the following chapters are based on the fundamental principles of a patient-centered care approach that has been successfully implemented in human pediatric medicine modified for veterinary use with dogs and cats, including the following:[2,3]

1. Observe carefully and assess the pet's emotional state.
2. Plan ahead.
3. Be flexible.
4. Increase predictability.
5. Maximize patient choice and control.
6. Avoid triggering fear.

Observe Carefully and Assess the Pet's Emotional State

Observation of the animal at all stages of the veterinary visit is the foundation of effective Low Stress Handling®. The animal's body language will provide the information needed to make an appropriate plan for handling. Watch how they move around the room and interact with their caregivers and team members. Does the animal willingly approach or hide under the bench? What does their body language communicate about their emotional state? Do not approach or touch the animal yet. For dogs, toss treats. For cats, open the carrier and drop a few treats inside. Reassess. What is the animal communicating now?

In this book, you will learn how to observe an animal to formulate an individualized handling plan and educate caregivers about their pet's emotional well-being. The importance of reframing a pet's behavioral response as fearful or stressed, rather than "bad" or "dangerous for the staff," is also covered. Understanding that a reactive pet is scared, engages the caregiver's compassion, rather than inducing anger or embarrassment, and can help smooth the way for other interventions, such as sedation, if needed.

Plan Ahead

Set patients up for success by avoiding potential triggers of fear or stress that may occur before leaving home, such as desensitizing and counterconditioning a patient to their carrier or car rides. Entering the building, approaching the reception desk, and waiting in the lobby before entering the examination room also affect a pet's overall experience.

For patients with a known history of fear or anxiety, planning begins as soon as the appointment is made. Instructing caregivers ahead of time to wait in their car reduces accidental encounters with other animals, traffic, and congestion in the waiting room. Arrange special accommodations for animals who are more comfortable being examined outside the hospital. Make plans to provide appropriate sedation for the patient prior to their veterinary visit if needed.

Documenting the individualized needs and plans for each pet allows future visits to go more smoothly. Customer care representatives can remind caregivers to administer prescribed pre-visit medications. During the examination, knowing distraction preferences (e.g., toys or treats), familiar cues, and preferred examination location (e.g., the bottom of the carrier, floor, or table) helps to quickly win the pet's trust and avoid unnecessary trial and error, which can increase stress.

Be Flexible

Flexibility of a plan is as essential as the plan itself. The need to remain attentive and flexible throughout the pet's care in every aspect of their hospital experience is emphasized. At each step of a veterinary appointment, continuously assess and reassess the animal's body language and behavior.

A previously successful approach to a pet's visit is a good guideline, but allowances should be made for any changes needed for their comfort. An animal presenting for a painful wound may behave differently than they did for their annual examination. Dogs and cats change their behavior as needed in response to their immediate environment, their handling, and their own pain and discomfort levels. Throughout every chapter, you are reminded to observe body language and their response before and during each new interaction so that you can adjust your plan.

Increase Predictability

Anytime we face a situation without knowing what to expect, anxiety is elevated. Imagine being a student again, entering finals week. All you are told is that your first exam is at 9 am on Monday. You are not told which class the test will be for or what material you will be tested on. You do not know how long you have to complete the exam. You are just told that after some time, a proctor will come and collect the paper. What a frightening thought! Dogs and cats may not understand all the words we use, but our actions help them anticipate what we are going to do. Knowing what to expect decreases stress.

In this book, we discuss handling plans that limit disruption of flow, such as moving animals around the facility and having all equipment readily available to avoid leaving the area and returning multiple times. Techniques are outlined instructing handlers to keep a hand gently resting on the animal at all times while examining, handling, and restraining. Removing and replacing hands with each new step can startle the animal due to unexpected "attacks" on new body parts. Slow movements and, when possible, movement in one direction telegraph your intentions to the patient, allowing you to assess the patient's response and helping the animal to anticipate your next move.

Maximize Patient Choice and Control

Choice and control are a central theme throughout the book. Being able to choose whether to participate allows animals to feel in control of what is happening to them. Maximizing patient choice is perhaps the most important aspect of reducing stress and anxiety.[4]

Genuine cooperation cannot occur in the absence of choice. Force, which deprives animals of choice, can vastly increase their anxiety and fear. Physically manipulating animals into position is more apt to induce an attempt to escape and to increase the risk of a defensive response. Animals are more likely to volunteer to participate in their care if given the option.[4] This book addresses ways in which handling can be made more palatable to patients so that they will choose to opt in, or at the very least, choose not to opt out.

Invite Cooperation

Positive and rewarding interactions (e.g., eating high-value treats, play, petting, praise) are important ways of winning a pet's cooperation. However, a positive interaction is only helpful if it is positive for that individual. Remember the expression, "One man's treasure is another man's trash." Petting may be valuable for some patients but fear-inducing for others. Even animals that enjoy petting in some contexts frequently do not appreciate it when under stress.

For most dogs and some cats, food is the most appreciated positive interaction. While food preferences can vary, stress may impact a dog or cat's appetite. Team members can provide options between different food items or toys, and it is essential to observe the animal's body language to assess positive interactions. Does the animal approach or shy away from each offering? Throughout this book, we demonstrate the use of food, toys, play, and other enjoyable interactions as distractions and rewards, all in line with a reward-based approach that inspires dedicated caregivers to initiate cooperative care training at home.

The judicious use of food is an important tool in Low Stress Handling®. Many veterinarians are reluctant to use food due to the fear of gastroesophageal reflux if sedation or anesthesia might be needed. However, studies have shown this risk to be minimal when dogs are fed a small meal prior to anesthesia.[5–7]

Handling and Restraint

Handling or restraint that is harsh, overly restrictive, or simply improper for the individual animal often results in worsening fear, more struggling for escape, and increased aggression. Strive to use the minimum amount of restraint needed for the individual animal. For some animals, this may be achieved by using familiar cues, luring them into position, or allowing the caregiver to offer treats.

An animal may respond to skilled and gentle restraint with an initial attempt to escape. With appropriate technique and adjustments, such pets may settle or quickly relax. It is important to avoid prolonged or repeated fighting or struggling. For these animals, a change in plan may be needed such as rescheduling, previsit medications, or sedation.

If an animal experiences fear at the veterinary hospital, the emotional experience may have lasting consequences. Many veterinary professionals have been taught to avoid sedation whenever possible for the sake of patient safety, time, and caregiver finances. Significant fear and distress distort physical examination and laboratory findings, delay healing, and risk the safety of both the pet and humans.[1] Furthermore, with a patient-centered approach, patient safety, time, and cost are improved with expedited use of sedation and chemical restraint rather than waiting and allowing escalation.[8,9]

Conclusion

Preventing and treating suffering in animals must involve a welfare-centered approach and requires that we look at our examination and treatment process as part of animal welfare.[10–12] Dr. Yin recognized this is accomplished through an understanding of the animals' physical and emotional states, and the effects our interactions have upon them. This book details the fundamental principles and techniques that contribute to a Low Stress Handling® philosophy, while providing a positive experience for everyone involved.

References

1. Gouin, J. P., & Kiecolt-Glaser, J. K. (2011). The impact of psychological stress on wound healing: methods and mechanisms. *Immunology and Allergy Clinics of North America*, 31(1), 81–93.
2. Lerwick, J. L. (2016). Minimizing pediatric healthcare-induced anxiety and trauma. *World Journal of Clinical Pediatrics*, 5(2), 143–150.
3. Kathleen, L., Meert, K. L., Jeff Clark, J., et al. (2013). Family-centered care in the pediatric intensive care unit. *Pediatric Clinics of North America*, 60(3), 761–772.
4. Moscarello, J. M., & Hartley, C. A. (2017). Agency and the calibration of motivated behavior. *Trends in Cognitive Sciences*, 21(10), 725–735.
5. Ioannis, S., Timoleon, R., & Dimitris, R. (2009). The effect of pre-anaesthetic fasting time and type of food on gastric content volume and acidity in dogs. *Veterinary Anaesthesia and Analgesia*, 36(6), 539–546.
6. Tsompanidou, P., Robben, J. H., Savvas, I., et al. (2021). The effect of the preoperative fasting regimen on the incidence of gastro-oesophageal reflux in 90 dogs. *Animals* (Basel), 12(1), 64.
7. Savvas, I., Raptopoulos, D., & Rallis, T. (2016). A "light meal" three hours preoperatively decreases the incidence of gastro-esophageal reflux in dogs. *Journal of the American Animal Hospital Association*, 52(6), 357–363.
8. Howell, A., & Feyrecilde, M. (2018). *Cooperative Veterinary Care*. Wiley Blackwell.
9. Döring, D., Roscher, A., Scheipl, F., et al. (2009). Fear-related behavior of dogs in veterinary practice. *Veterinary Journal*, 182(1), 38–43.
10. Bigras-Fontaine, C., Bazin, I., & Desmarchelier, M. (2022). Clinical relevance of rectal temperature in cats showing marked signs of stress during routine veterinary visits. *Proceedings of the American College of Veterinary Behaviorists Veterinary Behavior Symposium*, 11.
11. Moody, C. M., Mason, G. J., Dewey, C. E., et al. (2020). Getting a grip: cats respond negatively to scruffing and clips. *Veterinary Record*, 186(12), 385.
12. Riemer, S., Heritier, C., Windschnurer, I., Pratsch, L., Arhant, C., & Affenzeller, N. (2021). A review on mitigating fear and aggression in dogs and cats in a veterinary setting. *Animals*, 11(1), 158.

Author: Stephanie Borns-Weil DVM, DACVB

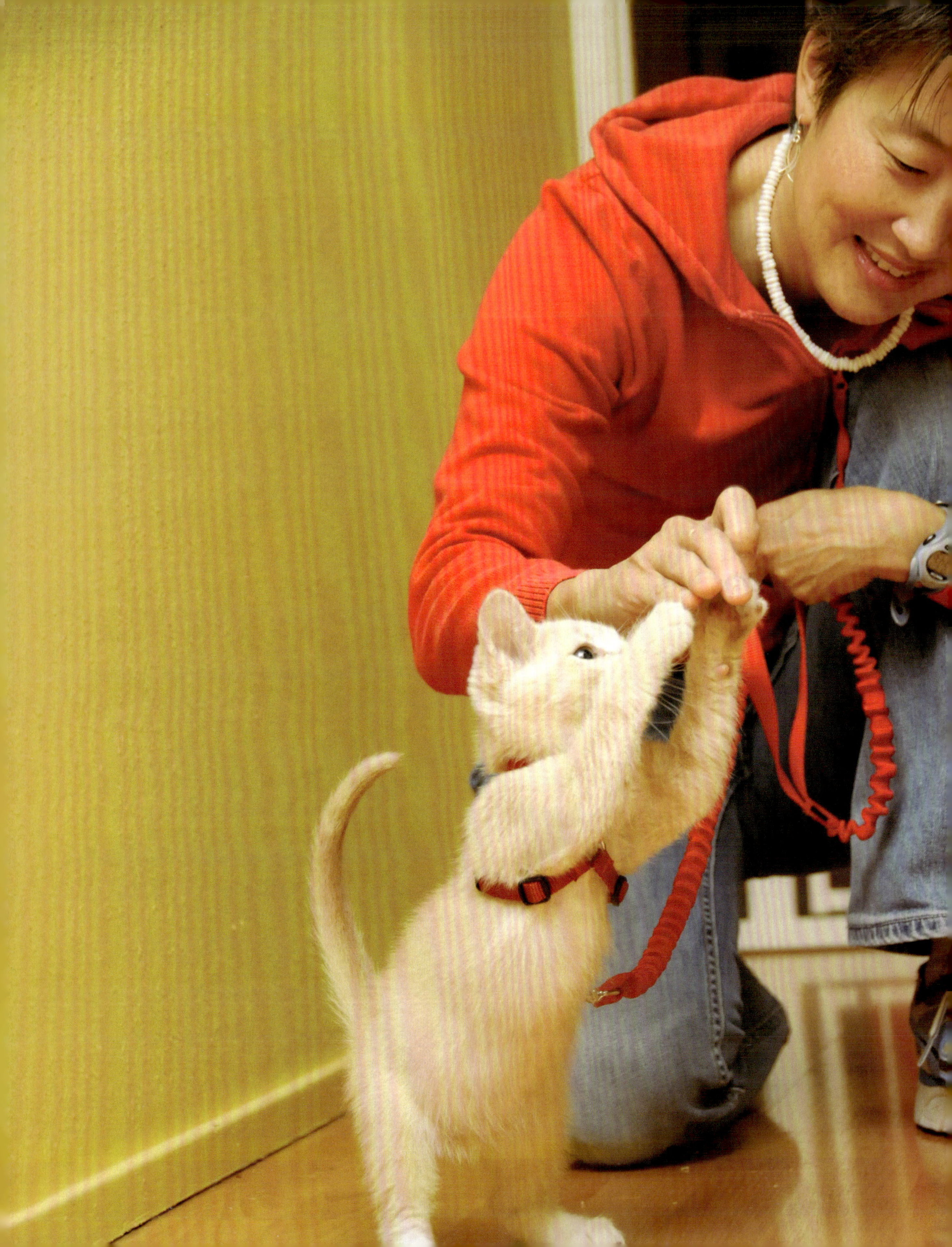

CHAPTER 1

Low Stress Handling®: A Part of Everyday Practice

"Humane and safe physical restraint is the use of manual or mechanical means to limit some or all of an animal's normal voluntary movement for the purposes of examination, collection of samples, drug administration, therapy, or manipulation. The method used should provide the least restraint required to allow the specific procedure(s) to be performed properly, should minimize fear, pain, stress and suffering for the animal, and should protect both the animal and personnel from harm. Every effort should be made to ensure adequate and ongoing training in animal handling and behavior by all parties involved, so that distress and physical restraint are minimized. Where appropriate, the animal should be acclimated to the restraint method/device before use to mitigate fear and distress. In some situations, chemical restraint may be the preferred method. Whenever possible, restraint should be planned and communicated prior to its application."

—The American Veterinary Medical Association

1.1 Introduction

The evolution of the second edition of this book, Dr. Sophia Yin's *Low Stress Handling® and Behavior Modification of Dogs and Cats*, reflects the ever changing and advancing knowledge in the field of animal behavior. Since the publication of the first edition of this book, there have been considerable developments in the understanding of animal emotions, welfare, cooperative care, and the impact of choice on emotional states.

Initially planned as a simple revision, the new edition of this book has transformed into a completely new work. This signifies a fresh chapter in the ongoing evolution of Low Stress Handling®. The updated material showcases the latest research and practices in the field, emphasizing the deepened understanding of animal emotions and welfare. It also highlights the importance of cooperative care, where animals are active participants in their own care, and the role of choice in influencing an animal's emotional state.

By presenting this updated material, this new edition serves as a campaign, urging all those involved in animal care to embrace these evolving principles and practices. The hope is that by doing so, the lives of animals and the people who care for them will be significantly improved, continuing Dr. Sophia Yin's legacy and vision.

1.2 History of Low Stress Handling®

The concept of Low Stress Handling® revolutionized the approach towards animal care, particularly in veterinary and shelter environments, thanks to the pioneering work of Dr. Sophia Yin, a veterinarian, animal behaviorist, and scientist. Her research, in collaboration with colleagues, highlighted the similarities between human and animal experiences of stress. This understanding brought to light the significant impact of emotions on animal health and their response to handling.

Prior to this shift in understanding, traditional animal handling and veterinary care practices often neglected the emotional states of animals. While effective in their practical objectives, these methods frequently led to an increase in stress, anxiety, and fear in animals. These negative emotional states often led to behavioral problems and complicated various medical procedures, such as examinations, venipuncture, catheter placements, and diagnostic tests.

Low Stress Handling®, emerging from this newfound understanding, places emphasis on minimizing negative emotional responses. Rooted in a deeper comprehension of animal psychology and behavior, this approach advocates for handling practices that are sensitive to both the emotional and physical well-being of animals, thereby strengthening the bond between animals and their caregivers.

Table 1.2.1: Sophia Yin's Ten General Principles of Low Stress Handling®

Principle 1:	Start with a comfortable environment.
Principle 2:	Prevent the animal from pacing, nervous or excited movements, squirming, or attempts to escape.
Principle 3:	Provide proper support with hands, arms, and body to ensure the animal feels secure and balanced.
Principle 4:	Move deliberately and slowly with animals that are nervous, scared, or confused to avoid triggering resistance or escape behaviors.
Principle 5:	Learn to control animal movement in any direction with appropriate hand and body placement.
Principle 6:	Wait until the pet is relaxed before starting a procedure.
Principle 7:	Use the minimal amount of restraint necessary for each individual animal.
Principle 8:	Avoid prolonged (more than two seconds) or repeated fighting or struggling.
Principle 9:	Use distractions and rewards when appropriate.
Principle 10:	Adapt handling and technique based on the animal's response and adjust methods accordingly.

1.3 How to Use This Book

Low Stress Handling®, Restraint, and Behavior Modification of Dogs and Cats, originally a comprehensive photographic guide with 1600 images, has undergone a substantial evolution in this latest edition. This updated version showcases a wide variety of photographs from individual contributors, veterinary teaching hospitals, emergency, specialty, and referral clinics, as well as private general practices. It comprises a mix of both new and original images, with numerous photos revised to showcase current practices and to demonstrate techniques on animals that appear less stressed. Still widely used in veterinary education worldwide, this new edition is full of real-life scenarios and examples of how to use Low Stress Handling® techniques in various animal care contexts and settings.

This book is organized to provide a logical progression of topics starting with foundational concepts such as communication and team building. It then explores the early development of puppies and kittens, focusing on training and learning. Subsequent sections examine how emotions affect behavior and how to foster a low stress hospital environment. Later chapters address navigating hospital environments, employing various handling techniques, using emergency tools, and integrating Low Stress Handling® into the euthanasia process. Throughout, key concepts are frequently revisited across different chapters to reinforce fundamental ideas, ensuring that readers not only comprehend the theoretical foundations of Low Stress Handling® but can also practically apply these principles in real life veterinary and animal care situations.

Originally designed for veterinary professionals, this book's core principles can be applied across all aspects of animal care. The latest edition is intended to be comprehensive, highlighting the book's applicability in a diverse range of animal care settings. This inclusive approach ensures that Dr. Yin's innovative work in animal handling reaches beyond veterinary settings, offering invaluable insights and guidance to a diverse group, from animal care experts to caregivers. By doing so, the book not only continues her legacy but also expands the audience that can benefit from her original teachings and these new concepts.

1.4 Low Stress Handling®: A Part of Everyday Practice

Dr. Yin's teachings revealed that while Low Stress Handling® techniques might require initial preparation, these techniques do not have to be time consuming or labor intensive. Small changes in how team members interact with animals can lead to significant impacts in their emotional well-being and overall health. The following are two real-life examples that not only show the practical application of Low Stress Handling® techniques in everyday practice, but also how easy they are to implement.

Willy: The Low Stress Handling® Approach

Willy, anticipating a delightful beach day, was unexpectedly brought to the veterinary hospital. The word "R-I-D-E" typically signaled exciting times of chasing seagulls, frolicking in the surf, and playing fetch by the sea with his caregivers. He was surprised when the anticipated fun ride ended up at the veterinary hospital, and his anxiety started mounting. Yet, as he exited the car and entered the building, his initial anxiety began to melt away. At the entrance, homemade bandanas were available, and Willy was gently fitted with one after a light application of pheromone spray was applied to it.

The examination room was designed for comfort, with soothing music playing in the background and a non-slip mat strategically placed on a platform, positioned away from the door in the center of the room. Nearby, a water bowl and an assortment of toys were accessible, offering him the choice to engage with them if he desired.

The veterinary technician entered the room quietly and greeted Willy by tossing a few treats behind him. This strategy encouraged Willy to turn away, find, and enjoy the treats, before turning around and venturing closer for more. Following this approach, the veterinarian engaged Willy in a similar manner, thereby fostering a positive association with the new environment and the people in it.

For the examination, Willy's caregiver engaged him in a familiar game using nose "touches" to ease his nerves. He was then guided to the platform, where the familiar "step up" cue was given. Willy stepped up onto the platform anticipating the reinforcement that always followed.

On the platform, Willy stood eagerly, as the veterinary technician skillfully used a Low Stress Handling® standing hold. This method provided stability with minimal restraint, enabling the veterinarian to examine him comfortably and safely. Willy was familiar with this technique from previous visits. To further ease the process, Willy's caregiver offered an additional distraction: Willy was allowed to lick yogurt off a lickable mat, which had been prepared at home the night before specifically for this appointment. The distraction helped keep him relaxed and engaged during the examination.

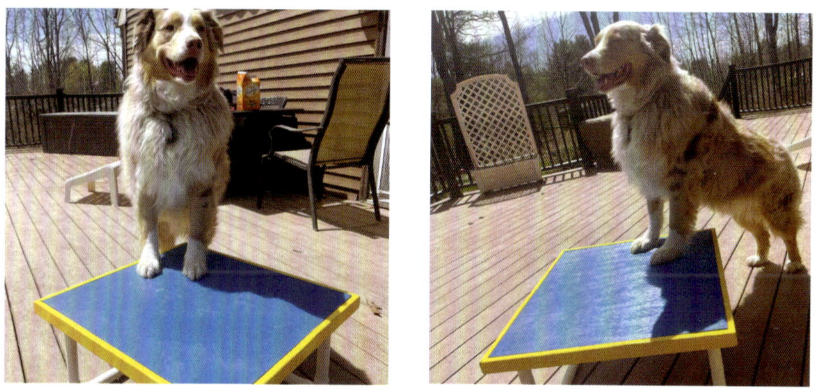

Figs. 1.4 A, B: Step up onto a platform is a behavior learned during prevention and intervention visits.

Administering vaccines and drawing blood from Willy's hind leg were uneventful. Willy remained relaxed and cooperative, not

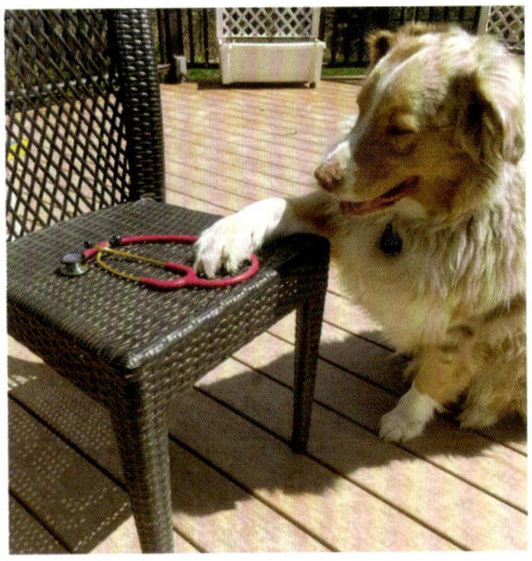

Fig. 1.4 C: Targeting a stethoscope is another useful behavior learned during prevention and intervention visits.

even flinching during the procedures. At the end of the appointment, he was free to leave the platform at his own pace. After stepping off the platform, Willy picked up a ball on the floor and approached the veterinarian, his stub of a tail wagging softly, his body relaxed, asking for her to throw the ball, which she happily did.

Cassidy: The Low Stress Handling® Approach

Cassidy, who seldom ventures out of the house, sensed something unusual was happening. Unbeknownst to her, Cassidy's caregiver had given her a favorite treat, tasty turkey wrapped around a gel cap of gabapentin, two hours earlier. While the car ride initially caused her some anxiety, the warm towel scented with pheromones and a cover over her carrier helped soothe her. She eventually realized they were headed to the veterinary hospital, but this visit was a little different than anything she had experienced in the past.

After their arrival at the veterinary hospital, Cassidy and her caregiver waited in the car until a text message indicated their room was ready. Her carrier, comfortably supported and still wrapped in the pheromone-infused towel, was then carried inside. Once in the room, the carrier was gently placed on the floor, and instead of hands reaching in to pull her out, the door was opened by her caregiver, giving Cassidy time to exit when she was ready.

After carefully observing her surroundings for a few moments, Cassidy decided to cautiously emerge from her carrier. With the room quiet and free of loud noises and sudden movements, she gradually became more at ease. As she explored the space, Cassidy noticed a soft blanket thoughtfully laid out on a bench next to her caregiver. Deciding it was a safe and comfortable spot, she chose to jump up and settle there.

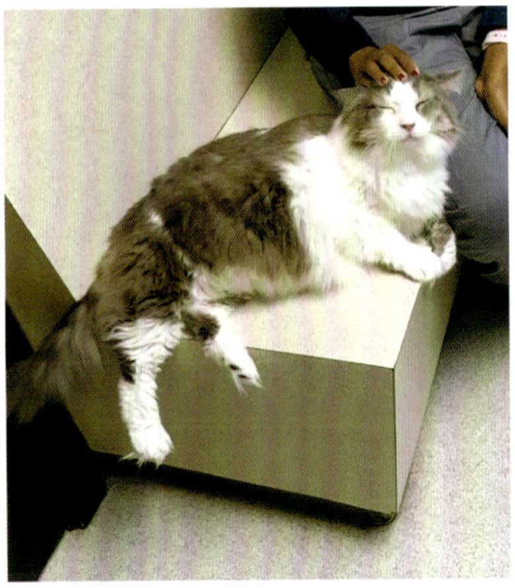

Fig. 1.4 D: Giving cats a choice of location for examination and procedures can help them feel more relaxed and comfortable. (Photo courtesy of Sierra Mitchell)

A member of the veterinary team entered the room and approached Cassidy slowly, speaking in a soft tone and moving deliberately to avoid startling her. When offered a lickable treat, Cassidy accepted and began to enjoy it. While she was preoccupied with the treat and receiving gentle strokes from her caregiver, the veterinarian managed to conduct the examination effortlessly, without causing Cassidy any distress. Even during vaccinations, Cassidy remained oblivious and continued to enjoy her special treat.

Although bloodwork was not required for this visit, the veterinarian provided contact information for a local veterinary technician who specialized in behavior and cooperative care training.

This technician would help Cassidy's caregiver with training specifically geared towards preparing Cassidy for her next annual wellness examination, scheduled to include venipuncture and blood pressure measurements.

By prioritizing Cassidy's comfort, letting her choose her examination spot, and employing the use of distractions, the veterinary team successfully turned what could have been a stressful encounter into a relaxed and collaborative experience. Furthermore, a strategy was laid out for future visits to maintain the Low Stress Handling® methods established during this visit.

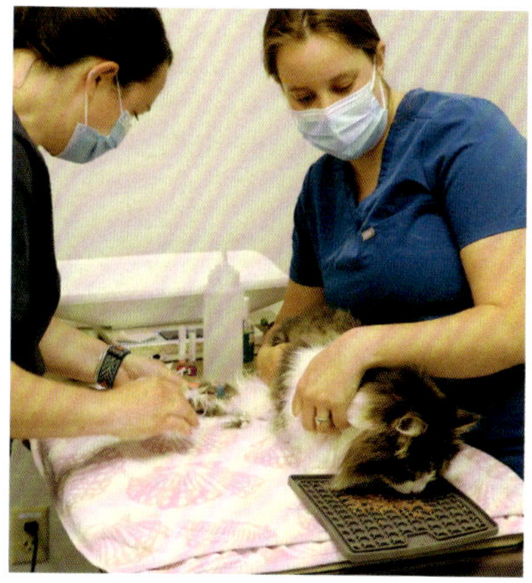

Fig. 1.4 E: Example of distractions and cat preference of positioning for venipuncture. (Photo courtesy of Portland Veterinary Emergency and Specialty Care - Bryan Oliver)

1.5 Conclusion

Building upon Dr. Sophia Yin's foundational teachings, this book is the culmination of a collaborative effort involving many authors and reviewers over a span of nearly four years. Throughout its development, characterized by several revisions and reorganizations, it has been a significant journey of learning and growth for everyone involved.

The new edition of this book is specifically designed to deepen the reader's understanding of animal behavior, welfare, learning processes, and emotional states. It focuses on fostering critical thinking skills essential for adapting to unexpected situations or deviations from standard handling protocols. As a comprehensive resource, the book extends beyond traditional educational materials, inspiring readers to open their minds and think "outside the box" to enhance the quality of life for both animals and their human caretakers.

Author
Christine D. Calder DVM, DACVB

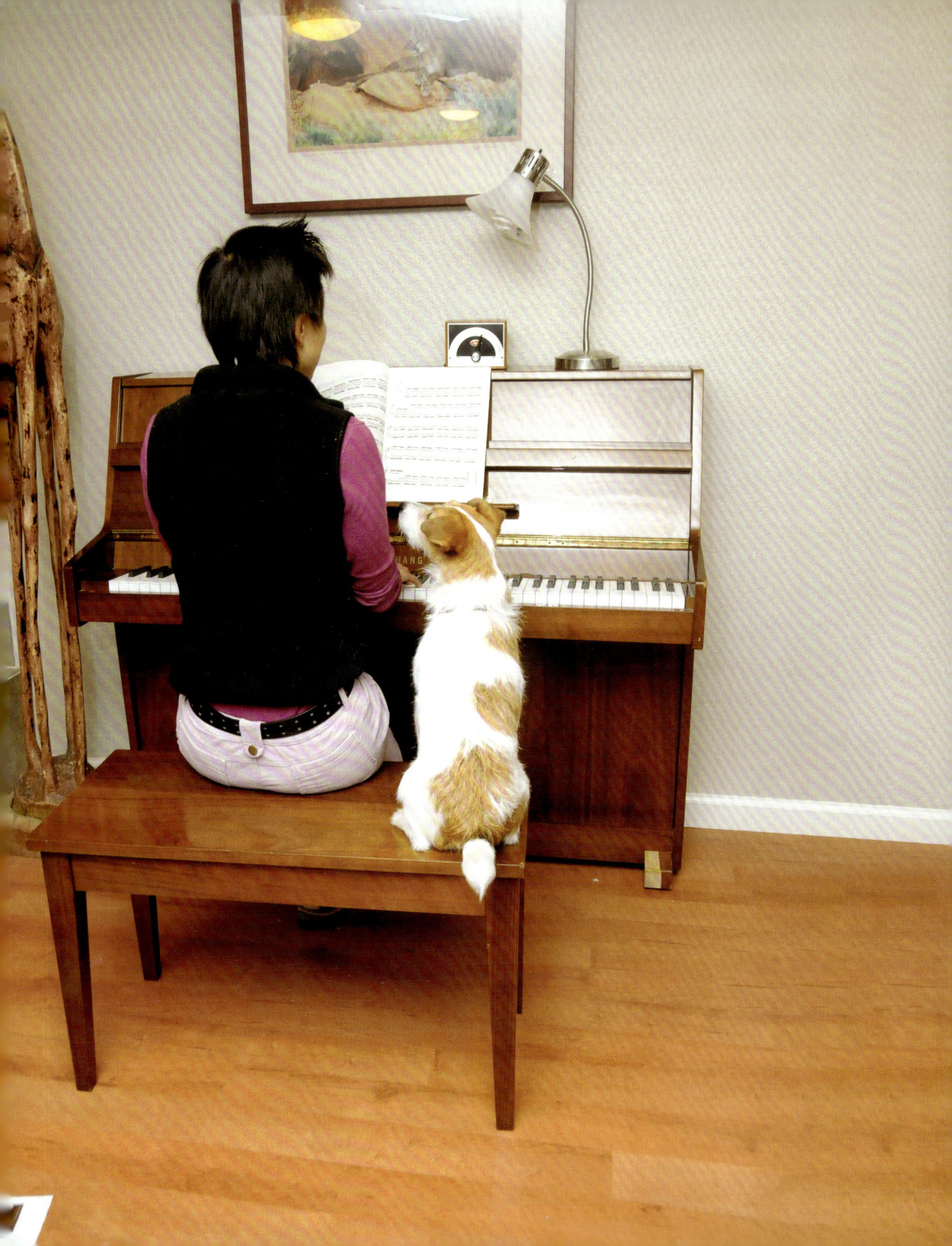

CHAPTER 2

Communication: Talking About Low Stress Handling® with Team Members and Clients

2.1 Introduction

Low Stress Handling® improves both patient and team member safety and helps prevent emotional and behavioral distress in animals. Although foundation skills such as animal handling, body language awareness, and responsiveness are crucial, implementing low stress ideals goes further. Equally important to the success of the low stress team is the ability to communicate with coworkers and clients about the importance of using these methods.

This chapter will discuss the importance of how to talk with team members about using Low Stress Handling® methods with their patients, implementing changes, and how to talk to clients about the use of medications to reduce fear and anxiety during veterinary visits.

2.2 Language Matters

Veterinary and other animal professionals generally seek out their career because of an interest in preventing and reducing pain and suffering in animals. Historically, these professionals are taught how to handle animals in a way that prevents human injury, yet with little regard to the emotional and mental welfare of the patient during handling. When people who are passionate about helping animals are required to handle animals using outdated methods (and essentially ignoring emotional distress), it can be harmful to the emotional health of the humans involved. As a result, animal professionals may "harden their hearts" in some ways to protect their own welfare.

Language and Labels Matter

One of the ways that animal professionals might attempt to protect themselves is by using certain kinds of language. Describing patients as fractious, difficult, aggressive, mean, naughty, spoiled, untrained, fear biters, etc., may lead to a culture of adversarial relationships between people and pets. Some might tell themselves, "Fido is just a little jerk," to allow themselves the ability to engage in strong physical restraint; however, such language or similar labels distances the professional from the emotional welfare of the animal. This emotional distance can have the appearance of protecting the team member's emotions on the surface. In actuality, the emotional distancing created by these labels undermines their ability to provide low stress care. Giving careful consideration to how patients are described or labeled is one way to direct the culture toward low stress goals.

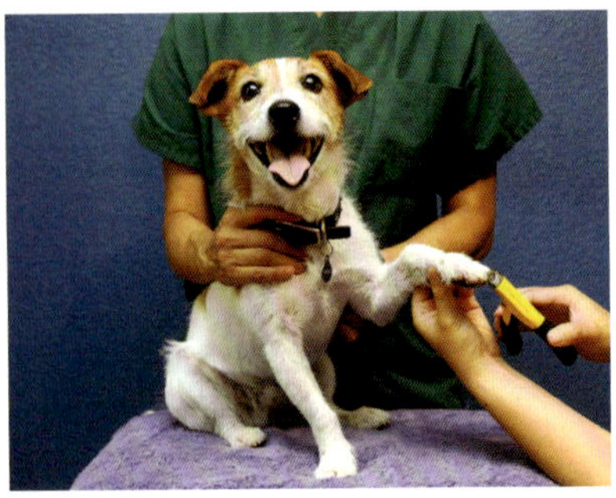

Fig. 2.2 A: Consider how patients are described or labeled to direct the culture towards low stress goals.

Consider describing an animal's observable individual behaviors. Instead of referring to a specific animal as being fearful or stressed, say that they are "showing" signs of fear, anxiety, or stress, or that they "appear to be experiencing" fear, anxiety, or stress. This distinction may seem small, but it is an important one. By assigning a specific emotional state to an animal, one is presuming to know the animal's thoughts. In truth, people can never know the exact thoughts of animals because they do not share the same verbal language. Instead, describe the behaviors observed, and categorize them accordingly as needed.

Using Common Language Among Team Members

Several stress scales are available which describe body language and may be used to provide guidance when a different handling strategy may be appropriate. Each level presented on the scale should be accompanied by images to help identify which behaviors are observed, and which stress level correlates with these signs.

Consider an example of a dog that needs to have an ear flushing performed because of otitis. The dog struggles for more than three seconds when restraint is attempted. He averts his gaze and moves away upon seeing the ear cleanser bottle. When restraint is attempted again, the dog crouches low, places his tail between his legs, and flattens his ears against the sides of his head. The situation may be described as: "I tried to hold Fido to flush his ears, but he would not cooperate and was being difficult." The low stress alternative way to describe this would be: "Fido is showing signs of moderate stress when I attempt an ear flush. I am concerned about continuing and would like to try something different." The first script represents a more confrontational approach to working with the patient, assigning a judgment to the animal's behaviors. The second script offers a description free from judgment and includes steps for the procedure while also protecting the pet's emotional health. By changing out labels with alternative descriptions in medical records and patient notes, teams can show empathy and improve their hospital's culture.

Table 2.2.1: Common Labels and Alternative Phrases to Use for Patients

Common Labels	Alternative Phrases
Fractious Difficult Mean Will Bite Caution Use Muzzle Spoiled Badly Behaved Naughty Wiggly Uncooperative	Shows signs of stress Shows signs of fear Description of <specific body language signs> Need pre-visit medications Needs sedation Does best with <success strategy notes>

2.3 Talking to Team Members

In the veterinary hospital setting, team members and veterinarians each have their own routine way of doing certain tasks. Support staff observe and learn each preference while working together to meet everyone's needs. For many medical therapies, this can be appropriate, but a unified team approach is needed when handling patients.

Low Stress Handling® provides a synchronized approach while accounting for the emotional welfare of each animal. Utilization of these methods improves body language awareness and allows for the creation of individualized handling plans. This knowledge empowers team members to intervene and advocate for ethical animal handling by others.

It is somewhat rare for hospitals to have an entire team comprised of professionals equally committed to Low Stress Handling® unless it is a certified facility. Therefore, conflict can occur among team members if others feel patient welfare is being compromised. Commitment to a Low Stress Handling® mindset starts with recognition and understanding of how to apply it; however, getting buy-in from all team members may be challenging. Efforts to unite the team are important because by doing so, they are more likely to work together towards a common goal of protecting patient welfare.

2.4 The Emotions of Change and Communication

Making the decision to provide Low Stress Handling® requires understanding and acceptance that the previous methods were less than ideal. An emotional struggle can occur in animal professionals passionate about reducing and reversing pain and suffering in animals. As an animal advocate, it can be difficult to realize their actions have been potentially harming patients while trying to help them. This realization can lead to emotional distress, manifesting as defensiveness, confrontations, avoiding conversations, or discounting the validity of these methods. The first step in making changes involves having constructive conversations to understand the potential emotional toll on others.

Completing the Story

Completing stories is satisfying for the brain. Experiencing a story with a beginning, middle, and end stimulates release of oxytocin and cortisol.[1] This happens whether the entire story is presented, or only one part of the story is provided because the brain fills in the rest by making an assumption. It does not matter if the story is true or false; the brain works to create a logical circle of information to understand what is happening.

Consider this interaction:

Team Member A walking through treatment sees Team Member B scruffing and stretching a cat for a cystocentesis.

Member A: "Can I help with that?"

Member B: "Nope. I've got it. He's spicy but this won't take long."

Member A is thinking: *What is B doing? This is not ok and I just want to help. Why is B doing that? Do they just not care? They probably don't care and just want to show the cat who is boss.*

Member B is thinking: *A thinks I don't know how to do my job. They are so nosy. Why can't they just mind their own business?*

Completing each of these stories with assumptions will give both A and B a release of oxytocin and cortisol. This thought process probably all happened subconsciously, without either person being fully aware of the occurrence.

Consider the assumptions A and B made about one another; both explaining the other's actions in a negative light. Whether the stories created and completed were true or not, the versions of each person's internal story will impact how they feel about each other, and how they interact with each other in the future.

Completing the Story

The core concepts here are:

1. Stories result in hormone release within the brain which is satisfying or reinforcing.
2. Only one part of the story is needed to promote the completed response.
3. Both true and false versions will result in the completion response and subsequent hormonal changes.

Understanding How Thoughts Influence Communication

Implementing Low Stress Handling® means staying curious about people's emotions and being aware of the way brains complete stories through assumptions hundreds of times a day. Fortunately, just like learning about using body language to identify signs of stress, it is also possible to gain awareness of personal thoughts and assumptions, and how these influence communication skills with others. The work of Dr. Brené Brown is an excellent guide for creating a foundation to achieve a more positive story. Dr. Brown's research suggests starting with the basis that every person is doing the best they can with the tools available to them.[2–4]

The concept of always assuming people are doing their best with the tools they have can be very difficult. Dr. Brown's research supports the idea that it does not matter if an assumption is true or false, but rather how making a specific assumption makes a person feel. In her writing, Dr. Brown described the first time she was confronted with this assumption, causing her to feel angry and self-righteous. She provided examples ranging from laziness to even cruelty and how everyone can make different assumptions depending on their perspective.

Judgmental feelings can be harmful to one's self-esteem, satisfaction, happiness, and even safety over time. When a person is in judgment, that person builds mental walls which block communication. Barriers to communication can be especially harmful when trying to implement changes among team members, encouraging them to try something new, different, or difficult. This is particularly important when such conversations also require team members to accept that their prior actions may have been harmful. Communication skills need to contain an elevated level of openness and generosity since feelings of generosity tend to override feelings of judgment.

Most people are doing the best they can with the tools they have at that moment. According to Dr. Brown, it is also important to consider what those tools are, how they may change, and why these matter. The concept of tools encompasses not only physical things like shelter, food, money, time, and technical skills, but also freedom from physical and emotional pain and fear, along with sufficient knowledge, communication, and critical thinking skills, history of safe communication partners, self-esteem, self-worth and so much more. A person's tools encompass physical, intellectual, and emotional capital.

Emotional Capital

What is emotional capital? For example, consider most veterinary team members' understanding of how to handle a fearful feline patient during a veterinary visit. This patient may accept, tolerate, or allow a certain amount of physical contact during the visit. This cat's tolerance level is influenced by factors other than the visit itself, such as being placed into a carrier, riding in the car, waiting in the lobby, hearing dogs bark and phones ring, smelling all the odors and getting pulled from the carrier prior to the exam. Each factor encountered requires spending some emotional capital. How much capital remains after this payout will dictate the cat's behavior for the remainder of this visit.

The same is true for people. A certain amount of emotional capital is available at any given time and influenced by factors both within and outside the person's control. Through the generation of good habits, funds are deposited into their emotional capital account. While under their control, the overall emotional bank account of a person will have a better balance, allowing them to invest more in colleagues, patients, and clients.

Dr. Brown's work shows us that assuming others are doing their best makes a big deposit in our own emotional capital account. Fulfilling our biological need for stories with generous assumptions improves our mental health, even if the assumption is a myth instead of fact. Being aware of the many stories we complete each day and choosing generous assumptions is a valuable skill because building up a team to embrace Low Stress Handling® methods requires a great deal of emotional capital.

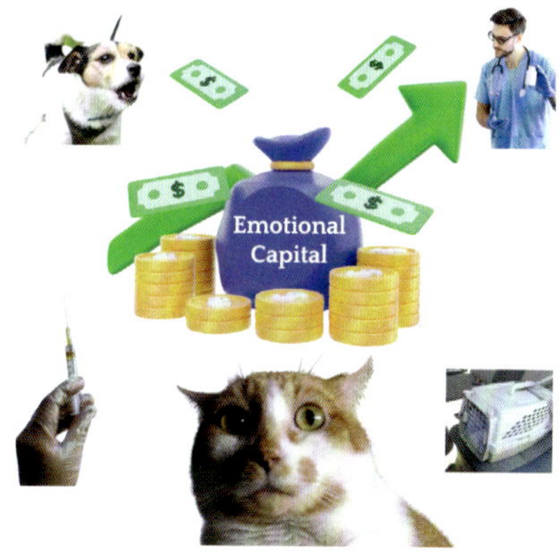

Fig. 2.4 A: A cat's emotional capital for a veterinary visit may be influenced by other factors in the environment.

How to Change the Story to Benefit Emotional Welfare

Revisit the conversation between Team Member A and B. Previous assumptions used to complete their stories have been replaced with more generous assumptions.

> Member A: "Can I help with that?"
>
> Member B: "Nope. I've got it. He's spicy but this won't take long."
>
> Member A's brain works to complete the story. *B probably isn't sure what else to do and is doing the best that they can at this moment. I can ask them about helping in a different way before the next cat appointment.*
>
> Member B's brain is also going to work to complete the story. *A is trying to help and I appreciate it. They are really skilled with cats. I should ask them about it later so I can up my game.*

In this example, A and B still both receive a release of oxytocin and cortisol. However, they will be free from the negative emotional strain that comes from completing stories in a judgmental way. Generous assumptions set them up for open communication moving forward.

Practicing generous internal assumptions is a skill that helps forward progress feel easier, even in a difficult situation. When one team member can make generous assumptions and communicate well but their partner is not as skilled, certain phrases can be used to facilitate this process, allowing the skilled member to be authentic and transparent. When practicing, Dr. Brown suggests using these phrases:

- **I'm curious about:** For example, "I'm curious about how I can be more helpful to you so that we can reach the goal of Low Stress Handling® together."
- **Tell me more:** For example, "Tell me more about what you have experienced and what you would find most helpful."
- **That has not been my experience:** For example, "That has not been my experience in such a situation. Can we talk about alternatives?"
- **Help me understand:** For example, "Help me understand the problem step-by-step. I'm listening and want to learn."
- **Walk me through that:** For example, "Walk me through that so I can understand more clearly."

2.5 Meeting Team Members Where They Are

Every journey together begins with a first step. When implementing change, leaders can start by first meeting team members at their physical, mechanical, emotional, and intellectual skill level. Goals can then be set. Providing a feasible progression to these goals takes into account the starting point of the learner, the end goal, and the motivating factors for the learner. A breakdown of steps between the starting point and the goal can then be outlined. For example, if the goal is ***scruff-free care***, but the team still sometimes uses scruffing to restrain and handle cats, telling the team that scruffing is now prohibited will not succeed as a stand-alone recommendation. This recommendation doesn't meet the collective team where they are, and it does not provide a feasible progression to the end goal. Consider the following alternative plan, using a breakdown of goal-oriented steps:

Goal: Scruff-Free Care

Starting point: Some team members scruff cats for certain procedures.

Progression:

1. Investigate with the team to learn more about when and why scruffing sometimes occurs. Use statements such as, "I'm

curious about how we can work together towards our scruff-free goals. Walk me through the thought process when you use scruffing techniques so that I can understand."

2. Identify a starting point based on team feedback. For example, if the team shares that they use scruffing when cats show signs of significant stress or are in the red stress scale category, focus on solutions for this one situation first.

3. Provide a replacement behavior. Give the team a structure to follow when in this situation. For example, "If you identify these body language signs, pause the procedure, and determine the necessity of continuing. Proceed once the patient is more relaxed or medication has been given."

4. Offer a secondary replacement behavior. For example, if the team shares that they use scruffing specifically for medial hindlimb venipuncture, recommend an alternative method for this procedure instead. Teach this procedure step-by-step during a team training event or individually until every team member has received the knowledge, skills, and supervised practice that they need to be confident in its use.

5. Make a plan for observation and positive support feedback. Communicate with the team that individual observations will occur, and positive feedback provided to help everyone collectively meet the goal. Transparency about observing and providing positive feedback is important since people often feel self-conscious when being watched. Under observation, people may feel pressure; therefore, they may have negative feelings about feedback and fear they will make a mistake. Coaches should be selected based on their ability to provide positive feedback and navigate conversations for change. Throughout the process, provide team members an opportunity to share their concerns about the change and coaching in a safe environment. For example, choose a narrative such as: "If you have concerns, I would like to hear them throughout this process. Please share them with me this way: [select what works best for the team]."

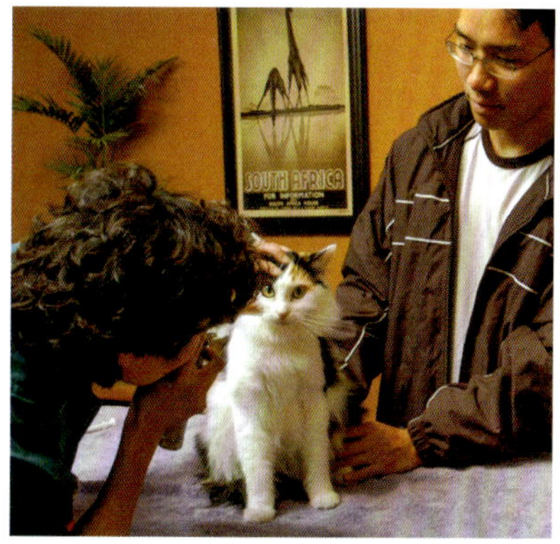

Fig. 2.5 A: Provide a replacement behavior to give team members a structure to follow.

6. Determine when to reconvene. Schedule a date and time to meet with the team as a whole or individually. Consider using statements such as: "Tell me about your experience implementing the scruff-free techniques. How is it going?" During this meeting, address concerns and support all efforts towards the end goal.

7. Endpoint: Scruffing is no longer used for medial hindlimb venipuncture or for "red" cats. Once this endpoint is achieved, the process can be repeated for the next goal regarding scruffing.

Insisting on global change or changing too much at once can create intense pressure on team members and overwhelm them. It is normal to feel frustrated when using a stepwise approach; additionally, if team members are asked to do more than what they realistically can at any given time, progression may not happen, and change will not occur.

2.6 Welcoming Clients

Pet caregivers, particularly those who have a long history of seeking veterinary care, have come to expect their pets to show signs of stress and fear during veterinary visits. Surveys show that up to 58% of cat caregivers avoid scheduling veterinary appointments due to perceived patient stress.[5] Even clients who do not have strong veterinary care relationships are exposed to the ideas that stress and fear are normal in the veterinary hospital. Exposure occurs through social media, online videos, television programming, entertainment, and general media presence, as well as stories from friends and family. These clients will either avoid care, when possible, to preserve the emotional welfare of their pet, or they will seek care with the expectation that their pet will show signs of fear and stress. When clients accept that signs of stress and fear during veterinary visits are normal, it can present some challenges when modifying practice methods to align with Low Stress Handling®.

Guidelines used for team member communication also apply to clients. When working with pet caregivers, an internal mental dialogue occurs, on either a conscious or subconscious level. This internal dialogue includes assumptions and efforts to complete stories. By practicing generous assumptions both mentally and verbally during the interaction with clients, communication dynamics and client compliance improve.

In many cases, clients will be grateful to see that the team is practicing Low Stress Handling® methods with their pets. This gives an opportunity for them to witness firsthand the care and concern each team member shows not just for the physical health, but also for the emotional health of each patient in their care. When team members verbalize behavioral observations and their adjusted response, client awareness is elevated regarding the importance of this type of care.[6] Below are a few scenarios of how simple communication can demonstrate empathy and improve client perception about the value of care.

Offering Treats to a Dog in an Examination Room

Visualize the dog: he walks slowly with an outstretched neck, carefully sniffing at the treats. The dog quickly snatches a treat from the team member's hand and retreats under the caregiver's chair to consume the treat. It would be obvious to a team member trained in Low Stress Handling® methods that this pet is showing elevated signs of fear, anxiety, and stress. Instead of offering treats from the hand, one strategy is to roll the treats away for the dog. If the dog then chooses to approach, roll another treat. While this interaction may take only a few seconds, the observation and skills highlight this team member's empathy which may not be immediately obvious to the client. This provides an opportunity to discuss the pet's fear, opening the lines of communication between the team and client.

Example script: "See how Rex is leaning backwards and stretching his neck out to get the treat from my hand, before moving away

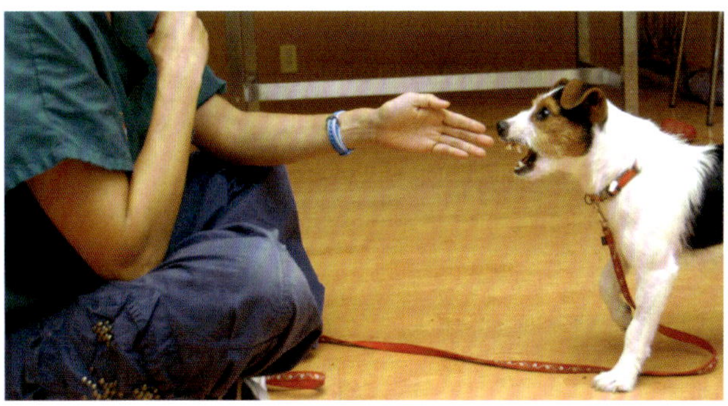

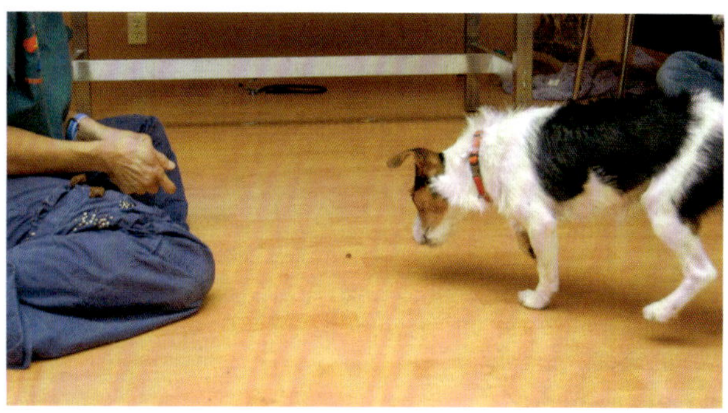

Figs. 2.6 A, B: Reduce stress by rolling treats away instead of handing them directly to a dog.

and eating it? This shows me Rex is worried about me, the environment, or both. I'm going to roll the treats away from me to see if he shows signs of relaxing when I feed him a different way."

Allowing a Cat to Sniff a Stethoscope Before Auscultation

A cat arrives in their carrier, the carrier is placed on the floor, and the door opened. After many minutes of history taking, it becomes clear the cat does not want to exit the carrier and is huddled at the back of the carrier, away from the door, ignoring any gentle attempts at introduction from the team member. The team member prepares to remove the lid of the carrier, and a warmed pheromone-sprayed blanket is placed over the cat to allow hiding when the lid is removed.

Although this cat is not growling or showing obvious signs of fear, anxiety, or stress from the caregiver's perspective, a team member trained in Low Stress Handling® might recognize the nervousness seen in the cat before approaching slowly to auscultate with a stethoscope. Here is another opportunity to communicate with the client that the pet's emotional welfare is equally as important as their physical welfare.

Example script: "Fluffy is experiencing fear and anxiety and trying to hide as a result. By leaving her in the bottom of the carrier and giving her a blanket to hide under, we can allow her to cope with her fear and anxiety and still move forward slowly with attempts at the physical examination within the carrier bottom."

Team members frequently make dozens of small adjustments during an interaction with a patient to minimize stress, all of which may be invisible to the client. Sharing insight with clients about providing such care builds a relationship between team members and clients, ensuring that the pet's emotional welfare will be accounted for in all future interactions.

2.7 Clients Who Are Uncomfortable with Low Stress Handling®

Some clients will not be comfortable with Low Stress Handling® methods and techniques. They may have their own beliefs about appropriate pet behavior, a long learning history with other veterinarians who handled their pet differently, or they may simply not share the team's goal to protect emotional welfare in animals.

Even when presented with clients who do not share the same level of commitment, it is acceptable and appropriate for animal care professionals to maintain their boundaries and commitment to these methods. Keeping an open mind, practicing generous assumptions, and having a plan for these conversations will help diminish team member stress levels when these clients are present. Offering appropriate care recommendations and adhering to Low Stress Handling® principles are the correct course of action. Maintaining boundaries about care may present a moral concern for animal care professionals new to this approach. Concerns may occur that the pet will suffer if the client is unwilling to authorize care while some clients may covertly or openly suggest that any suffering is the team's fault.

Preparing in advance with practice scripts improves everyone's welfare in these situations and may prevent difficult situations entirely. For example, consider these two responses to a client when their dog shows signs of fear, but the caregiver insists on vaccinating him:

> "I will not forcibly hold Rex down to vaccinate him. We don't do that here."
>
> *Versus:*
>
> "We are committed to Low Stress Handling® techniques. Rex's signs of fear have risen beyond an acceptable level, so let's pause and make a new plan."

Both examples share the same essential information; the provider is setting a clear boundary regarding manual restraint to administer a vaccine. The first script is closed-ended, creating tension between client and provider. The second script focuses on Rex's welfare and opens the door for open communication.

Helpful phrases include:

- “As we have learned more, we have updated our methods . . . ”
- “Low Stress Handling® keeps my team and patients safe, and that’s really important . . . ”
- “Decreasing your pet’s stress today preserves my ability to provide care for them in the future . . . ”
- “By allowing your pet’s stress level to increase today, they are at a greater risk for stress at their next visit . . . ”
- “I am in veterinary medicine because I love animals. Low Stress Handling® lets me show that care and concern in every way, every day . . . ”
- “Increased stress can cause changes in your pet’s test results and delay healing . . . ”

Make a list of reasons why commitment to provide Low Stress Handling® is important, both for the pet and for the veterinary team. Next, take a few minutes to turn these reasons into a series of statements which feel authentic to the team, are easy to remember, and can be delivered to clients with honesty, sincerity, and conviction. Creating a worksheet outlining possible scenarios and role playing can be used during team training.

2.8 The Medication Conversation

Embracing Low Stress Handling® methods results in increased dispensing of anti-anxiety medications and sedation. Whether it is oral medications administered before a visit, added to a hospitalized pet’s treatment plans, or injectable medications for procedural sedation and general anesthesia, practicing Low Stress Handling® will, by necessity, increase a professional’s use of these important tools.

Particularly early in the process, some team members may disagree with the administration of these medications. In addition to the emotional reasons discussed earlier, they may feel that sedation indicates poor handling and restraint skills, anticipate client refusal of treatment due to additional costs, or fear that the medications could pose a physical risk to the animal. While physical restraint could cause physical and emotional injuries to both the pet and the team, the result may be more costly for the hospital compared to sedation. For example, additional team members might be needed to help restrain each pet.

Conversations about medications with clients and among team members set the tone for the entire hospital. These conversations are perhaps one of the most crucial keys to successfully adopting these methods and techniques.

Table 2.8.1: Alternative Scripts for Medication Conversations

Different Methods	Low Stress Handling® Method
"Mrs. Smith, we will try to clean Fido's ear. If he can't hold still, we will need to sedate him. I can call you with an updated cost if we need to pursue sedation. If you don't allow us to sedate, we can do our best to clean it without sedation and see how it looks in a few days."	"Mrs. Smith, Fido has an infection in his right ear, and it needs to be flushed all the way to the eardrum. His ear is red and painful, so before treatment, the doctor would like to give him medications to reduce his pain and ease any anxiety he may experience. This will also allow us to thoroughly flush his ear so we can get him feeling better quickly. Is that alright with you?"
"Mr. Tip, Bowser is limping because he injured his leg, and I need to take a radiograph. Some dogs will let us take them while awake, but others will not. We will try without sedation first, and I will call you if he won't let us."	"Mr. Tip, Bowser needs a radiograph of his leg. See how he moves and looks away when I touch it? He is telling me that it hurts and that he is uncomfortable with me. I would like to give him pain medicine and something to help him relax so we can help him feel better."
"Ms. Blake, let me grab another assistant to hold Fluffy still for her blood draw. She is a wiggly kitty, and it will be tricky to get her sample."	"Ms. Blake, thank you for bringing Fluffy in for bloodwork. See how she flattens her ears a bit and moves away when she sees the syringe? This blood test is not urgent, and stress can change the blood test results. May I send you home with some calming medications, and have you bring her back for her blood draw in a few days?"

The first step in this conversation is to identify how these medications are used to treat fear, anxiety, stress, and pain. Using terms such as stress reducers, fear reducers, calming medicines, and relaxation medications helps clients understand their importance. The second step involves creating scripts to highlight the positive aspects of these tools for both the team and the veterinarian-client-patient relationship (VCPR). Table 2.8.1 shows examples of script replacements for common situations in which medications may be prescribed.

In these three examples, the same information is provided to the client. The left column undermines the skill of the veterinary team and the emotional capital of the pet. The right column clearly communicates how medications enhance and standardize care. Scripts like these improve the culture within the hospital and demonstrate to the client how deeply the veterinary team cares for their pet. Effective and open communication with clients and team members makes all the difference when it comes to implementing Low Stress Handling®.

2.9 What If These Communication Strategies Don't Work?

In rare circumstances, upholding the importance of Low Stress Handling® methods may result in a team member or client switching to another hospital for employment or veterinary care. While it can be disappointing to lose a team member or client, nurturing a Low Stress Handling® culture and prioritizing the physical and emotional welfare of pets is imperative. Not every hospital is the right fit for every team member or client. The goal should be to build the best team, foster client relationships, uphold a gold standard of welfare, and accept the occasional departure of an employee or client without compromising ethics.

2.10 Conclusion

Helping animals, and addressing their physical needs and emotional health, while working in a community of like-minded individuals, is truly a gift. Sharpening communication skills, not just with pets, but also team members, colleagues, caregivers, and *ourselves,* promotes wellness and welfare for all. At its core, veterinary medicine is a people business.

2.11 References

1. Zak, P. (2013). *How Stories Change the Brain. Greater Good: The Science of a Meaningful Life*. 17, 1–4. https://greatergood.berkeley.edu/article/item/how_stories_change_brain. Accessed 4/28/2024.

2. Brown, B. (2015). *Daring Greatly: How The Courage to be Vulnerable Transforms the Way We Live, Love, Parent and Lead*. Penguin Publishing Group.

3. Brown, B. (2018). *Dare to lead: Brave work. Tough conversations. Whole hearts*. Random House.

4. Brown, B. (2015). *Rising Strong: The Reckoning. The Rumble. The Revolution*. Random House.

5. Volk, J. O., Felsted, K. E., Thomas, J. G., & Siren, C. W. (2011). Executive summary of the Bayer veterinary care usage study. *Journal of the American Veterinary Medical Association*, 238(10), 1275–1282. https://avmajournals.avma.org/view/journals/javma/238/10/javma.238.10.1275.xml

6. Bard, A. M., Main, D. C., Haase, A. M., Whay, H. R., Roe, E. J., & Reyher, K. K. (2017). The future of veterinary communication: Partnership or persuasion? A qualitative investigation of veterinary communication in the pursuit of client behaviour change. *PLoS One*, 12(3), e0171380. https://doi.org/10.1371/journal.pone.0171380

Author
Monique Feyrecilde BA, LVT, VTS (Behavior)

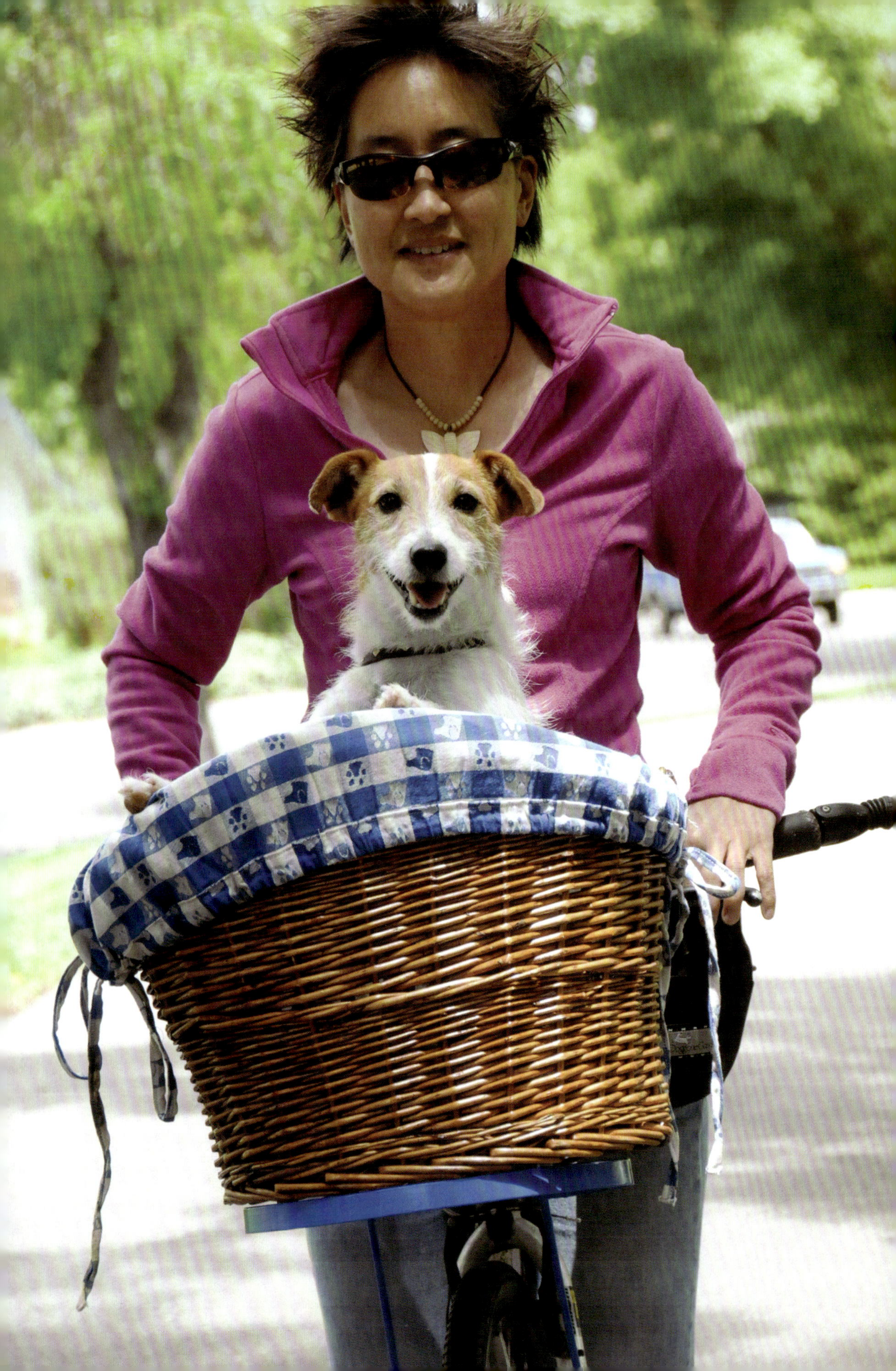

CHAPTER 3

Working Together to Build a Low Stress Handling® Pet-Centered Care Community

3.1 Introduction

Veterinary care is only one aspect of the multi-faceted lives of animals. Although animals spend a small proportion of their time under direct care of veterinary teams, the benefits of Low Stress Handling® and pet-centered methods apply to all aspects of their lives. Creating a *care community* is a good way to help meet a pet's needs. Not every animal care professional is aligned with Low Stress Handling® concepts, and veterinary professionals cannot always meet the needs of every pet (e.g., grooming, training, and boarding). By teaming up with other pet professionals who share the same philosophies, veterinary professionals can build networks throughout the community to meet the needs of pets and their caregivers.

When seeking out these professionals, clients often consult with the veterinary team. Therefore, it is the responsibility of the team to evaluate local service providers and to develop healthy working relationships with them, while educating clients on the importance of screening each provider. Because of this, veterinary hospitals are more likely to receive referrals and new patients, allowing for earlier detection and intervention when problems arise. When local professionals cannot be found in the community, many services, especially behavioral care, training, and coaching, can be found remotely.

Some hospitals have relatively informal referral processes in place, with team members familiar with other community members who provide these services. It is important that all team members be on the same page when making these referrals. Client care representatives should have a list of resources available that can be provided to ensure these referrals fall within the standards of the hospital's beliefs and ethics. This chapter provides guidelines for building your care community.

3.2 Providing Behavioral Care

Using a *detect-and-refe*r model is helpful for behavior disorders. This model is quite common in veterinary medicine at large. For example, most general practice veterinarians can identify a patient who is suffering from intervertebral disc disease but would refer the patient to a Diplomate of the American College of Veterinary Internal Medicine (Neurology) for specialized imaging or surgical care. The same model is effective for behavior concerns and referral to a Diplomate of the American College of Veterinary Behaviorists for diagnosis, prognosis, and a comprehensive treatment plan. For those pets that do not require referral, the veterinarian should provide recommendations for appropriate, welfare friendly trainer and consultant options.

Clients may not immediately consider contacting the veterinary team for behavior or training questions. Asking behavior and elimination questions during every history primes clients to ask the veterinary team for help when they detect a change in behavior or problematic behaviors. This strategy allows for earlier intervention and often a better prognosis.

Types of Behavioral Professionals

In the treatment of behavioral disorders, each professional has a potential role in the behavioral care for pets. Based on their credentials, skill sets, and experience level, some professionals fulfill more than one role in this process. Behavioral professionals include:

- **Veterinarian:** Veterinarians in general practice diagnose, prescribe medications, treat medical and behavioral conditions, and perform surgery.
- **Board-certified Veterinary Behaviorist:** A Diplomate of the American College of Veterinary Behaviorists (DACVB), is a veterinarian who has completed specialty training through a residency, contributed to research in behavioral science, published case reports, and passed a several days' long exam.

These specialists evaluate the mental and physical health of an animal, providing in-depth specialized care for all species.

- **Veterinary Technician:** Credentialed technicians support the veterinarian and maintain accurate medical records. They obtain patient histories, assist with examinations, collect lab samples, and communicate with clients by explaining the diagnosis and treatment plan prescribed by the veterinarian. Depending on their skill level, some technicians create and administer detailed training and behavior modification plans, including discussing prescribed medications and strategies for their administration.
- **Veterinary Technician Specialist:** Specialized technicians, VTS (Behavior), are certified through the Academy of Veterinary Behavior Technicians. For this certification, documentation of at least 4,000 clinical experience hours in behavior, a credentials evaluation, and passing a national board exam are required. Considered top-level experts in the field, these specialists can provide even deeper levels of support to the veterinarian for prevention and interventional treatments for behavior patients.
- **Applied Animal Behaviorist:** An applied animal behaviorist holds a master's degree or PhD in addition to passing a rigorous certifying examination. Certified applied animal behaviorists (CAABs) and associate certified applied animal behaviorists (ACAABs) can provide behavior modification and training for both prevention and intervention. CAABs and ACAABs cannot diagnose disorders or prescribe medications.
- **Behavior Consultants and Trainers:** Behavior consulting and animal training organizations are unregulated, or they are entirely self-regulated through individual certifying organizations. Different organizations require separate types of assessments. Some organizations require a lengthy educational program followed by examination, while others are dues-based membership organizations.

3.3 Evaluating and Networking with Fellow Veterinary Professionals

Creating a care community for collaboration starts by identifying local and remote options to support pets and their families. Providing the best service for pets and their families means establishing these relationships early before they are needed. Directories that list veterinary behaviorists (DACVB) and technicians certified as VTS (Behavior) are available on their respective websites: www.dacvb.org and www.avbt.net. Contact these specialists directly to determine availability of services, wait time, the referral process, and cost.

With relatively few veterinary behaviorists, the nearest board-certified veterinary behaviorist (DACVB) may be too far for feasible in-person referral. Most offer vet-to-vet remote consultations and some provide direct-to-client remote consultations depending on telemedicine laws. When regional referral is not feasible, inquiring through the website can identify who provides these services.

Some veterinarians are not board-certified but have practices limited to behavior or accept behavior cases within certain parameters. Consider networking within your community to identify these veterinarians. When contacting them, inquire about the types of cases they accept, wait times, cost, and scheduling process. Veterinarians who are not board certified may not have the same code of ethics as a DACVB. Therefore, it is important to discuss what methods they recommend for training and behavior modification before directing clients their way.

Technicians with a specialty in behavior are also few. For veterinarians seeking support with behavioral patients, a VTS (Behavior) can be an excellent resource. A number of these technicians do accept telemedicine and teletraining referrals for training, behavior modification, client education, and case support. Direct contact with the primary veterinarian will need to be maintained throughout the treatment.

3.4 Evaluating Trainers and Behavior Consultants

Unlike veterinary medicine, training and behavior modification services are unregulated. Individuals can advertise their services

Table 3.2.4 Common Behavior and Training Organizations

Professional	Designation	Degree Required	Written Exam	Practical Skills Evaluated	Continuing Education Requirement	Code of Ethics
Veterinary Behaviorist	DVM, DACVB	DVM, Residency	Yes	Yes	Yes	Yes
Veterinary Technician Specialist	LVT/CVT/RVT, VTS (Behavior)	Technician Credential	Yes	Yes	Yes	Yes
Certified Applied Animal Behaviorist	CAAB ACAAB	PhD MS	No	No	Yes	Yes
Karen Pryor Academy Certified Training Partner	KPA CTP	No	Yes	Yes	Yes	Yes
Certification Council for Professional Dog Trainers® Certified Behavior Consultant	CBCC-KA	No	Yes	No	Yes	Yes
Certification Council for Professional Dog Trainers®	CPDT-KA	No	Yes	No	Yes	Yes
Certification Council for Professional Dog Trainers®	CPDT-KSA	No	Yes	Yes	Yes	Yes
International Association of Animal Behavior Consultants	CDBC, CCBC, CHBC, CABC	No	Yes	No	Yes	Yes
Pet Professionals Guild: Accredited Training Technician or Professional Canine Trainer	PCBC-A PCT-A CTT-A	No	Yes	Yes	Yes	Yes
Pet Professionals Guild: Member	None	No	No	No	No	Yes

without fulfilling any formal requirements for knowledge, methods, or ethics. Caregivers may unknowingly assume any trainer or consultant with a business is accredited in some way.

Since all caregivers benefit from the services of these professionals, providing clients with guidelines on how to evaluate these professionals helps them choose the ones using evidence-based and humane training methods. Providing a welfare friendly lifestyle for pets means choosing humane training and behavior modification techniques which are effective and do not rely on the primary use of pain, fear, intimidation, or scarcity of resources to achieve training goals. Since prevention and early intervention start at a young age, those who offer puppy and kitten kindergarten classes should fall within these guidelines.

Veterinary Team Guidelines for Evaluation

Attending and directly observing classes is the best way to assess a trainer and the tools they use. Alternatively, published material and videos found on their website and social media pages help assess training philosophies and methods. When evaluating a trainer or consultant, consider:

1. **Positive Reinforcement First:** Positive reinforcement training is effective, creates lasting results, and preserves the relationship between the pet and caregiver. There is little risk for emotional or behavioral fallout when errors are made during the training process.

   During training and behavior modification, aversive tools are not appropriate. This approach creates more stress in the learner, decreases the number of behaviors the learner may offer, does not show the animal the correct answer quickly, and may increase stress, fear, and even aggression in some cases. Some other devices trainers may use are based on avoidance: shaker cans, squirt bottles, bean bags, throw chains, ultrasonic emitters, booby traps, static electric charge mats, and more.

   It is incredibly difficult to fulfill the criteria for effective punishment. Timing, frequency, intensity, and accuracy require immense skill to apply properly. In the overwhelming majority of cases, that skill is far better put toward positive reinforcement methods in the first place.[1–8]

   Not every consultant is committed to a welfare friendly lifestyle for animals, and not all are transparent about the devices and methods used. Ask which methods and devices a trainer or consultant uses before referring clients.

2. **No Guarantees:** Positive outcomes during training and behavior modification do not come with a guarantee. Training and behavior modification are dynamic processes dependent on many factors: emotional and physical health, skill level of client, trainer, or consultant, and more. Although training outcomes cannot be guaranteed, this does not apply to customer satisfaction policies.

3. **Open Door Policy:** Transparency is important. Trainers and consultants should be open to having their classes observed, although watching private sessions with paying clients might be inappropriate. This allows for verification of the methods and devices used, as well as evaluation of communication skills. Trainers should focus more on educating the caregiver than the pet. Some certification programs, such as the Karen Pryor Academy for Professional Dog Trainers, assess a trainer's teaching and communication skills before issuing a certification.

4. **Knowledge of Limitations:** A skilled professional understands the limitations of their knowledge and skills. Asking what types of cases the trainer or consultant accepts, and when they refer to a colleague, can streamline the process when looking to collaborate for a specific client. For example, some trainers or consultants may only work with one type of behavior, such as a certified separation anxiety trainer (CSAT), while others may not accept those cases at all.

5. **Protocols for Fearful, Anxious, and Stressed Pets:** Protocols should be in place for pausing, discontinuing, rescheduling, or restructuring sessions when a pet is showing signs of fear, anxiety, or stress during class.

6. **Check for Red Flags**: Examine photos on social media, websites, and marketing materials for pictures or videos of animals wearing aversive tools such as choke collars, prong collars, electronic shock, or vibration collars. Photos showing dogs in close proximity to one another, especially if they are on platforms, or down-stays should prompt a deeper look into the trainer's methods.[7]

Making the Referral

Check with trainers and consultants before referring animals with aggression and a bite history. These cases require prompt, streamlined referrals to professionals who have been confirmed in advance to accept them.

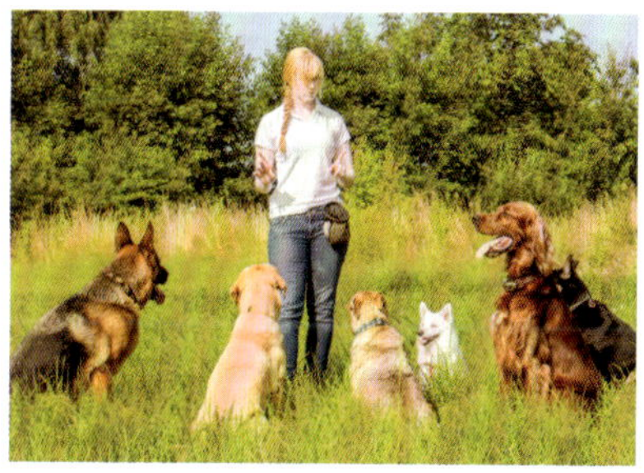

Fig. 3.4 A: Always check marketing photos for dogs training alongside each other, signs of stress (such as panting, looking away), and shock or vibration collars.

Table 3.4.2: Red Flag Terms

Red Flag Terms
Commands
Dominance
Alpha
Dominant Energy
Compliant
Submission
Alpha Roll
Dominance Down
Show A Dog Who's Boss
Make Them Submit
Doesn't Need Treats
Perfect
Guaranteed
Balance
Boot Camp

Important Vocabulary

When choosing a trainer or behavior consultant, check the text of their website, social media posts, and advertising for words like "dominance," "alpha," "command," "guaranteed," "balanced," or "boot camp," as these terms may indicate outdated training philosophies and methodologies. These beliefs and red flag terms can lead to recommendations that caregivers need to physically and emotionally intimidate or overpower their pets and that dogs are in competition or conflict with people.

Positive reinforcement trainers use words like "cue" instead of "command." These words have different connotations: cue is used when asking for behavior whereas command demands. In training, it is important to ask for behaviors and not demand them. Therefore, cue is more appropriate and indicates the trainer has a higher level of understanding learning theory and follows scientifically backed training methods.

Some trainers offer bootcamps which are often board-and-train facilities. Be cautious of this term as many of these facilities use punishment-based training techniques and aversive tools. In addition, the caregiver needs to be an integral part of the training process, which is not possible when they are not present. A few positive reinforcement trainers can be found offering this option; however, caregivers still need to be active participants since they also need training and will be the ones applying these concepts.

"Balanced" can be a tricky term. Some trainers and consultants who predominantly use punishment techniques in combination with rewards call this method balanced. Others utilizing rewards in addition to verbal interruptions, body blocking, or corrections for mistakes may also use the term balanced. A consistent definition for the term balanced is not available in the training world; therefore, this term should prompt further discussion about the tools and methods used.

Professionals who describe their methods as "Least Intrusive, Minimally Aversive" (LIMA) mean they work through a series of behavioral interventions utilizing primarily positive reinforcement first with negative reinforcement and positive punishment last, if at all. While punishment results in a change in the animal's behavior, it is difficult to perform successfully and can impair the pet's safety and welfare.

What is a Cue?

A ***cue*** is a signal to the learner that reinforcement is available if a certain criteria or condition happens. For instance, the word sit may be a cue that if the animal assumes a seated position, a reward will become available such as a treat, toy, or being released into the yard for play.

3.5 Evaluating Other Pet Professionals

Pet sitting, boarding, and grooming are other services caregivers may seek beyond veterinary care and training. These services can have a direct impact on the emotional health of the animal. When utilizing these services, it can be difficult for caregivers to assess the environment and human interactions that occur in their absence. Clients often ask the veterinary team to recommend boarding, pet sitting, and grooming options. Instead of direct referrals, the team can provide clients with a how-to list to evaluate and choose these businesses based on the criteria below.

Grooming

Clients often ask about grooming services for their pet. While veterinary hospitals may have a professional groomer on site, others do not. Therefore, knowledge about groomers and their handling skills in the community is important. Asking what methods are used can help caregivers choose groomers aligned with Low Stress Handling® methods. Some key questions to consider include:

- Are they comfortable with veterinary-prescribed medications to reduce anxiety during grooming?
- Are training or practice grooming sessions available to increase the pet's comfort level with the grooming process?
- Does the groomer recognize body language associated with fear, anxiety, and stress?
- What protocols are in place for pets who are showing distress during the grooming process?
- What safety measures are in place to prevent grooming-related injuries, both physical and emotional?

Groomers are a crucial part of the Low Stress Handling® community, and many pets visit the groomer more often than the veterinary hospital. Some organizations offer a certification course with an ethics pledge. Providing referrals for certified grooming options helps the veterinary team protect the emotional welfare of their patients on multiple levels, not just for veterinary care.

Least Intrusive, Minimally Aversive Method

LIMA does not justify the use of punishment in lieu of other effective strategies. The overwhelming majority of behavior change can and should be achieved through assuring the animal's needs for well-being are met (nutrition, physical health, exercise, social interaction), antecedent arrangement, management, positive reinforcement, reinforcing alternate desired behaviors, desensitization, counterconditioning, etc. Always ask a trainer or consultant which tools they use, and what they try first. Punishment is never an appropriate first intervention.

In-Home Pet Sitting and Home Away Sitting

In-home pet sitting can be a valuable service, especially for pets that are afraid and anxious when away from the home. Some pet sitters may hold an additional certification, such as one from Pet Sitters International (PSI®) or Fear Free® Pets. Both certification programs require a knowledge assessment and adherence to a code of ethics. Inquire about a pet sitter's level of education, first aid training, insurance status, and comfort level before providing a referral.

Since a stranger entering the home may be stressful, a meet-and-greet should occur in which the sitter comes to the home, learns important safety information, meets the pet(s), and performs a mock entry into the home. This test visit with the caregivers nearby gives an opportunity to arrange an entry routine that minimizes stress and suits the needs of the pet.

As an alternative to in-home services, some pet sitters offer home away sitting (care in their own home). This requires the pet to travel to the sitter's home. For this option, additional inquiries beyond those above should include a safety plan for interactions between visiting pets and the sitter's own pets (if applicable), what training methodology, if any, is used in the home, and plans for pets who show signs of distress.

In recent years, pet sitting apps have become available for choosing and scheduling both in-home and home away options. These apps list sitters, allowing caregivers to search by area, available dates, and other filtering data. As a result, it has become even more important for caregivers to carefully evaluate chosen sitters in advance since these apps provide little to no oversight regarding each individual skill level or certification. Because of this, veterinary teams should consider providing clients with a handout or tutorial to assess these sitters.

Pet Boarding

Boarding differs from pet sitting because it often occurs at a facility with a significant number of other animals. Not every animal will be emotionally suited to this option. The basic guidelines for pet welfare at boarding facilities are similar to those for at-home and home away sitting but should also include a facility visit prior to boarding.

Pet boarding centers should be chosen based on their open-door policy for visitation prior to boarding. The facility should be clean, well-maintained, and have a high staff-to-animal ratio.

Caregivers should inquire about any training performed during boarding, safety protocols, and a plan for pets that are fearful, anxious, or become distressed during their stay.

Dog Daycare

Dog daycare can be beneficial for some dogs; however, not all dogs will enjoy or benefit from the experience. Some veterinary hospitals provide this service. Credible daycares should include staff training for basic animal behavior, including body language interpretation and positive reinforcement methods to manage dog groups.

A high staff-to-dog ratio is important to maintain a minimally stressful environment. When this ratio is low, staff members may become overwhelmed and use aversives and punishment-based training methods. Dogs should be screened carefully, with protocols in place to evaluate stress levels during their stay.

Dog Walking

Having a dog walker can enrich the lives of many dogs. Some dog walkers may only walk one dog at a time while others juggle several or provide adventure services in which they take the dogs to an off-leash area, hiking trails, or private property for longer excursions. Like pet sitting services, dog walking apps are available.

As with pet sitters, dog walkers generally come into the home while the caregiver is away to collect the dog. A meet-and-greet session should occur prior to the first walk (see in-home pet sitting). Each walker should be carefully evaluated for the tools they use (e.g., collar, harness, etc.), training methodologies, the number of dogs walked at once, and their comfort level with dogs needing space, special handling, or other safety considerations.

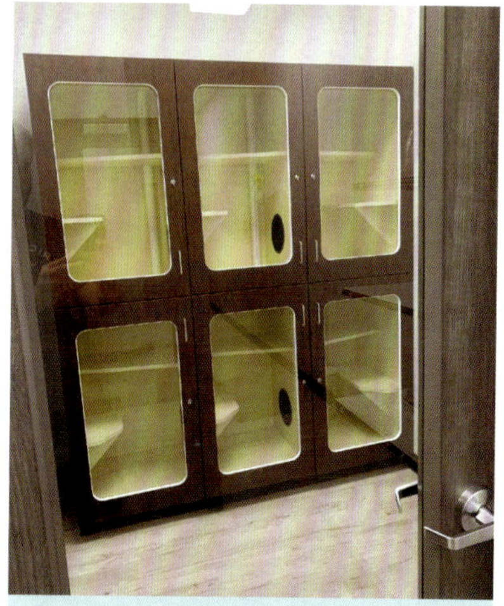

(Photo courtesy of Jennifer Le- A Couple of Vets)

When boarding cats, special considerations should be made and how a facility houses their cats.[3]

Criteria to look for should include:

- Cages should not be near dog facilities, preferably out of hearing range.
- Cage layout should be such that cats can not see other cats.

3.6 Conclusion

Veterinary professionals are in a unique position to enhance the lives of people and pets in their care. Creating a care community allows veterinary teams an opportunity to protect the welfare of their patients. Through education and referral to specific providers, the veterinary team helps clients choose groomers, trainers, and other common services to improve their pets' quality of life and protect the human-animal bond.

3.7 References

1. Feyrecilde M. (2024) *Cooperative Veterinary Care.* Wiley Blackwell

2. AVSAB. (2019) Position Statement: How to choose a trainer. *The American Veterinary Society of Animal Behavior*. Accessed 11/1/2022. https://avsab.org/wp-content/uploads/2021/08/AVSAB-Humane-Dog-Training-Position-Statement-2021.pdf

3. Taylor, S., St Denis, K., Collins, S., Dowgray, N., Ellis, S. L. H., Heath, S., Rodan, I., & Ryan, L. (2022). ISFM/AAFP Cat friendly veterinary environment guidelines. *Journal of Feline Medicine and Surgery*, 24(11), 1133–1163.

4. Martin, D., Shaw, J. (2023) *Canine and Feline Behavior for Veterinary Technicians and Nurses*. Wiley Blackwell

5. Herron, M. E., Shofer, F. S., & Reisner, I. R. (2009). Survey of the use and outcome of confrontational and non-confrontational training methods in client-owned dogs showing undesired behaviors. *Applied Animal Behaviour Science*, 117(1-2), 47–54.

6. Wise, Janee, (2022) Exploring relationships between dog training approaches and aggression, fear, and dog-owner relationship *CUNY Academic Works.* https://academicworks.cuny.edu/hc_sas_etds/968

7. Masson S, de la Vega S, Gazzano A, Mariti C, Pereira GD, Halsberghe C, Leyvraz AM, McPeake K, Schoening B. (2018) Electronic training devices: discussion on the pros and cons of their use in dogs as a basis for the position statement of the European Society of Veterinary Clinical Ethology. *Journal of Veterinary Behavior*, 25, 71–75.

8. Edwards, P. T., Smith, B. P., McArthur, M. L., & Hazel, S. J. (2023). Implementing stress-reducing veterinary care: perceptions of Australian veterinary professionals working with dogs. *Anthrozoös*, 36(4), 555–578.

Author
Monique Feyrecilde BA, LVT, VTS (Behavior)

CHAPTER

4

The Process of Learning and Changing Behavior

4.1 Introduction

Learning can be functionally described as a change in behavior resulting from experience or mechanically defined as changes within the organism due to such experiences.[1–3] However, learning is a dynamic and complex process that occurs on a cellular level, affecting both the neurochemical and anatomical makeup of the brain.[3] This process enables an organism to adapt their behavior to patterns observed in the environment, all while processing sensory input to acquire, retain, and recall information.[1,2] Many behavior problems are rooted in fear, anxiety, and frustration. As such, a combination of management, training, and behavior modification is needed. To understand the reasons behind certain behaviors and how to modify them, comprehending the basics of learning theory is essential.

4.2 How Animals Learn

The study of how animals learn and adapt to their environments reveals two fundamental types of learning: non-associative and associative learning. These two forms of learning are foundational in understanding animal behavior and cognition, each playing a role in how animals interact with their surroundings.

Stimulus

Anything the nervous system perceives through sight, sound, touch, smell, or taste. ***Stimuli*** is the plural of stimulus.

Non-Associative Learning

Non-associative learning is a basic form of learning that does not involve making direct associations but influences how an animal responds to individual stimuli.[3,4] The animal's perception and behavior can increase or decrease upon repeated exposure. There are two forms of non-associative learning that permit an animal to adapt to its environment: habituation and sensitization.[3,4]

Habituation

Defensive reactions play a key role in survival when faced with surprising or novel stimuli, giving time for the brain to assess their significance.[4] *Habituation*, the simplest form of learning, often leads to a decrease in response to a sensory stimulus over repeated exposure, including aversive ones.[3,4]

The intensity of the stimulus and repeated frequency determine the rate of habituation.[4] However, habituation might be temporary, and spontaneous recovery, also known as *dishabituation*, could occur, returning to the initial fear response.[4] This is more likely to occur with a high intensity stimulus over short intervals as opposed to a lower intensity stimulus exposure over longer intervals.[4]

Sensitization

In contrast to the habituation process, *sensitization* is an increase in response to a sensory stimulus over repeated exposure.[3,4] This typically occurs when escaping or avoiding the repeated stimulus is not possible.[4] Sensitization results in a heightened, almost hyper-focused reaction, hindering the ability to ignore the stimulus.[4]

Most research on habituation and sensitization centers around aversive events. However, this type of learning also occurs with nonaversives.[4] For instance, while initial engagement with a new toy may lead to

Example

Habituation

Imagine a caregiver uses an anti-bark collar as a training tool to discourage barking. The first time the dog barks and receives a mild shock, the dog might startle and stop barking briefly due to the unexpected sensation and discomfort from the shock. However, if the shock remains at the same mild intensity and is applied each and every time the dog barks, the dog might start to bark again even after feeling the shock. This is because the dog becomes ***habituated*** to the sensation, recognizing it as non-threatening or at least something they can tolerate. Over time, the less intense shocks lead to quicker habituation, and the dog no longer startles and just continues to bark. Habituation is why these types of aversive devices are ineffective and unnecessary.

Sensitization

Returning to the same example of the anti-bark collar: the first time the dog barks and receives a mild shock, they might startle and stop barking momentarily due to the unexpected sensation and discomfort. If the shock remains at the same mild intensity and is frequently applied every time the dog barks, instead of becoming accustomed to it, the dog might become more reactive. This is ***sensitization***. Each subsequent shock, even if mild, might amplify the dog's distress and protective emotions (anxiety, fear, or frustration). Over time, the dog does not just react to the sensation of the shock but might also start to react anxiously to situations or stimuli associated with the shock, such as the sound of the collar beeping before the shock or even the action of putting the collar on. In this case, due to the inability to escape or avoid the stimulus, an intensified and hyper-focused response occurred instead, thus hindering the dog's ability to ignore or tolerate the stimulus. Sensitization is why these devices are ineffective, unnecessary, and inhumane.

disinterest over time due to habituation, there is also the potential for hyperfocus or even compulsive like behavior with the toy due to sensitization.[4]

Associative Learning

Unlike non-associative learning, associative learning occurs when two stimuli or events become linked.[3,4] This principle of association traces back to the Greek philosopher Aristotle in 350 BC.[4] He recognized the importance of *contingency*, or close proximity in time, for one event to be linked to another.[4] The closer the events occurred together, the more likely one was to lead to the thought of the other.[4] Associations do not necessarily rely on logic.[4] They can be formed based on *temporal contingency*, indicating how close they are in time, or *spatial contingency*, referring to how close they are in location.[4]

While Aristotle's findings were based off human observations, Ivan Pavlov, a famous Russian physiologist, and Edward Thorndike, an American student of psychology were the first scientists to research how these associations were acquired by animals.[3,4] Independently, their research provided the foundation for both *classical* and *operant conditioning*, which often occur simultaneously.[3,4] With conditioning referring to a type of learning where the timing (contingency) of events is important, animals learn both from natural interactions within their environment and from human manipulation of stimuli or consequences.[4]

Ivan Pavlov, a Russian scientist, is best known for his experiments with drooling dogs and ringing bells. He demonstrated that an evoking stimulus (food) can be repeatedly paired with a neutral stimulus (bell) to create the same response (drool) as the evoking stimulus. The dogs subconsciously learned to drool in response to the bell even when no food was present. Pairing stimuli is one way to modify behavior. This is known as ***classical conditioning***.[4]

Edward Thorndike earned his Ph.D. in Psychology with his thesis titled "Animal Intelligence," based on experiments using mazes and puzzle boxes he created. At the time, it was believed that in order to solve a problem, an animal first had to understand it. Using chickens, dogs, and cats in his experiments, Thorndike proposed that an animal's level of intelligence was based on their ability to solve these puzzles through the process of ***trial-and-error*** or ***instrumental learning***. He concluded that all animals learn in a similar manner. Thorndike was the first scientist to study operant conditioning within behaviorism, which is learning behaviors through interaction with the environment.[4]

B. F. Skinner, an American psychologist best known for his work with lever-pressing rats and pecking pigeons, developed a new research tool known as the Skinner Box, inspired by Edward Thorndike's puzzle boxes. Unlike Thorndike, Skinner introduced the concept of ***shaping***, where reinforcements are given for approximations toward the desired behavior, rather than waiting for the full behavior to occur. The Skinner Box was designed with levers that the subject could manipulate, which removed the necessity for researcher intervention during reinforcement.[3,4] Through his experiments, Skinner demonstrated that an animal's behavior could be strengthened (increased) or weakened (decreased) based on the consequences that followed the behavior. He termed the impact of this response-reinforcer relationship on behavior as ***operant conditioning***.[4] Changing consequences is one way to modify behavior.

Spatial contingency is defined as the consistent association between a *specific location* and a *subsequent event*.[4] For example, if a cat receives a treat from the pantry every time they enter the kitchen, they will start to run to the kitchen or become alert when they hear the pantry door, in hopes of getting a treat. This behavior occurs because the cat has learned to associate the sound of the pantry door opening with receiving treats.

Temporal proximity is defined as the occurrence of *two events* closely together in *time*.[4] For instance, when a dog sees their caregiver pick up their leash, they usually go for a walk shortly thereafter. Due to the repeated close timing between seeing the leash and the beginning of the walk, the dog starts to show excitement and anticipation at the sight of the leash, expecting that a walk is about to happen. This association between the leash and the walk is established because they consistently occur one right after the other.

Classical Conditioning

Classical conditioning, also known as Pavlovian conditioning, involves the pairing of two stimuli to create the same involuntary response.[3,4] It is considered stimulus-stimulus-response learning (S-S-R). Involuntary or unconscious responses can include any reflexive physiological changes such as heart rate, blood glucose level, salivation, and emotions. During classical conditioning, a stimulus (unconditioned

Example

Example of classical conditioning: Imagine a young puppy named Max. The first time Max goes to the veterinarian, he has no idea what a stethoscope is. As the veterinarian approaches Max with the stethoscope, the puppy feels anxious about the unfamiliar environment, the different smells, and the unfamiliar people handling him. When the veterinarian uses the stethoscope to listen to Max's heartbeat, the coldness and pressure of the instrument might make him a little uncomfortable and more anxious.

After a few more visits where the same sequence happens, Max begins to associate the sight of the stethoscope with the feeling of anxiety and the overall experience of the veterinary visit. Now, whenever Max sees what he thinks is a stethoscope, even outside the veterinarian's office, he might show signs of anxiety or discomfort, anticipating the feelings he has come to associate with it. The stethoscope, initially a ***neutral stimulus (NS)***, has become a ***conditioned stimulus (CS)*** that evokes an anxious ***conditioned emotional response (CER)*** in Max due to its association with veterinary visits.

Now let's look at the same example of Max and the stethoscope from a different perspective:

The first time Max goes to the veterinarian, he has no prior association with a stethoscope. As the veterinarian approaches Max with the stethoscope, his caregiver presents him with a tasty treat. Max eats it and enjoys the treat. While the veterinarian uses the stethoscope to listen to Max's heartbeat, Max continues to eat treats that his caregiver is giving him.

After a few visits where this process is repeated, Max begins to associate the sight of the stethoscope with the yummy treat that his caregiver provides, forming engaging emotions. Now, whenever Max sees a stethoscope, even outside the veterinary office, he might wag his tail or show signs of excitement, anticipating the treat he has come to associate with it.

This is also an example of ***classical conditioning***; in this instance, the stethoscope, initially a ***neutral stimulus (NS)***, has become a ***conditioned stimulus (CS)*** that evokes engaging emotions and an expectant ***conditioned emotional response (CER)*** in Max, due to its association with treats given by his caregiver during veterinary visits.

stimulus or US) that initiates a response (unconditioned response or UR), is paired repeatedly with a neutral stimulus (NS) until it becomes a conditioned stimulus (CS) and creates that same response. That response is then called a *conditioned response (CR).*

Emotions can be classically conditioned to create a *conditioned emotional response (CER).*[3,4] Definitive measurements of emotional states are not possible, but observable body language provides insight.

Taste Aversion

Taste aversion is a distinct type of classical conditioning with unique features. Unlike typical conditioning that needs several pairings of stimuli, taste aversion often occurs through *one-event learning*. This means that just one instance of pairing a specific taste with sickness can create a lasting dislike for that taste. This kind of conditioning is also unique in its ability to handle long delays between the taste (neutral stimulus) and the sickness (unconditioned stimulus), sometimes for several hours. This challenges the usual idea in classical conditioning that the stimuli need to be close together in time. Taste aversion has real-world importance. Animals, including humans, can develop dislikes for foods linked to past sicknesses, even if the sickness appears hours later. This serves as an important survival mechanism to avoid harmful substances. However, in long-term illnesses, it can cause animals to avoid foods they connect with their clinical signs, leading to possible nutritional deficiencies and other health issues. Therefore, taste aversion shows the complexity and adaptability of learning in animals, suggesting that classical conditioning can work in ways different from what was traditionally thought.

Classical Counterconditioning

Classical counterconditioning is a behavior modification technique used to change an emotional response to a particular stimulus by associating it with an opposing or desired response.[3,4] In this process, a stimulus that previously elicited a protective emotion is consistently paired with a positive or desirable stimulus, in an attempt to replace the protective emotions with engaging ones.[3–10] Classical counterconditioning is often used in conjunction with desensitization.

Fear Conditioning

Emotionally driven reactions prompt behaviors that involve either interaction with the environment (engaging emotions) or self-preservation (protective emotions). Fear, anxiety, pain, and frustration can lead to a temporary yet adaptive emotional arousal, marked by physiological and behavioral reactions that ensure the animal's safety. However, when these reactions are experienced repeatedly or over prolonged periods, they can become maladaptive, resulting in distress and suffering. This is called ***fear conditioning.***[5–10]

Is the Animal Stubborn or Just Not Food Motivated?

Delaying reinforcement can sometimes motivate animals to try harder. When trainers frequently reinforce only familiar behaviors, they usually see just those behaviors repeated. However, trainers who are not consistent with reinforcement might find the animal losing interest, leading to the mistaken belief that the animal is stubborn or not motivated by food. If this is occurring, breaking the behavior down into smaller steps and reinforcing each step often leads to the animal learning the goal behavior more quickly and staying engaged in the process.[4]

Operant Conditioning

Operant conditioning involves conscious behavior that occurs due to a consequence.[3,4] It is considered response-stimulus (R-S) learning. When the consequence occurs during a behavior or immediately following a behavior (contingency), the animal can associate the two events.[3,4] Predicting consequences helps an animal determine what behavior to display in a certain context. Consequences can be *added (+)* or *removed (–)* and they can serve as *reinforcement (R)* or *punishment (P)*.[3,4,11] When aspects combine, they form the four processes (contingencies) of operant conditioning (sometimes called four quadrants).[3,4]

Positive Reinforcement (+R): *Adding* a desirable consequence with the goal of *increasing* future behavior.[11]

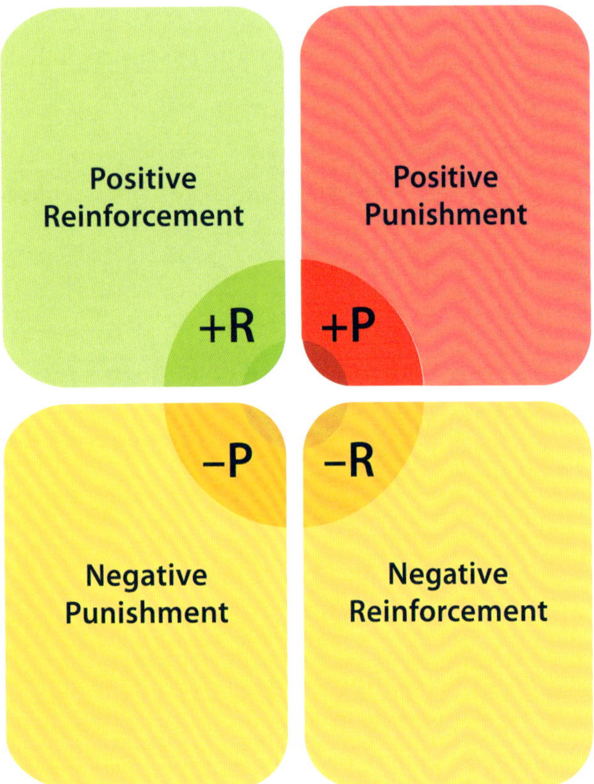

Fig. 4.2 A: The four consequences (contingencies) of operant conditioning.

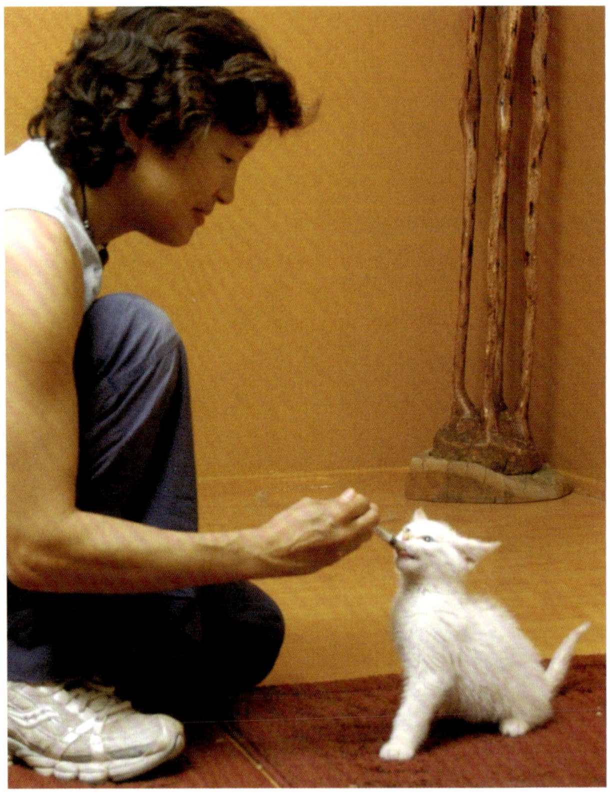

Fig. 4.2 B: Positive Reinforcement. The kitten sits and is fed a treat. If sitting increases in the future, giving (positive) the treat (desirable) acts as reinforcement.

Negative Reinforcement (–R): *Subtracting* or removing an undesirable consequence with the goal of *increasing* future behavior.[11]

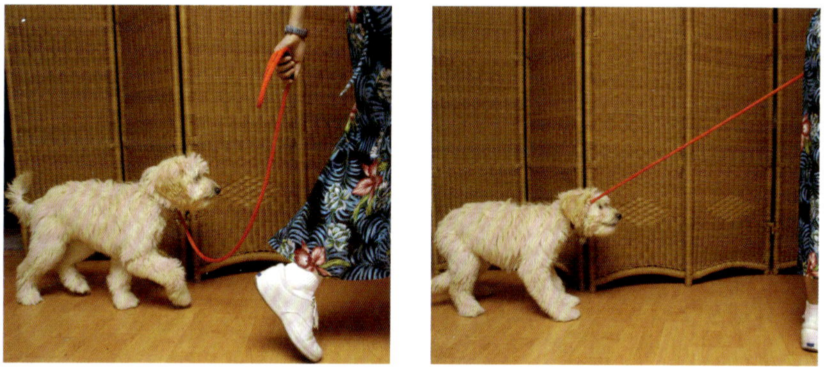

Figs. 4.2 C, D: Negative Reinforcement. The dog moves forward, and the leash loosens. If the dog moves forward in the future, the removal (negative) of leash pressure (aversive) acts as reinforcement. Moving forward to avoid leash pressure will likely occur again.

> ***Negative reinforcement*** is often confused with ***positive punishment*** because they both involve an undesirable or aversive consequence. Remember the intended goal: ***reinforcement*** increases the frequency of a behavior and ***punishment*** decreases that frequency.

Positive Punishment (+P): *Adding* an undesirable or aversive consequence with the goal of *decreasing* future behavior.[11]

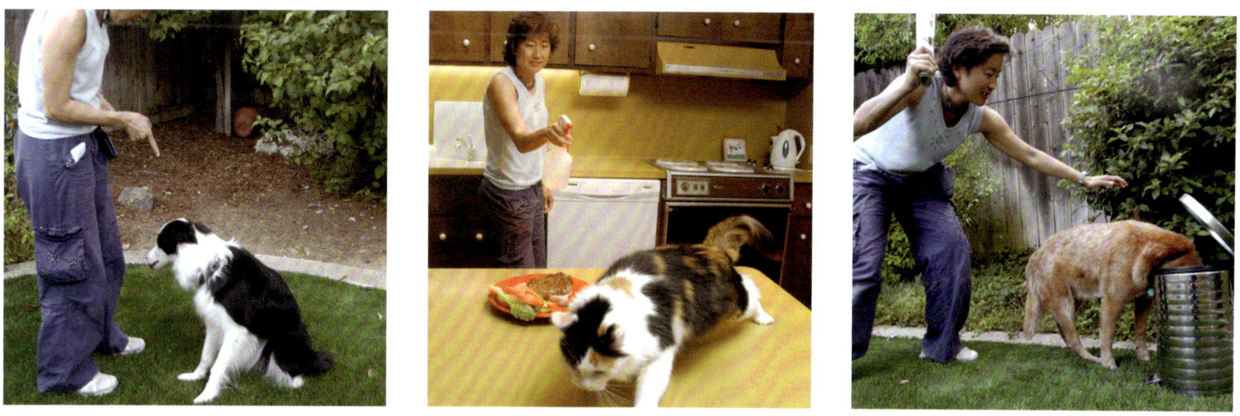

Figs. 4.2 E–G: Positive punishment. The animal performs an undesired behavior and a threatening tone of voice or gesture, sprayed water, grabbing, and hitting (aversive) are applied (added) by the person. If the unwanted behavior decreases in the future these consequences act as punishment.

Increasing or *decreasing* a behavior refers to not just the frequency of occurrence but also the intensity, duration, speed of onset, speed of performance, and overall look of the behavior.

Perils of Punishment

Positive punishment is ***NOT*** recommended due to the high risk of pain, protective emotions (fear, anxiety, frustration), and defensive behaviors (including aggression).

The animal determines what is desirable or undesirable in any given context, not the person. Whether a consequence is reinforcing or punishing can only be determined by observing if future behavior increases or decreases.

Negative Punishment (–P): *Subtracting* or removing a desirable consequence with the goal of *decreasing* future behavior.[11]

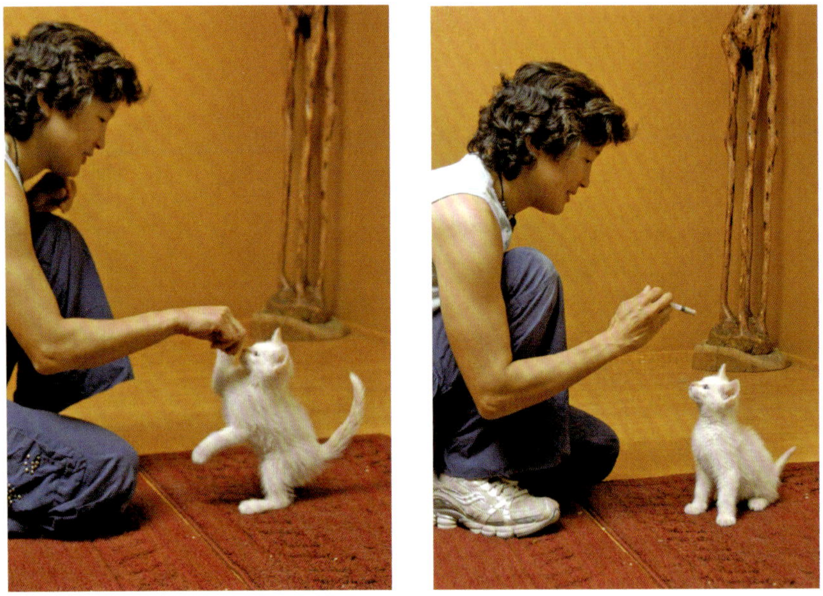

Figs. 4.2 H, I: Negative punishment. The kitten's paw grabs the hand holding food (undesired behavior). The hand with food is withdrawn (subtracted). If the paw grabbing behavior decreases in the future, the removal of food (consequence) acts as punishment.

Displacement and Conflict Behavior

Displacement behaviors are behaviors that are typical for the species but exhibited out of context.[12] Conflict behaviors can occur during motivational or decision-making struggles.[12] Both are the result of *confusion*, *stress*, *frustration*, or *anxiety*.[12]

Even with careful planning and skilled implementation, learning new behaviors can be stressful. The inconsistency in training, due to mixing reinforcement and punishment techniques or using ineffective reinforcers, reduces predictability and affects communication. Recognizing displacement and conflict-related behaviors, as well as observing subtle changes in body language, helps identify potentially stressful environments and interactions. Once these are recognized, adjustments can be made to the training plan to improve the learner's comfort level.

4.3 Three-Term Contingency

The three-term contingency, also known as the ABC model, refers to:

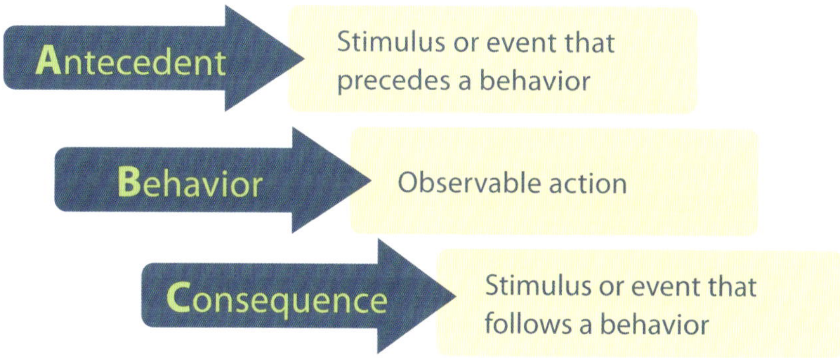

Fig. 4.3 A: The Three Term Contingency or ABC's of Behavior. (Illustration courtesy of Sherrie Yuschak)

Identified as a *behavior unit*, this concept of evaluating behavior is credited to B. F. Skinner.[17,18] He introduced this model as part of his development of operant conditioning theory.[18] In operant conditioning, behaviors are learned and modified based on their consequences, and the three-term contingency helps describe and analyze the relationship between the environment and behavior.[3,4,17,18] The ABC model has since become a foundational concept in applied behavior analysis (ABA) and is widely used in various fields, including education and therapy for individuals with autism and other developmental disorders.[18]

Antecedents

Antecedents (A) help an animal determine the appropriate behavior and when to perform it.[17] Within the behavior unit, the antecedent indicates what consequence is likely to follow and helps the animal predict the behavior's success.[17] Humans can provide antecedents such as a verbal cue to sit, while the environment offers antecedents such as a litterbox indicating where to urinate.

Behavior

In the ABC model, B stands for *behavior*, which refers to the specific action or response exhibited by an individual following an antecedent and before a consequence.[17]

Common Displacement and Conflict Behaviors[13–16]

- Licking lips when not eating (dogs)
- Scratching or licking fur (dogs and cats)
- Yawning (dogs)
- Sniffing the ground/object (dogs)
- Shaking off when not wet (dogs)
- Mounting (dogs)
- Blinking (cats)

Yawning

Given the stimulating veterinary environment, if a pet yawns during a visit, it is unlikely that they are tired or bored. Since yawning is out of the typical context of sleep, it is likely indicative of confusion or stress.

Consequences

Consequences (C) help an animal determine why they should repeat a behavior.[17] Because they are part of the three-term contingency, a consequence influences the meaning of the antecedent and determines whether a behavior is likely to be repeated or not. Humans can provide consequences such as yelling when the pet spills the trash, and the environment offers consequences such as lying in a sunbeam provides warmth.

Example

Applying the ABC Model

Antecedent (A): A human approaches the dog's food bowl while the dog is eating.

Behavior (B): The dog bares their teeth, growls, and snaps at the human.

Consequence (C): The human retreats and leaves the dog and their food alone.

Behavior Analysis and Functional Assessment

Animals behave to achieve consequences that meet their needs. *Applied Behavior Analysis* is an applied science that is used to change behavior by determining the function or purpose of a behavior through a *Functional Assessment.*[19,20] Understanding the relationship between a behavior and its antecedent, and how the behavior varies with different consequences, provides insight into the function that behavior serves.[17,19,20] This knowledge can be used to modify behavior.[19,20]

When evaluating behavior using the ABC (antecedent, behavior, consequence) method, it is important to operationalize the behavior.[19] To *operationalize* means to define the behavior in terms that are *clear*, *observable*, and *measurable*.[19] This way, any observer, regardless of their personal viewpoints or interpretations, can consistently identify the behavior.

Example

Applied Behavior Analysis

Every time a cat hears a can open, they run into the kitchen, meow for food, and rub up against the person's legs. The sound of the can opening serves as an ***antecedent***, signaling to the cat that food might be available. Running into the kitchen, meowing, and rubbing against the person's legs are the cat's ways of expressing their desire for food. This is the ***behavior***. If the cat is fed, this ***consequence*** reinforces the behaviors of running, meowing, and leg-rubbing, making it more likely for the cat to repeat the same behaviors the next time they hear the can opener.

On the other hand, if the cat does not receive food after several instances of the can opening, these behaviors might decrease over time because the expected consequence of receiving food is not consistently delivered.

Functional Assessment

Antecedent (A): The cat hears the sound of a can opener or the opening of a food can.

Behavior (B): The cat quickly runs to the kitchen and begins to meow and rub up against the person's legs.

Consequence (C): The cat receives the food from the opened can and eats it.

Antecedent Arrangement

Antecedents are plentiful within the environment and include anything the animal perceives before a behavior.[17,19,20] Reducing distractions helps in focusing on the necessary information. Antecedents can be strategically arranged to elicit a goal behavior.[17,19,20] Determining where to train, how props should be placed, where the person should sit or stand, and the position of the animal are some basic considerations.

Animals tend to orient towards people and food so placing any props (needed for the goal behavior) in front of the person and between the animal sets up the ideal opportunity for prop interaction.

4.4 Teaching Animals

Teaching animals diverse behaviors enables more choice and cooperation during daily life. Positive reinforcement training focuses on generating behaviors desirable for both humans and animals. Key skills to effectively teach an animal using positive reinforcement include *observation*, *timing*, and *reinforcement*.

Before a behavior can be reinforced, it first needs to occur. Several positive reinforcement techniques can be used to generate behavior including *luring, targeting, capturing, and shaping*. Choosing a method depends on the goal behavior, its intended usage, the animal and person's skill set, and the time frame. Creating a plan before starting a session helps maximize success. Training efficiency is gained when goal behavior occurs frequently. Short, two-to-three-minute sessions, a few times per day are all that is needed.

Example

Operationalization of the Behavior

Consider the behavior of a dog being aggressive.

- ***Non-operationalized description:*** The dog is aggressive. This is ***subjective*** as aggressive could mean different things to different people.
- ***Operationalized description:*** The dog bares its teeth, growls, and snaps at a person within a distance of two feet. This is a more ***objective*** description of the behavior.

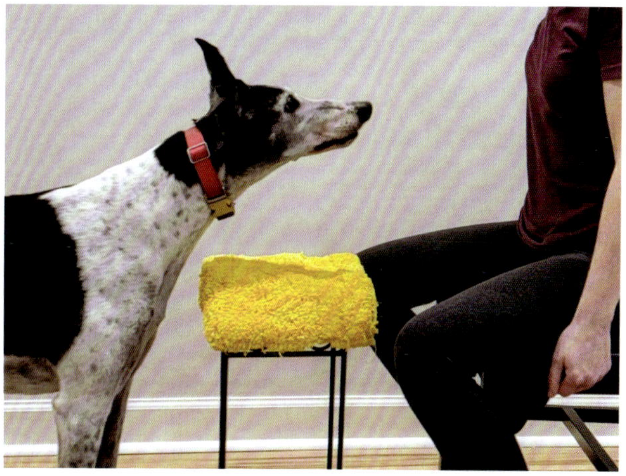

Fig. 4.3 B: The target prop is in front of the person and close to their feet. The dog is likely to approach the person and line up with the prop. (Photo courtesy of Sherrie Yuschak)

Changing Behavior

When experiencing confusing, obnoxious, or unwanted behavior, remember this behavior serves a purpose for the animal. Identifying the Antecedent, Behavior, and Consequence (ABC) of that specific behavior helps to understand its function. A behavior modification plan can then be developed to manipulate either the antecedent or the consequence, to achieve a different behavior from the animal.[19,20]

Luring

Lures come before the behavior, but they are also the reinforcer.[4] Food and toy lures are used most often when training animals. They entice the animal to do a behavior by presenting partial access to the lure. Once the behavior is achieved, they get the lure. Using a lure may seem simple but it does require skill. A lure must be chosen that is interesting but doesn't distract the animal from recognizing the behavior and consequence.[4] The lure must remain accessible to the animal to prevent frustration or disinterest. Lures should be faded after a few reps, to prevent reliance on the lure before offering the behavior.

When an animal is shown a reinforcer before performing a behavior, it is sometimes termed a *bribe*.[4] Labeling this as such is anthropomorphic, attributing human traits to animal behaviors. A lure is different from a bribe. In training, the presence of a reward acts as a conditioned stimulus signaling an upcoming reward or as a cue for a specific response.[4] Many trainers avoid lures because they might result in an animal that only responds when they see

Reinforcement and Observation

The goal of ***reinforcing*** a behavior is to increase its occurrence. Animals perform behavior all the time. Careful ***observation*** helps the person identify the behaviors they would like to reinforce.

Motivational Conflict

Using a food lure to guide an animal toward a frightening situation can intensify fear, create ***motivational conflict***, and potentially result in the animal avoiding that food in the future. Instead, use a different technique to increase the animal's comfort and use food as the reinforcer.

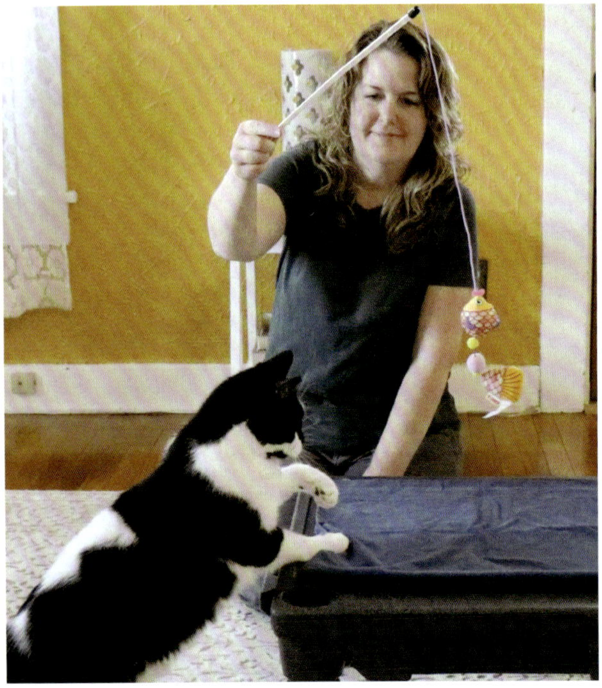

Fig. 4.4 A: A feather toy is used to lure the cat onto a platform for cooperative veterinary care. (Photo courtesy of Tara Fisher)

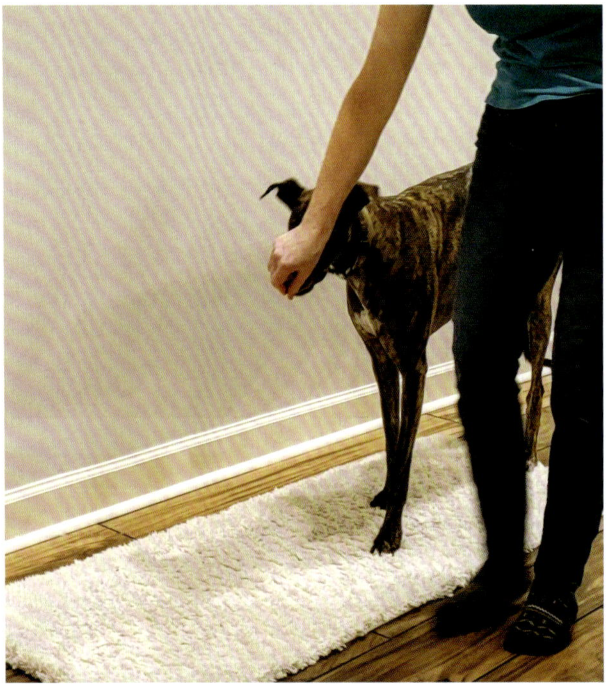

Fig. 4.4 B: Notice how the lure is in contact with the dog's mouth. This ensures the animal and lure move together to minimize frustration. (Photo courtesy of Sherrie Yuschak)

the reward. This could reduce their interaction with the environment and, as a result, limit their ability to learn new things.[4] However, in veterinary hospitals and other animal care settings, lures can help position animals without physical handling, especially when known behavioral cues are inconsistent or unknown.

Targeting

Targeting teaches an animal to electively place their body part on an object or person (such as a hand). This behavior is extremely useful for shaping many different cooperative care behaviors. Portable target props can be placed on other objects to shape a new behavior. The target can remain the cue for the specific behavior, or a different cue added. Fluent target behavior can help an animal focus and easily gain reinforcement, and pleasure, in uncertain scenarios.

All targeting related behaviors allow the animal to initiate the interaction instead of the person or object touching them. Once fluency is achieved, if the animal is unable to interact with the target on cue, or if they discontinue their interaction, this can indicate emotional or physical discomfort. Adjustments should be made before proceeding. Engagement with the target can improve communication and increase choice for the animal.

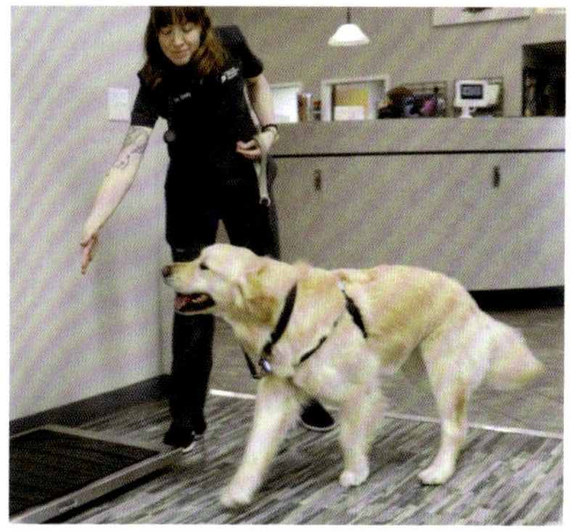

Fig. 4.4 C: This dog has learned to follow a target onto the scale. (Photo courtesy of Tara Fisher)

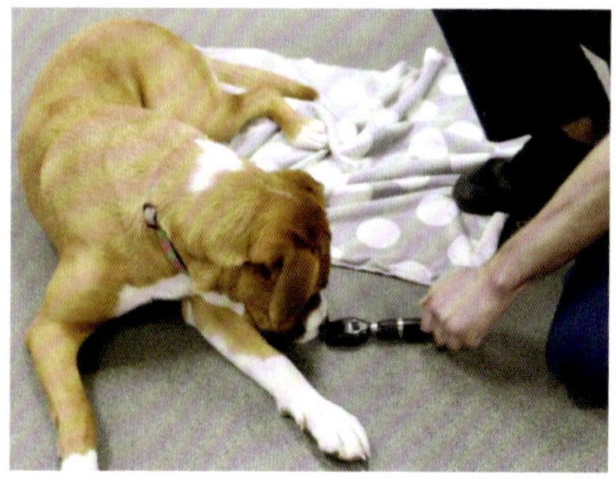

Fig. 4.4 D: This dog is targeting an ophthalmoscope before an eye exam. (Photo courtesy of Tara Fisher)

Targeting Tips and Pitfalls

- Targeting should not be used if the animal appears fearful or avoidant.
- The presentation method and location should be emotionally and physically comfortable for the animal.
- The target needs to be easily identified by the animal.
- Target manipulation skills are needed to ensure success and prevent frustration.

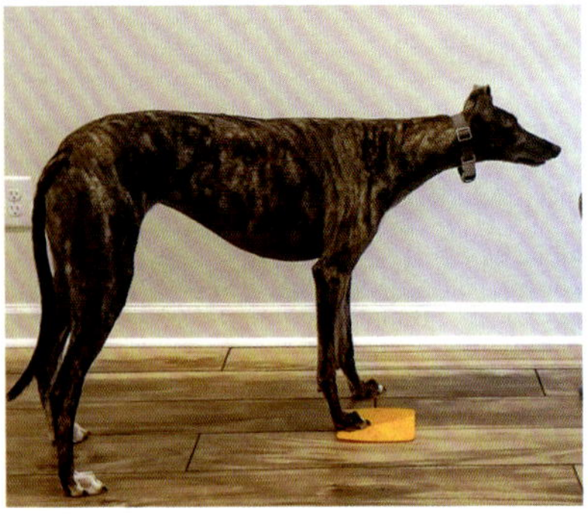

Fig. 4.4 E: An easy to identify, portable target was used for this dog's paw behavior. It can be moved to different locations to build fluency or shape new behaviors. (Photo courtesy of Sherrie Yuschak)

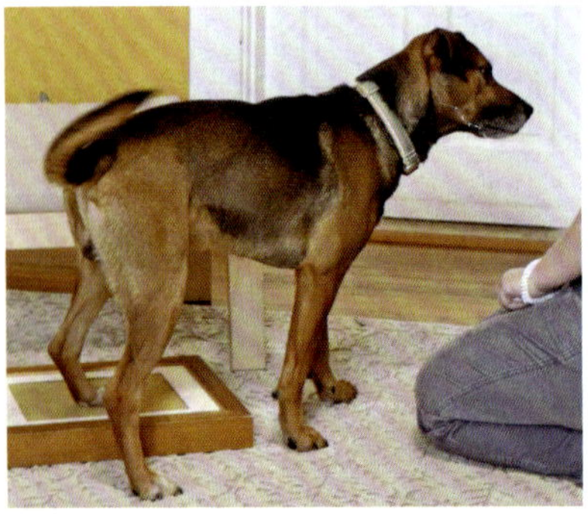

Fig. 4.4 F: Front or hind paw targeting can be used to shape self-filing of nails. (Photo courtesy of Tara Fisher)

Types of Targeting

Nose Targeting

Nose targeting can be used like luring but provides additional benefits over food lures. The animal's behavior causes the reinforcer (food) to occur instead of a human bribing the animal to do the behavior (with food).

- Exploration of objects, the environment, grooming and veterinary tools
- Placing the head in a certain position for examination, medication, or grooming
- Holding the head still (and thereby the body) for a blood draw, or other treatment
- Placing the nose/muzzle into an object such as a muzzle or inhaler

Paw Targeting

- Exploration of objects, the environment, grooming and veterinary tools
- Placing the paws/leg in a certain position for nail trim, venipuncture, or grooming
- Holding the paw still (and thereby the body) for examination and treatment
- Stepping onto an object such as a scale, platform, or mat
- Stepping, walking, and paw placement for mobility or neurological examinations
- Stepping, walking, and paw placement for physical therapy exercises and fitness
- Self-filing of nails
- Self-wiping of paws
- Putting paw/leg inside a body harness

Chin Targeting

- Placing the head in a certain position for examination, medication, or grooming
- Holding the head still (and thereby the body) for a venipuncture, teeth brushing
- Shaping step for relaxation on a mat

Eye and Ear Targeting

- Examination, cleaning, medicating, and grooming

Shoulder or Hip Targeting

- Examination or treatment through a safety barrier (protected contact) such as a mesh carrier, metal grate, or fence
- Intramuscular (IM) sedation

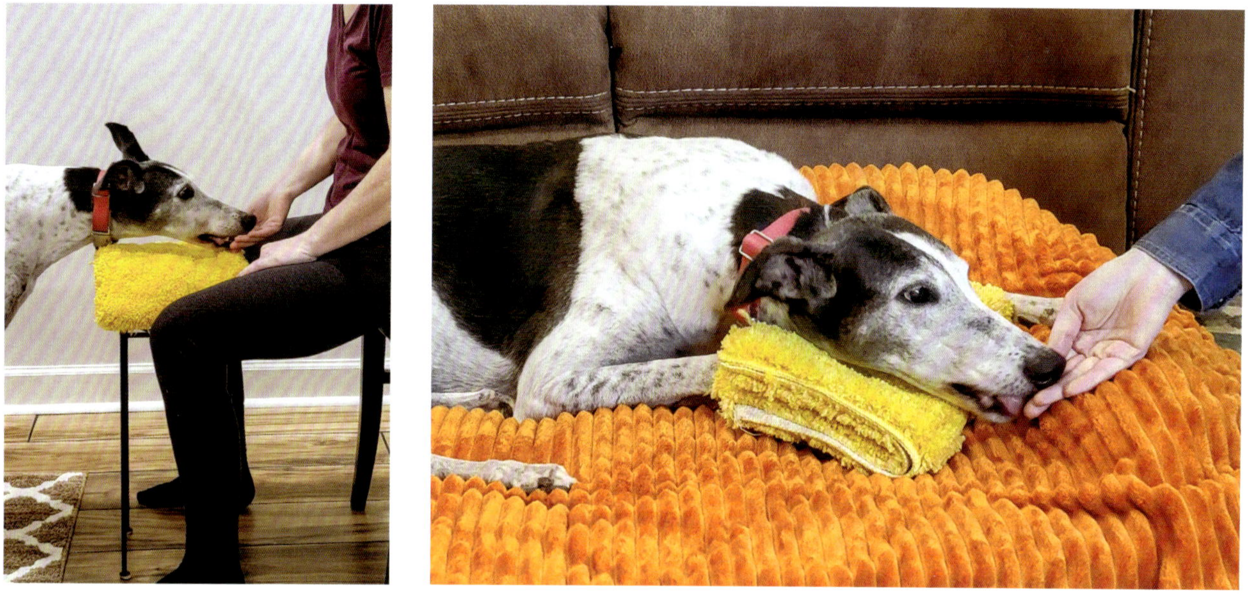

Figs. 4.4 G, H: A soft, portable target is used for this dog's chin. Adjusting the location of the target can gain different cooperative care applications. (Photos courtesy of Sherrie Yuschak)

Capturing

Capturing refers to reinforcing spontaneously offered behaviors. It can be used to teach behaviors that are difficult or challenging to teach using other methods. It is most effective when a goal behavior is naturally offered, occurs frequently, can be observed, and anticipated. Capturing can be the sole training technique or the first step in shaping new behaviors. Choosing which behaviors to capture depends on the individual animal, goal behavior, and the environment in which it will occur.

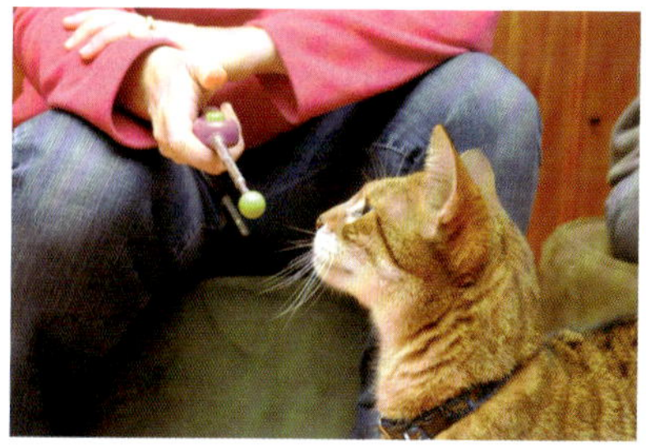

Fig. 4.4 I: A cat is taught to touch (target) their nose to the green ball at the end of a target stick.

Example

Capturing Examples

Urination

When the puppy squats to urinate outside, mark as soon as the urine stream finishes, then immediately follow with a treat. Urination behavior is ***captured***, and the outdoor environment becomes a future prompt (antecedent) to urinate.

Eye Contact

Animals naturally turn toward, move toward, look at, or otherwise pay attention to people, especially if they anticipate a potential reinforcement. Orienting toward a person is a great behavior to ***capture***. This behavior is useful in many scenarios, such as when the animal is seeking interaction, ready to receive a cue, or disengaging from a concerning stimulus.

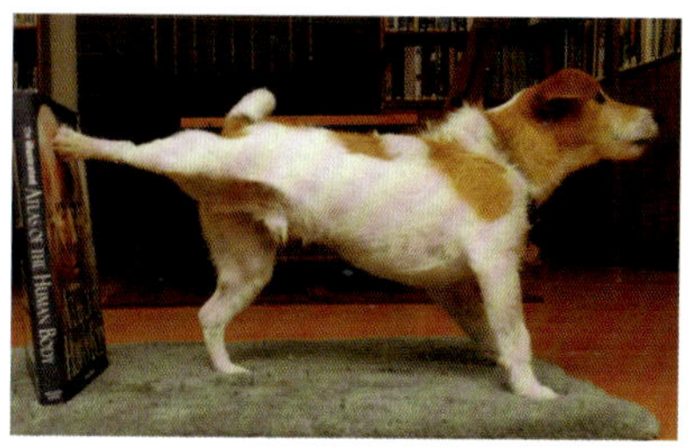

Fig. 4.4 J: Dr. Sophia Yin taught her dog, Jonesy, to target an object with his hind foot.

Relaxation on a Mat

Teaching an animal how to relax on a mat by first targeting specific body parts, such as the nose, chin, or feet, can later be used to modify behavior in different situations or environments. This approach helps create a positive conditioned emotional response to the mat, which then facilitates relaxation in new or distracting environments. By rewarding small steps towards the desired behavior, called ***shaping***, fewer errors occur, the learning process is accelerated, and a higher rate of reinforcement is achieved.

Example

Shaping

Goal Behavior: Lying on a mat

Antecedent: Fluffy, non-slip rug, placed in front of the person's feet

Reinforcement Strategy: Clicker. Toss the treat behind the dog to enable the next approach.

Approximations:

- Dog steps toward the mat. Mark then treat.
- Dog looks at the mat. Mark then treat.
- Dog places one paw on the mat. Mark then treat.
- Dog places two paws on the mat. Mark then treat.
- Dog places three paws on the mat. Mark then treat.
- Dog places four paws on the mat. Mark then treat.
- Dog sits on the mat. Mark then treat.
- Dog lies down on the mat. Mark then treat.

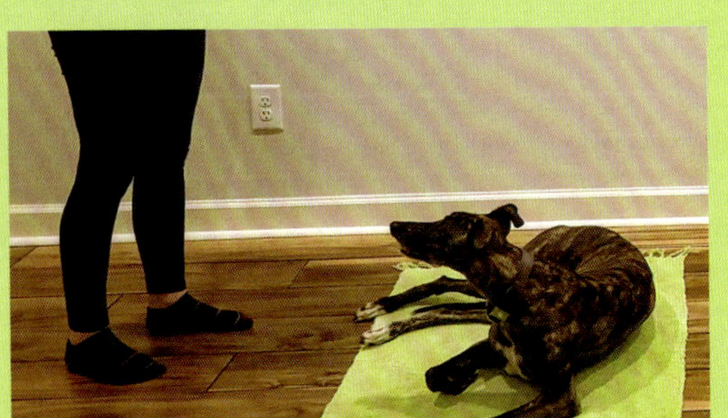

Photo courtesy of Sherrie Yuschak

Shaping

Shaping is a technique that reinforces small approximations toward a goal behavior.[4] Almost any behavior can be shaped, and the training techniques mentioned above blend well with shaping. Splitting a behavior into tiny, achievable steps is a critical component of shaping success.[4] The number of steps necessary depends on many factors, including the individual animal's needs and skill set. A reinforcement should be received every few seconds to minimize periods of waiting for the animal to offer new behavior.[4] This helps decrease frustration and speed up the learning process.[4] An effective shaping plan includes planning for the antecedent arrangement, acute observations, good timing, and an appropriate reinforcement schedule.

4.5 Creating Reliable Behavior

The success of animal training relies on maintaining newly acquired behaviors. This process involves introducing cues for behavior identification, using markers for accurate communication, and developing behavior ***fluency***. Beginning in low-distraction environments before gradually progressing to more challenging environments helps improve reliability. This approach ensures a dependable response to specific cues (stimulus control) and the adaptation of behaviors to various contexts (*generalization* and *discrimination*), ultimately achieving consistency of the behavior in different settings.

Adding in a Cue

Cues are information about which behavior to perform and an opportunity to receive reinforcement.[4] Sometimes the word *command* is used interchangeably with the word *cue*. However, command is more of an order or demand, and noncompliance is often followed by punishment. To best pair a cue with a specific behavior, teach the behavior first. Once the behavior is offered repeatedly and predictably, add the cue immediately before the behavior occurs. This process helps make sure that the cue acts as an effective antecedent for a specific behavior with a predictable consequence. Cues can be anything such as a particular word, a person's body or hand movements, sights, sounds, scents, sensations, and tactile (body) touching. A cue should only be associated with one specific behavior, able to be administered consistently each time, and easy to give by all people interacting with the animal.

Criteria

Criterion is a term that describes the specific behavior necessary to gain reinforcement. Preplanning and clear identification of the goal criterion lets the trainer know whether to click (and treat) or not. Shaping uses tiny shifts in criterion to meet the end behavior goal. ***Criteria*** are plural and include multiple aspects of behavior. Effective shaping steps focus on one criterion at a time.

Building Fluency

Fluency is the reliability and quality of behavior performance in response to a cue. Fluent behavior is *predictable* (animal responds correctly eight out of ten times) and is *functional* to its intended use. Fluent behavior can serve as communication from the animal. If they are unable to respond, their emotional or physical discomfort should be assessed. Fluency aspects include *precision* (consistent appearance), *latency* (time between cue and response), *speed* (performance time), *distraction* (environmental stimuli), *duration* (maintaining behavior), and *distance* (from the person or prop). Each aspect of fluency is shaped individually. When they can all be combined, a behavior is said to be fluent.

Adding a Cue: Before adding the ""sit" cue, the behavior of sitting in front of a person must first be captured. For example, a cat receives a treat every time they are observed sitting. After several repetitions, the person can start to anticipate when the cat will sit. Now, when the cat starts to sit, the person says "sit." As predicted, the cat sits and is reinforced. Thus, the cue "sit" is successfully paired with the sitting behavior.

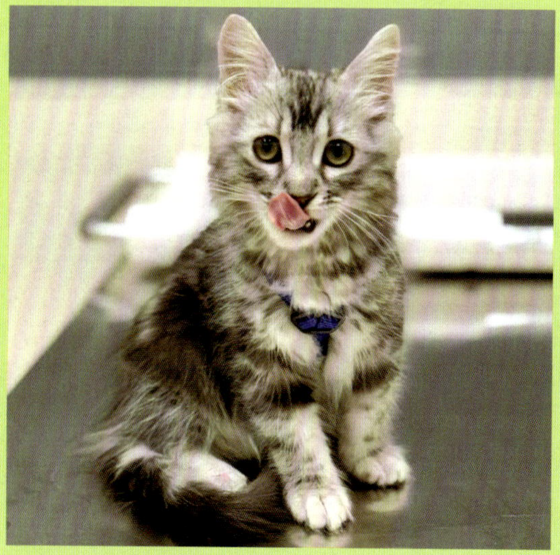

Photo courtesy of Monica Henderson

Stimulus Control

Stimulus control refers to the ability of a cue (stimulus) to reliably predict a behavior. When control over the stimulus (cue) is achieved it means the animal will respond to a specific cue paired with that behavior, every time it is cued. Once a behavior is placed under stimulus control, the behavior will not be offered if it was not cued, a different behavior will not be offered to that cue, and the behavior will not be offered for a different cue. Training sessions can be planned to teach stimulus control and ensure cues are reliable.

Generalization vs. Discrimination

Generalization, also known as proofing, can be included within fluency.[4] It refers to an animal's ability to exhibit a specific behavior across various environments and contexts.

Before generalization can occur, an animal must be able to differentiate between cues, accounting for various environmental factors such as words and body gestures, to achieve a dependable and functional application of that behavior. This process of differentiation is called ***discrimination***, or what some call placing a behavior under ***stimulus control***.[4]

Example

Placing a Cue Under Stimulus Control

Scenario: The desired behavior is for a cat to sit when given a verbal cue "sit."

Stimulus Control is Achieved When:

1. The cat sits every time they hear the cue "sit."
2. The cat does not sit unless they are specifically given the "sit" cue.
3. When cued to "sit," the cat does not offer an alternative behavior, like lying down.
4. When a different cue is used like "down" the cat does not sit.

Explanation: In this scenario, the behavior (sitting) is reliably under the stimulus control of the specific stimulus (the "sit" cue), and not any other stimuli or cues. This means the behavior has been effectively placed under stimulus control.

4.6 Reinforcer Types and Reinforcement Schedules

Reinforcement is a consequence of behavior.[3,4,19,20] During training, the reinforcer can be delivered to the animal strategically to set up the next behavior. The consequence of the previous behavior

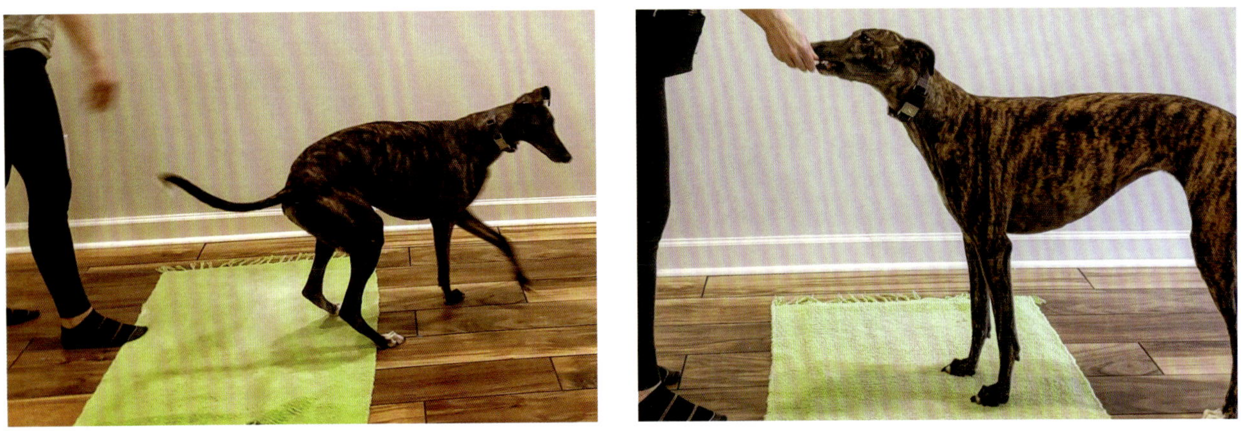

Figs. 4.6 A, B: When a person and a mat (antecedent) are in front of the dog, and the dog steps on the mat, a click occurs, and the treat (consequence) is tossed behind the dog. The dog turns around to face the person and mat again then steps on the mat. The tossing of the treat helps set up the next repetition of stepping on the mat. (Photos courtesy of Sherrie Yuschak)

then becomes part of the antecedent for the next behavior. This increases training efficiency because it keeps the session focused on goal behavior.

Reinforcement Types

Reinforcement can be divided into two different categories depending on how they are achieved.[4] They can be primary or secondary reinforcers.[3,4]

Primary Reinforcers

Primary reinforcers (unconditioned reinforcers) are things innately reinforcing and often biologically necessary for life such as food, water, shelter, sleep, sex, and more. The animal does not have to learn to desire this type of reinforcer.[3,4]

Secondary Reinforcers

Secondary reinforcers (conditioned reinforcers) are created by pairing a neutral stimulus with a primary reinforcer.[3,4] Through classical conditioning, the animal learns the value of the secondary reinforcer.[3,4] If the pairing decreases in frequency or without effective timing the secondary reinforcer will lose its association.[3,4] Money is a secondary reinforcer for humans. It is paired with primary reinforcers such as food and shelter and therefore money's value is learned.

> **Choice and Control**
>
> ***Choice***, which provides animals with the opportunity to ***control*** their environment and achieve a desired outcome, is a basic need and a ***primary reinforcer***.[20]

Marker Signals

To be effective, the reinforcement must occur during or immediately following the goal behavior.[3,4] Observing when the behavior is about to occur is important but if the primary reinforcer is delayed, learning will slow.[4] Instead, a signal can be conditioned as a secondary reinforcer and used to mark the exact moment the goal behavior occurs.

Using a marker is like taking a picture of a behavior. It captures the moment a behavior occurs and transfers it into the memory file. The best markers are easy for the animal to perceive but are neither startling nor scary. They should be distinct, devoid of any other meaning, easy to deliver, very fast, and consistently paired with the primary reinforcer. Choosing an appropriate marker depends on the sensory perception and preferences of both the person and the animal, as well as the intended goal behavior and the environment.

Markers

A ***marker*** can include a clicker, the word "yes," a thumbs-up, or a finger tap on the shoulder for animals that are hearing or visually impaired.

A clicker is a common marker. After every click, a primary reinforcer, such as food, is delivered to maintain the associations formed during classical conditioning between the clicker and the marker. Learning how to handle the clicker and deliver treats requires some practice before working directly with the animal. Deciding on which hand to use for the clicker and for treat delivery, and where to secure the treat pouch (or which pocket to use) comes first. The hand holding the clicker can rest at the person's side, and the treat delivery hand should remain still, in a position away from the treat pouch (such as near the belly button), except when actively delivering a treat. This helps the animal distinguish the connection between the click and their own behavior.

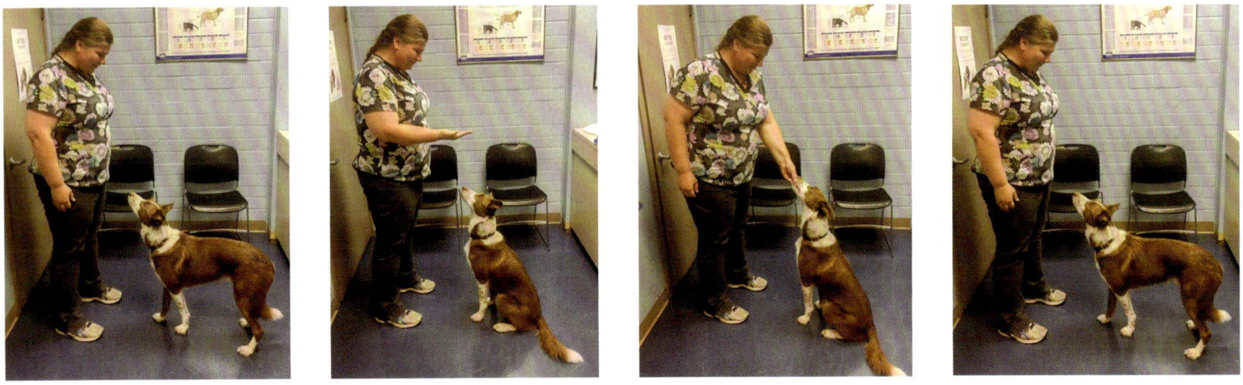

Figs. 4.6 C–F: Both hands are neutral at the person's side. The right hand can hold the clicker and give the sit cue. When the right hand clicks, the left hand reaches into the treat pouch, feeds the treat, and then both hands go back to the neutral position. A verbal marker or tongue click was used in these photos. (Photos courtesy of Monique Feyrecilde)

Using Treats

Smaller treats are preferred over larger ones during training sessions due to their ability to maintain an animal's interest and provide frequent reinforcement opportunities, especially when learning new behaviors.

Large, frequent rewards can lead to ***satiation*** (a feeling of fullness), causing an animal to lose interest in the training session.

Reinforcement Schedules

A reinforcement schedule identifies which instance of correct behavior will be reinforced.[3,4] Several different schedules exist with the goal of impacting behavior.[3,4] Some schedules require an advanced skill set to plan and implement effectively. Basic continuous reinforcement and intermittent reinforcement schedules will be discussed.

Continuous Reinforcement Schedule

A continuous reinforcement schedule strengthens behavior quickly and provides clear communication since every correct response is reinforced.[4] This schedule is best when teaching new behaviors, shaping for fluency, or working with a challenging behavior.[4]

Intermittent Reinforcement Schedule

Correct responses are reinforced some of the time when using an intermittent reinforcement schedule.[4] There are two dimensions: *Ratio* or *Interval* and *Fixed* or *Variable*.[4] Within these dimensions, there are four types: Fixed Ratio (FR), Fixed Interval (FI), Variable Ratio (VR), and Variable Interval (VI).

- ***Ratio:*** Number of responses necessary to gain reinforcement. Creates relatively rapid behavior change.
- ***Interval:*** Time duration after which the first response is reinforced. Creates relatively slower behavior change.
- ***Fixed:*** Predetermined and unchanging throughout the program. Can be a ratio (number of responses) or interval (length of time). Creates more persistent behavior, slower to be suppressed by extinction.
- ***Variable:*** Reinforcement fluctuates around a preset average (animal never knows which instance will be reinforced). Creates more persistent behavior, slower to be suppressed by extinction.

Three Key Principles of Reinforcement

1. Ratio schedules produce a higher rate of response and are less resistant to extinction than interval schedules.
2. Fixed schedules result in more pausing after a reinforcement is delivered and are less resistant to extinction than variable schedules.
3. Regardless of the reinforcement schedule, a lower rate of reinforcement leads to a less intense response during training but increases resistance to extinction after extensive reinforcement.

Matching Law

Matching Law demonstrates that animals will choose to perform the behavior that results in reinforcement more often. This is helpful to behavior change. Consistently reinforcing desired behaviors while reducing reinforcement for unwanted behaviors helps solve behavior problems.

Example

Matching Law

The Matching Law in behavioral economics suggests that the rate of a particular behavior is directly proportional to the rate of reinforcement for that behavior, compared to other available behaviors.

Behavior: A cat sits on the table after dinner, which occurs once per day.

Plan: Reinforce the cat every time they sit on the dining room chair, which occurs four times per day.

In this scenario, sitting on the chair is being reinforced four times as frequently as sitting on the table. According to the ***Matching Law***, this cat is more likely to choose the behavior (sitting on the chair) that is reinforced more frequently, meaning the cat will probably sit on the chair more often than on the table as long as all other conditions remain the same.

4.7 Changing Behavior

Behavior modification employs various methods to change emotional and subsequent behavioral responses to a stimulus or scenario. To be most effective, a detailed behavioral and medical history, along with a comprehensive treatment plan, is required.

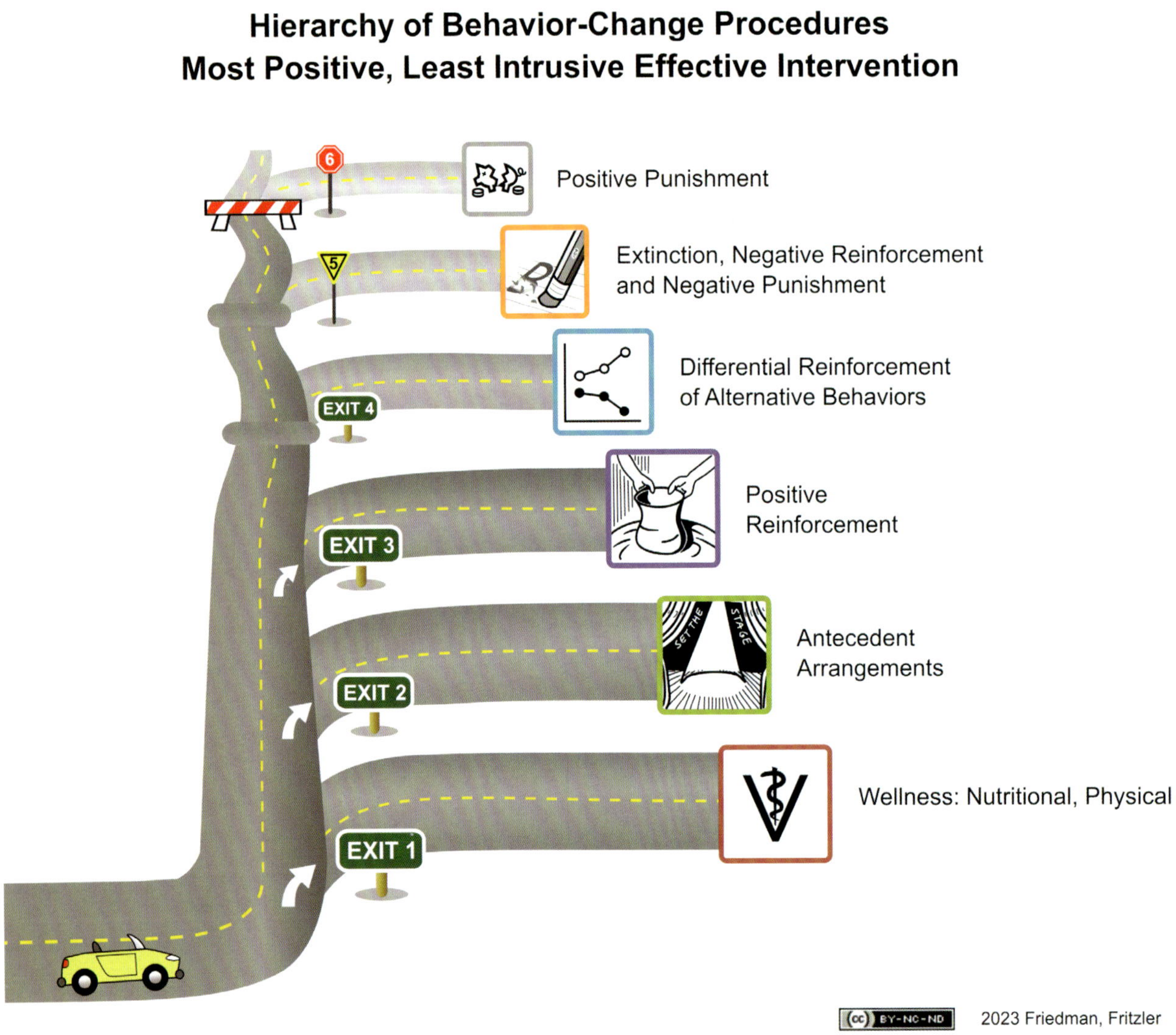

Fig. 4.7 A: Hierarchy of Behavior-Change Procedures. This graphic provides a visual representation of ranking modification methods to enable behavior change. (Illustration courtesy of Susan Friedman and James Fritzler)

The success rate for changing behavior is influenced by the animal's needs, the current knowledge and skills of the individuals involved, behavior goals, and available resources. A good understanding of body language, including displacement behaviors, is essential so adjustments can be made based on feedback from the animal. Although each animal is an individual, there are several ways to effectively modify behavior. Utilizing the most positive, least intrusive, effective solution should always be the priority.[20,21]

Procedures to Modify Behavior

Exit 1: Meeting Basic Needs

Meeting an animal's physical and emotional needs is the first step in the behavior modification process and is fundamental to ensuring their overall welfare and well-being.[20] While the categories of needs are the same for every animal, there variations based on the species and individual. Adaptations to the animal's environment and lifestyle, as well as addressing any medical conditions, should occur before proceeding with other behavior modification techniques.[20]

Addressing an animal's fundamental needs, including wellness, nutrition, and physical care, is essential for all behavior modification programs and indicates good welfare. Measuring welfare can be subjective, so guidelines like The *Five Freedoms of Animal Welfare* offer objectivity in determining if these needs are met.[22,23] These measurement guidelines, established in the 1960s due to concerns about livestock treatment in the UK, have since gained global acceptance emphasizing the importance of recognizing and addressing both the physical and emotional needs of animals.[22,23]

Over time, the perspective on animal welfare has evolved beyond the Five Freedoms.[23] When measuring welfare, professionals, ranging from animal welfare specialists to farmers and shelter workers, examine behavioral observations, health assessments, and physiologic factors such as stress hormone (cortisol) levels to provide a more comprehensive picture of an animal's emotional well-being and welfare.[23] Understanding and putting into practice these welfare measurements are fundamental. This comprehensive approach ensures that any changes to the animal's environment, lifestyle, physical, and emotional health are properly addressed, thus laying a solid foundation for effective behavior modification techniques.

Table 4.7.1: The Five Freedoms of Welfare

1	**Freedom from hunger and thirst**: by having readily accessible fresh water and appropriate nutrition to maintain health.
2	**Freedom from discomfort**: by providing an appropriate environment including shelter and a comfortable resting area.
3	**Freedom from pain, injury, or disease**: by providing adequate veterinary care.
4	**Freedom to express normal behavior**: by providing sufficient space, proper environment, and social interactions.
5	**Freedom from fear and distress**: by ensuring conditions and treatments which prevent mental suffering.

Exit 2: Antecedent Arrangements

Antecedents signal to the animal that a specific behavior, if performed now, will be reinforced.[20] Antecedents can be provided by a person as a cue or can come from the environment. Identifying and modifying or removing these antecedents is a straightforward and effective method for behavior modification.

Example

Antecedent arrangements

Antecedent arrangements: Food on the kitchen table (***antecedent***) results in the dog jumping onto the table (***behavior***) to get food (***reinforcer***). Removing the food (***antecedent***) can decrease the dog's jumping behavior. When using this procedure, other behavior modification methods should be added to maximize success such as management and reinforcement of an incompatible behavior.

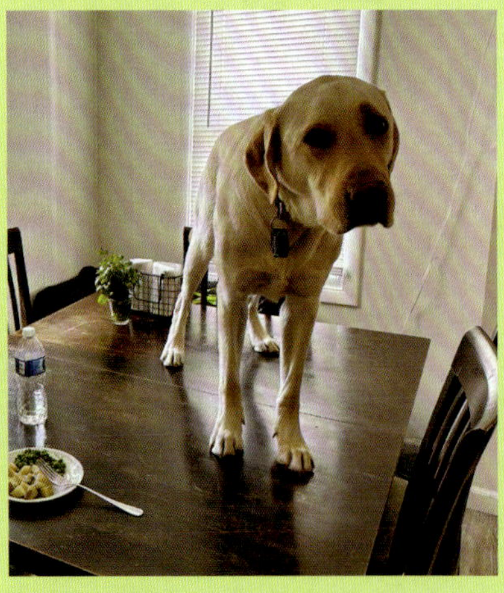

Fig. 4.7 B: This dog jumped on the kitchen table when food (antecedent) was present. (Photo courtesy of Deb McVicker)

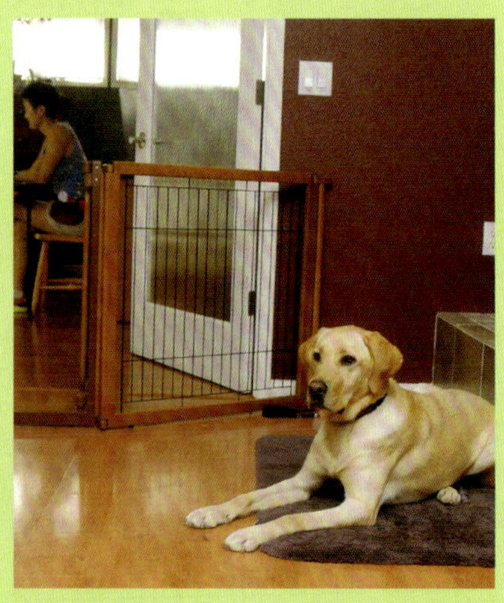

Fig 4.7 C: By removing access to the antecedent (food on the table), the behavior (jumping on the table) decreases.

Exit 3: Positive Reinforcement Training

Positive reinforcement is adding a desirable consequence with the goal of increasing future behavior. Communication and cooperation are necessary when humans and animals interact and live together. Increasing an animal's behavioral repertoire creates options for various contexts of everyday life such as preventing or managing unwanted behaviors. Animals learning with positive reinforcement are often more attentive to their caregivers, can have quicker response time to cues, show fewer fear related behaviors during training, and may have fewer behavior problems.[24–31]

Studies support that positive reinforcement is effective for all species, sizes, and breeds of animals and is an important part of a behavior modification plan.[24–33] This includes all types of behavior problems, even serious concerns such as biting, fighting with other animals in the household, running away, or predatory behavior.[29,34–36]

Note the Speed Bump Before Exit 4.

Exit 4: Differential Reinforcement of Behavior.

Differential Reinforcement of Alternative (DRA) and Incompatible (DRI) Behaviors are two methods for changing unwanted behaviors.[19,20] *DRA* focuses on reinforcing a specific *alternative* behavior to replace an undesirable one, while *DRI* involves reinforcing an *incompatible* behavior that cannot physically be performed at the same time as the unwanted behavior. Since these techniques require the learning of a new behavior, pause and collect additional information before proceeding. These steps can be more intrusive and stressful than previous methods. Because the animal no longer receives reinforcement for unwanted behaviors, they must learn a new behavior instead.

DRA vs. DRI

Differential Reinforcement of an Alternative Behavior (DRA) is the reinforcement of a specific alternative behavior to replace an unwanted one.

Differential Reinforcement of an Incompatible Behavior (DRI) takes place when the animal is reinforced for a behavior that cannot physically be performed at the same time as the unwanted behavior.

YIELD: PROCEED WITH CAUTION

Exit 5: Extinction, Negative Reinforcement, and Negative Punishment

The path diverges at this point, indicating that aversive techniques and their consequences should never be used in behavior modification or training.[24–33,37–40] Once this point is reached, referral to a board-certified veterinary behaviorist may be needed to evaluate

Example

Differential Reinforcement of an Alternative Behavior (DRA)

A cat has developed the habit of walking across the computer keyboard whenever their caregiver is typing, in an attempt to gain attention. Recognizing this, the cat's caregiver decides to employ a ***Differential Reinforcement of Alternative behavior (DRA)*** strategy. Therefore, instead of giving attention to the cat when they walk across the keyboard, the caregiver will deliberately ignore this behavior and walk away. However, when the cat chooses to lie down beside the keyboard without disrupting the typing, rewards will be given for this preferred behavior. Over time, the cat will learn that lying next to the keyboard is a more effective way to receive attention than walking on it.

In this scenario, lying beside the keyboard becomes the ***reinforced alternative behavior***. The caregiver, employing the DRA method, could have chosen to reinforce another behavior that was not disruptive to typing, such as the cat sitting on a designated mat or playing with a specific toy, and still have been successful. Adding food, a primary reinforcer, would also have been beneficial.

Example

Differential Reinforcement of an Incompatible behavior (DRI)

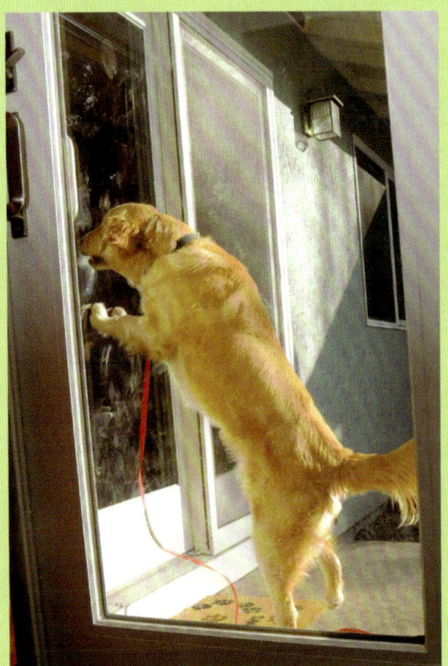

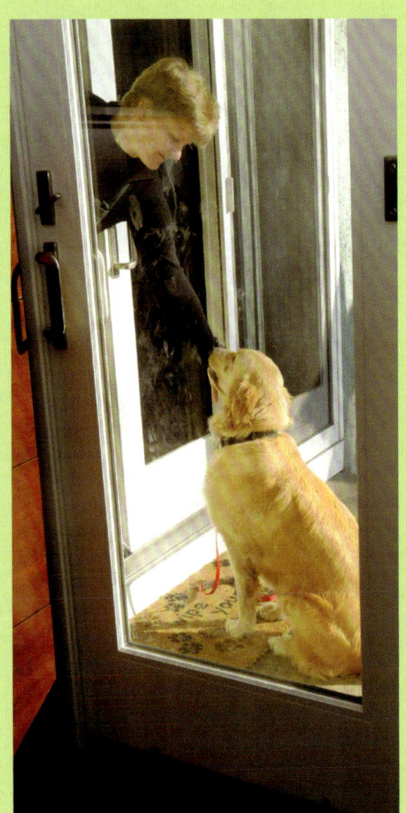

In this example, a dog has developed the behavior of jumping on the door as a signal of their desire to come inside when the door is shut. A functional assessment identifies the shut door as the antecedent, jumping on the door as the behavior, and the opening of the door, which allows the dog to come inside, as the consequence. To modify this behavior, ***Differential Reinforcement of an Incompatible (DRI)*** behavior is employed.

Initially, the dog is taught to respond to a visual hand signal for 'sit' using positive reinforcement. Once the dog consistently responds to this cue, the person uses the hand signal to encourage the dog to sit before opening the door. Gradually, the hand signal is phased out, and the closed door itself becomes the cue for the dog to sit to signal their desire to enter. Through the application of DRI, the dog has learned that sitting, rather than jumping, will cause the door to open, allowing entrance into the house.

the animal's overall medical and emotional health. At this appointment, the caregiver's goals can be reevaluated, a diagnosis made, and comprehensive treatment plan created.[41,42]

Animals naturally avoid aversive (unpleasant) experiences and seek reinforcement. Using aversive consequences may be effective at suppressing or eliminating unwanted behavior temporarily, but since fear, intimidation, or pain is part of the process, the animal must problem solve to decrease, avoid, or escape the punishment, resulting in long term emotional damage.[26,28–29,31–33,38–40]

Protective emotions (fear, pain, frustration, confusion) often occur when aversive tools and techniques are used, therefore, behavior modification goals should be geared towards promoting engaging emotions, not correcting mistakes or suppressing undesirable behavior.[29,31,33-37–41,43–44] Techniques that are never recommended for behavior modification include flooding, extinction, negative reinforcement, and punishment.

Extinction

Extinction of a behavior occurs when a previously reinforced behavior no longer gains reinforcement.[3,4,45] As soon as reinforcement stops, extinction begins, and the frequency of the behavior should decline. While using extinction may appear to be an ideal way to eliminate unwanted behavior, it often proves to be a slow and tedious process that is challenging to implement. Moreover, it can pose dangers to both individuals and animals and negatively impact their welfare. A more effective approach is to prevent and manage the repetition of unwanted behaviors while reinforcing desired behaviors.

Extinction Burst

An ***extinction burst*** is a term used to define the escalation of unwanted behavior that occurs when an animal no longer receives a reinforcement for a particular behavior.[3,4] Other unwanted behaviors often occur too, as the animal tries harder before giving up (if they do). This is likely the result of confusion and frustration.

Example

Jumping

This person is folding their arms and looking away from the puppy that is jumping on them, ignoring the puppy in the hope that it will teach the puppy not to jump up.

Although the theoretical goal of ignoring this behavior is to ***extinguish*** the jumping, this method is not optimal and often proves ineffective because:

- Other types of reinforcement may be maintaining the jumping behavior (e.g., the action of jumping itself could be enjoyable).
- The technique of ignoring is often applied inconsistently. For instance, at times the dog is ignored, while at other times, they may receive mixed responses, such as being petted, pushed down, or even punished.
- Simply ignoring the behavior does not provide an alternative, acceptable behavior. Instead, the dog must trial and error different behaviors until something else is eventually reinforced.
- Ignoring the behavior could intensify the jumping or lead to other unwanted behaviors.
- Ignoring the behavior can be risky or dangerous for both the person and the animal.

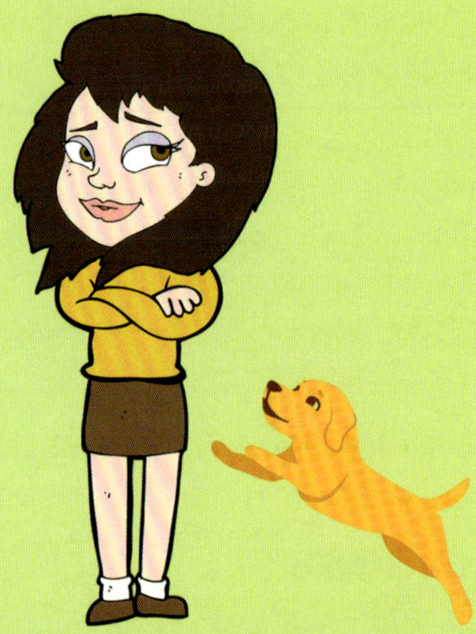

(Illustration courtesy of Jessica Benoit)

Negative Reinforcement (-R) and Negative Punishment (-P)

Negative reinforcement is subtracting or removing an undesirable consequence with the goal of increasing future behavior while negative punishment is subtracting or removing a desirable consequence with the goal of decreasing future behavior.[11] If negative reinforcement is chosen, the intensity of the aversive matters. Physical or emotional distress can occur as the animal attempts to remove the aversive stimulus and gain relief. Additionally, with negative punishment the inability to achieve reinforcement can result in frustration, confusion, anxiety, and fear. Because of this, neither technique should be used for behavior modification.

STOP

Exit 6: Positive Punishment, Aversive Tools, Techniques, and Their Consequences

At this exit, there is a roadblock, stop sign, and vanishing road to indicate that positive punishment is not necessary, not recommended, and should never be used for behavior modification.

Positive punishment is the addition of something unwanted or aversive to decrease or stop future behavior.[11] The animal's behavior serves a purpose for the animal: to gain reinforcement (something they need or want). When their behavior is punished, they cannot achieve the desired outcome, leading to unpleasant emotions (protective emotions) and a feeling of lack of control.[5–10,46] Punishment focuses on stopping behavior instead of reinforcing existing behaviors or teaching the animal new behaviors. The animal's behavior repertoire shrinks which limits choices in everyday life. Use of punishment can increase the risk of fear and anxiety related behavior problems as well as posing a physical injury risk to the animal.[38]

Criteria of Punishment

The use of punishment in animals is detrimental to both the animal and the person administering the punishment, who is also negatively impacted. Although punishment can be effective in some cases, it must meet certain criteria:

1. ***Timing:*** Punishment must occur immediately after the unwanted behavior.
2. ***Consistency:*** Punishment must be applied each and every time the unwanted behavior occurs.
3. ***Intensity:*** Punishment must be intense enough to deter the behavior from repeating, without causing physical discomfort, anxiety, fear, frustration, or distress (i.e., protective emotions).

Meeting these criteria can be challenging, and punishment often leads to numerous potential side effects, such as emotional distress, pain, and injury. For these reasons, positive punishment is never appropriate for behavior modification or training. It is unnecessary; positive reinforcement techniques are much more humane and effective.

Table 4.7.1: The chart lists several ways punishment negatively impacts the person who punishes and the animal who is punished. (Illustration courtesy of Sherrie Yuschak)

Potential Risks of Punishment	
Person Applying Punishment	**Animal Being Punished**
Escalation of intensity if results are inconsistent	Increased usage if results seem effective
Time and money spent to remedy side effects or further modify behavior	Physical pain and negative impact from physiological stress responses
Negative emotions, such as guilt, fear, or embarrassment	Emotional pain: confusion, frustration, fear, anxiety
Risk of losing the pet due to relinquishment, rehoming, or euthanasia	Less opportunity to gain reinforcement through new skills
Limitation of skillset, rather than building new techniques	Fewer choices and lack of control
	Increase or new unwanted behaviors (risk for more punishment)
	Avoidance of interaction
	Decline in quality of social bonds
	Risk of neglect or loss of home due to relinquishment, rehoming, or even euthanasia

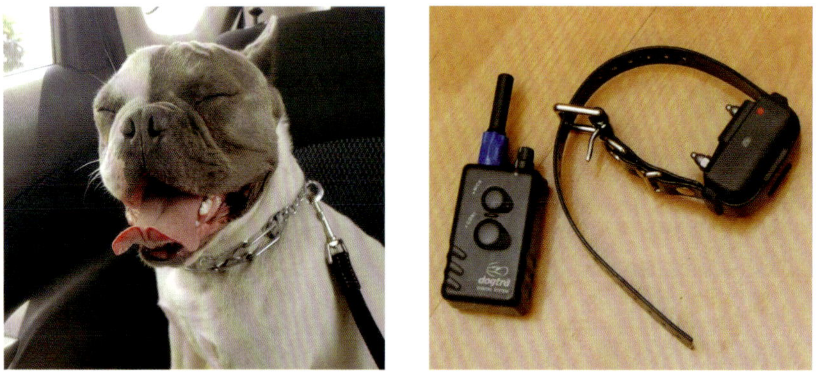

Figs. 4.7 D, E: Choke, prong, and electronic shock collars use positive punishment and negative reinforcement to change behavior. These tools should not be used because they can result in physical pain, injury, and emotional distress.

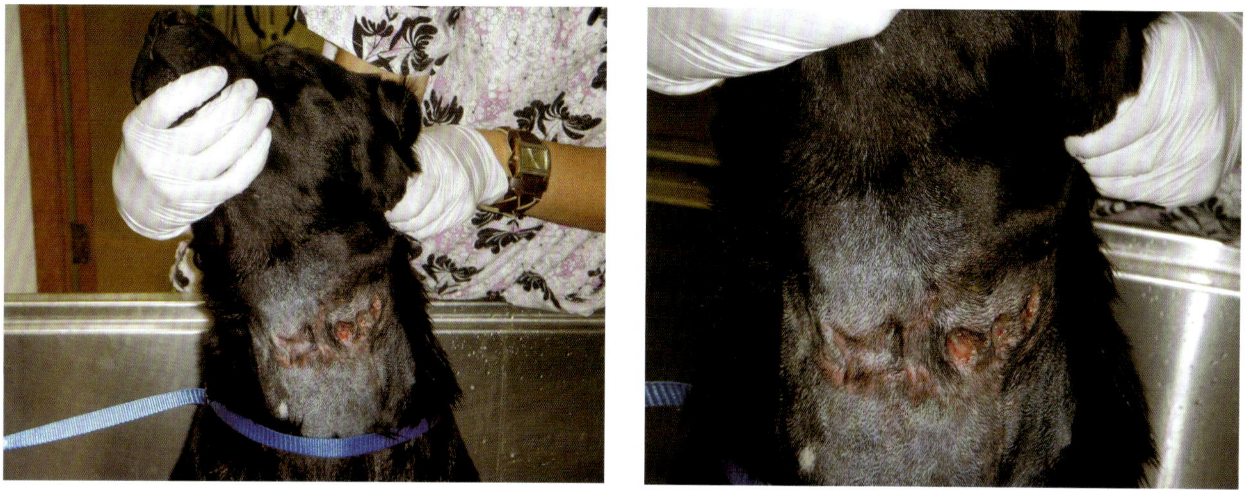

Figs. 4.7 F, G: Use of aversive tools such as electronic collars can result in physical and emotional injuries.

Although using fear, intimidation, or physical force to stop an animal's behavior may seem simple and easy, fulfilling the criteria for effective punishment is challenging. Even with perfect implementation, the risk of negative side effects from punishment remains high.[38]

Dominance and Pack Theory Training Debunked

Starting in the 1940s, the term *alpha* was assigned to the wolf who controlled and led the pack, based on research and publications by behaviorist Rudolph Schenkel and biologist David Mech.[46–51] Both men were studying captive wolves in a pack of unrelated individuals. Conflict and competition were observed and the wolf who repeatedly won altercations was labeled "alpha" and determined "dominant" while the other individuals in the pack were "submissive."[46–54]

This original wolf research became very popular and was adopted as insight into dog behavior by the public and dog trainers. It was assumed that since dogs were related to wolves, and wolves within a pack respect the alpha, a human could assume the role of alpha and pack leader. The goal was to create submission and prevent or punish unwanted behavior. Suggested ways to dominate dogs included shaking the dog by their scruff (scruff shake), rolling them onto their back (alpha roll), staring into their eyes, eating and going through doorways first.[52–54]

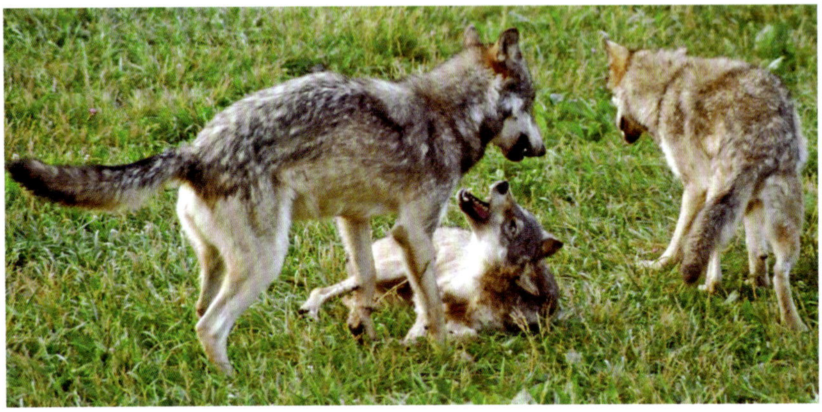

Fig 4.7 H: Wolves look like dogs, but their behavior and social organization are different. (Photo courtesy of WolfPark.org)

Dogs Are Not Wolves

Although wolves (*Canis lupus*) and the domesticated dog (*Canis familiaris*) share approximately 99% of the same DNA, they are different species. Dogs became domesticated over thousands of generations and exhibit behaviors very different from wolves.

The scientific study of dog behavior and learning theory does not support pack leader or dominance-based training methodology as an effective way to change behavior.[29] These methods and techniques damage the relationship between humans and dogs while increasing the risk of protective emotions and defensive behaviors.[38] Trainers and other professionals who promote these outdated ideas and concepts need to be avoided.

The Dominance Myth

Since the initial publication of this research and after 70 years of researching wolves in their natural environment, David Mech has updated his findings. He has learned that a linear social hierarchy does not exist within a wolf pack and has since replaced the term alpha with "breeding male," "breeding female," or "parents."[46–54]

4.8 Changing Emotional Arousal and the Fear Response

There is an ongoing debate in the dog training community regarding the effectiveness of positive reinforcement methods compared to punishment-based training, balanced training, and the use of aversive tools. Some argue that behaviors driven by fear, anxiety, and frustration, especially those deemed aggressive, can only be corrected with force, punishment, and corrections. However, this is not true.

Positive Reinforcement Techniques

Positive reinforcement techniques involve adding a stimulus to increase the likelihood of a behavior, a fundamental aspect of behavior modification. These techniques not only promote desired behaviors but also help prevent the development of protective emotions. While proponents of traditional and balanced training methods often argue that relying solely on positive reinforcement is inefficient, evidence-based research consistently highlights its effectiveness. This indicates that techniques based on punishment are not essential for successful training or behavior modification.

Example

Use of Punishment Techniques and Aversive Tools

Walking Equipment

Two individuals are taking their dog for a walk and using a remote electronic collar to administer corrections.

Environment and Protective Emotions

The dog, upon receiving the aversive stimulus from the collar, might not clearly understand which specific action triggered this pain and discomfort. As a result of the collar's use, the dog's body language indicates protective emotions (clear indicators of distress and fear). These indicators include a lowered posture, lack of movement, a tucked tail, ears drawn back, and a closed mouth. Over time and with repeated exposures, the dog could begin to make these associations, not just with the aversive stimulus of the collar, but with the entire environment of the walk itself.

Relationship with Caregivers

Meanwhile, the individuals delivering this form of positive punishment seem assured of its efficacy, as evidenced by their forward-moving body language. Their focus is primarily on the walk, not on the dog or their interactions with each other.

The Use of Positive Reinforcement Techniques

Let us revisit the scenario where caregivers walk their dog using positive reinforcement instead of a remote electronic collar.

Walking Equipment

In this scenario, the caregivers choose to use a front clip harness. This harness, with the leash clipped in front, effectively reduces the dog's pulling without causing fear or discomfort.

Environment and Engaging Emotions

During their walks, the caregivers remain alert and engaged. They reinforce the dog with treats when eye contact is offered. This method encourages the dog to focus on them despite the numerous distractions around them, like other dogs, people, strollers, bikes, or cars. Whenever the dog gets sidetracked, they employ the "touch" cue. This technique involves the dog touching a body part, such as a nose to their caregiver's hand, a behavior previously taught through positive reinforcement.

Working Around Distractions

To maintain the dog's engagement, they incorporate Leslie McDevitt's Control Unleashed® 1-2-3 Pattern Game. This game involves counting one, two, and three followed by a treat after three. A predictable routine, this game helps keep the dog focused, even in distracting environments. As the dog becomes accustomed to the game, he begins to anticipate the treat, often making eye contact at "one" or "two," before the count reaches "three."

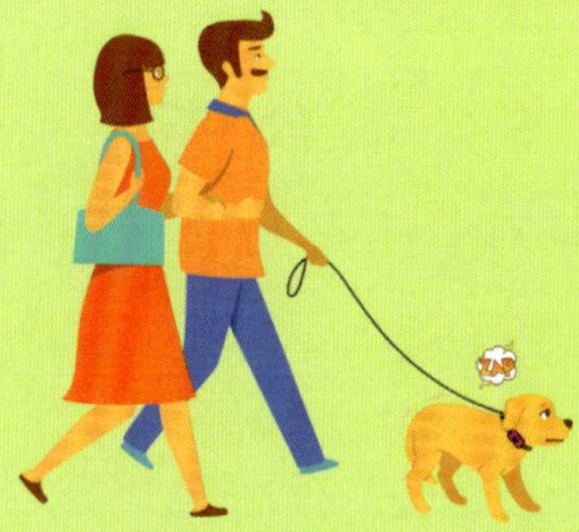

(Illustration courtesy of Jessica Benoit)

Relationship with Caregivers

This approach, in contrast to punishment-based methods, transforms the caregiver's role. They evolve from mere walkers to active participants in the dog's learning. Their deeper involvement allows them to be more responsive to the dog's needs and signals, thereby strengthening their bond. The walks become more enjoyable and fulfilling, showcasing how positive reinforcement and engagement are not only effective and humane training methods, but also enrich the overall experience for both the dog and the caregivers.

Systematic Desensitization and Counterconditioning

Systematic desensitization (DS) is often used to modify a specific fear response.[41,43] Desensitization involves exposure to fear inducing stimuli on a gradient.[41,43] This process is most effective when fears are identified, and a hierarchy is outlined from least to most intense. In some situations, systematic desensitization may not be possible because gradient exposure cannot be well controlled or other factors contribute to the threshold of a fear response.

Counterconditioning (CC) alters emotional responses, and when combined with desensitization (DS), it is more efficient. When paired correctly, the appearance of fearful stimuli will predict the offering of food, which is often used in this process. Changing behavior using this process relies on factors like stimulus intensity and distance. Each session should be structured to control these factors, taking frequent breaks in between sessions. During sessions, monitor the animal's body language for displacement and conflict behaviors. Avoid flooding and make sure the animal stays below their emotional threshold.

Refusal of Food

Fear, anxiety, frustration, and stress (protective emotions) can suppress appetite. If an animal refuses food during DS/CC, the procedure should be stopped. Further information should be gathered, and a new behavior modification strategy developed. A consultation or referral to a board-certified veterinary behaviorist is recommended.

Importance of Stimulus Presentation Order in Counterconditioning

When pairing a fearful stimulus with food to create a positive emotional response, the order of presentation is important.

Optimal Pairing:

- **Procedure:** First present the nail trimmers, followed by offering food to elicit positive emotions.
- **Outcome:** With consistent repetitions, the nail trimmers begin to evoke positive emotions.

Risky Pairing:

- **Procedure:** Offer the food first, then introduce the nail trimmers.
- **Outcome:** Over time, the food might become associated with the fear of nail trimmers. Consequently, the pet might avoid eating that food in future or similar contexts.

Note: *While offering food both before and during a fear-inducing event might distract the animal, it is not the most effective way to implement counterconditioning.*

Table 4.8.1. Desensitization and Counterconditioning Plan

Desensitization and Counterconditioning Plan
Step 1 Behavioral Assessment and Identification: • Identify the specific fear (e.g., sight of nail trimmers). • Observe the animal's positive emotional state and body language (e.g., relaxed muscles, gently taking treats, leaning toward the trimmers, engaged in the session). • Recognize subtle fear signs previously exhibited in the context (e.g., ears pulled back, looking away, yawning, pulling paw away). • Determine how to regulate the intensity of the fear stimulus (e.g., repositioning the trimmers, allowing the animal to approach or retreat). • Identify the preferred stimulus that induces a positive emotional state and desired body language (e.g., engagement, relaxed posture, leaning toward the trimmers). **Step 2 Developing a Controlled Exposure Plan:** • Establish the initial exposure level where no fear is detected, and only positive emotions and behaviors are evident. For instance, placing nail trimmers two feet away from the animal while observing a relaxed demeanor. • Plan controlled exposure levels ensuring the animal remains beneath their emotional threshold. For instance, having the trimmers two feet away, then one foot, then holding them. At each stage, the animal should display relaxed behavior and willingly engage with the trimmers. **Step 3 Plan Execution:** • Begin the session when the animal appears relaxed and below their emotional threshold. • Introduce the fear stimulus at its minimal intensity, followed by offering food. • Progress to the subsequent stimulus level only if the animal exhibits positive emotions and body language without any fear signs. • If any sign of fear is detected, revisit the previous step or adjust the plan accordingly.

Flooding

Flooding is an exposure technique used for fear-related behaviors. Unlike systematic desensitization, where the feared stimulus is presented gradually, flooding introduces the stimulus at its full intensity while preventing the animal from escaping or avoiding it.[3,4,55] Though the animal might stop showing outward reactions, emotionally withdrawing, the internal emotion of fear persists. Such behavioral reactions can include vocalizing and defensive behaviors (e.g., lunging and biting), along with physiological responses (e.g., urination, defecation, and anal sac expression). These responses not only indicate distress but also pose safety risks to nearby humans and animals. Due to the profound emotional distress inflicted and the removal of an animal's sense of choice and control, flooding is highly discouraged in behavior modification.

Example

Flooding

Physically Cannot Escape:

- A dog, afraid of baths, is placed in a tub with high sides and water already filled. The dog cannot jump out due to the high sides, and the water intensifies the fear.
- A cat afraid of strangers is held tightly in someone's arms during a loud party. The cat cannot wriggle free, and the noise and unfamiliar faces increase the anxiety.

Escape Route Is Uncertain or Perceived as Worse:

- A cat, scared of dogs, is placed in a room with a loose, unfamiliar dog. While the cat might climb or hide, the cat is uncertain if there is a safe spot where the dog cannot reach.
- A dog with a fear of loud noises is left in a yard during a fireworks display. Although the dog has the space to run, the dog does not know where to go to escape the frightening sounds, and running around the yard aimlessly might intensify the dog's distress.

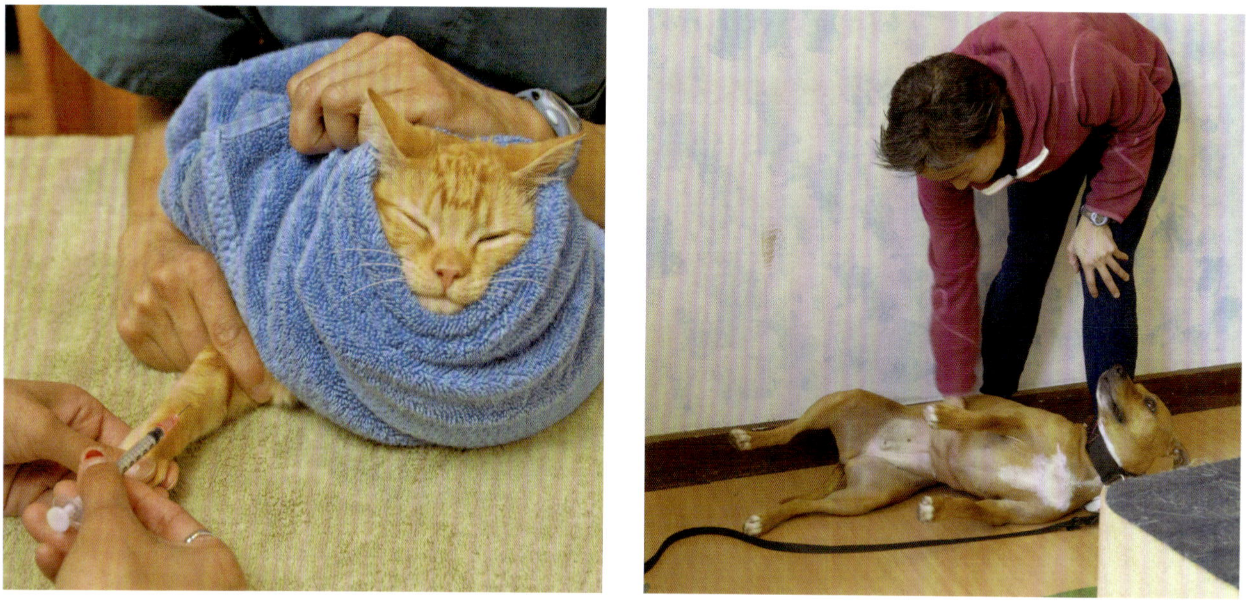

Figs. 4.8 A, B: The towel wrap is triggering protective emotions in this cat as evidence by the closed eyes, stiff body and ears rotated out and slightly flattened. In the second picture (B), the dog is rolling over with dilated pupils, a drawn, tight mouth, stiff forelimbs, and ears are back. Both are examples of flooding.

4.9 Introduction to Cooperative Care

Cooperative care empowers animals by offering them choices, control over those choices, and predictability during veterinary, grooming, and other husbandry procedures.[54–57] By teaching pets beneficial behaviors, it not only broadens their behavioral repertoire but also diminishes feelings of fear, anxiety, frustration, and distress (e.g., protective emotions).[5–10] This strategy provides enrichment, enhances overall wellness, and ensures that animals receive more comprehensive care that is both comfortable and safer for everyone involved.

Teaching an animal how to participate in their own care by adding predictable cues and building fluency can take some time and requires advanced training skills. The animal's repertoire of behaviors, the training skills of the caregiver and training professional, behavior goals, and available resources should be considered when deciding which behaviors to teach for cooperative care. Behaviors that can be adapted to many scenarios and those useful for frequent procedures (e.g., venipuncture) are beneficial. Positive reinforcement training is used to teach foundational behaviors before adding on the systematic desensitization and classical counterconditioning (DS/CC) procedures. Combined, these techniques can condition a positive conditioned emotional response to the veterinary environment and procedures.

Treatment Station

A treatment station designates a specific location where an animal can choose to engage in cooperative care activities. It is also a location where desensitization and counterconditioning techniques for veterinary care and grooming procedures are applied. Using positive reinforcement methods, a pet can be taught to step onto a platform, jump onto a table, or settle on a mat. Once this behavior is fluent, under stimulus control, and generalized to the veterinary environment, additional behaviors like chin targeting, lying on their side, or paw targeting can be incorporated.

A consistent location for care provides predictability and the pet can choose to get onto or off the station. The pet still receives food reinforcement if they choose to leave the station, emphasizing clear communication and affording them control over interactions, thereby making it evident that both choices are acceptable and available.

Remote Treat Dispensers

Remote-controlled or timed treat dispensers are useful at treatment stations and for cooperative care training. The machine can

Targeting and Cooperative Care

- a chin rest for an oral exam
- shaping a pet to lie on their side for a lateral saphenous venipuncture
- handling of feet for nail trimming

The Treatment Station

Choose a ***treatment station*** based on the preferences and needs of both the animal and the caregivers. This station should be in a low-distraction area that is comfortable, stable, and non-slip. The animal needs to be able to get on and off the station independently.

Cats may prefer elevated surfaces whereas a couch or floor-level station might be more appealing to small dogs or animals with mobility challenges.

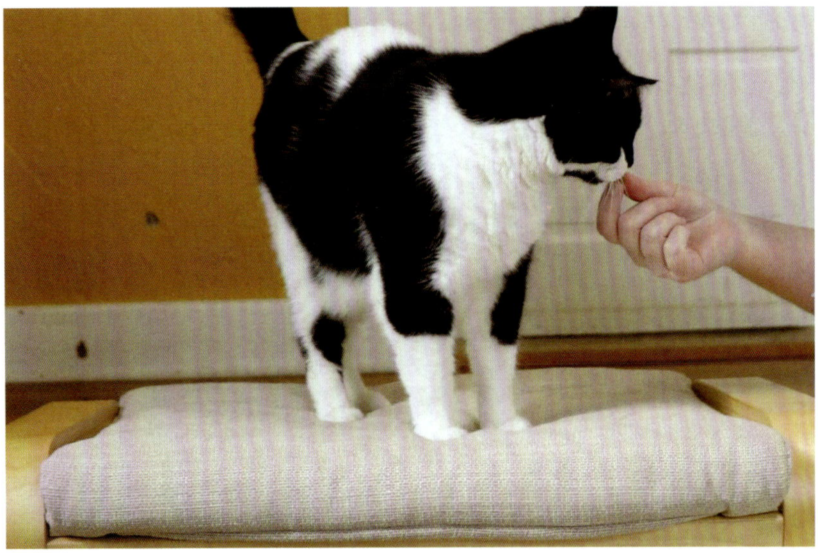

Fig. 4.10 A: An elevated station is a comfortable choice for this cat. (Photo courtesy of Tara Fisher)

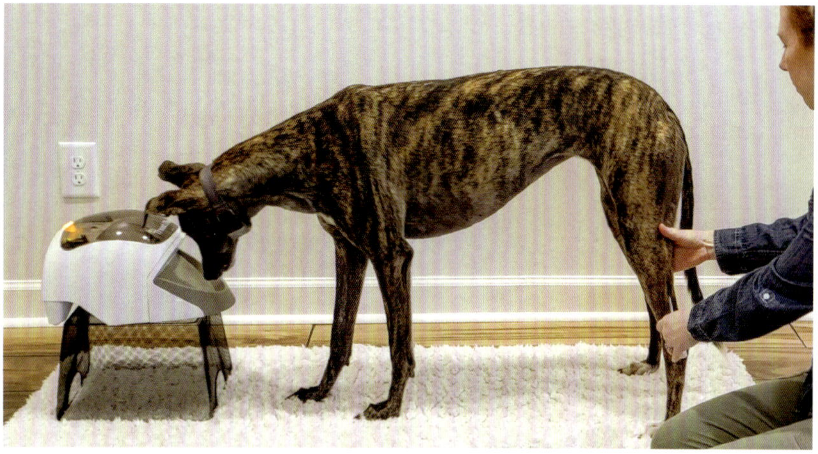

Fig. 4.9 B: Here a remote treat dispenser (Treat and Train®) is used for stationing, distraction, desensitization, and counterconditioning to a lateral saphenous venipuncture. Note: This dog is wearing a GPS device and not a correction collar. (Photo courtesy of Sherrie Yuschak)

deliver a treat for hands-free reinforcement and an adjustable time-interval setting is available to help build duration of stillness. Many devices offer a beep marker (like a clicker) before the treat releases, but the volume can be turned down or turned off if it startles the pet.

4.10 Conclusion

Every interaction between an animal and their environment creates associations among emotions, events, behaviors, and the outcomes of those behaviors. Empathy and compassion are built when people objectively measure behavior and understand how animals learn and the reasons behind certain behaviors. Behavior modification techniques can effectively change behaviors while simultaneously enhancing the animal's physical and emotional well-being. Positive reinforcement methods can be used to teach new behaviors and encourage cooperation between people and animals. Increasing knowledge about animal behavior and practicing training skills will lead to clearer communication, maximize everyone's choices, and contribute to the pet's overall well-being.

4.11 References

1. De Houwer, J., Barnes-Holmes, D., & Moors, A. (2013). What is learning? On the nature and merits of a functional definition of learning. *Psychonomic Bulletin & Review*, 20, 631–642.

2. Lachman, S. J. (1997). Learning is a process: Toward an improved definition of learning. *The Journal of Psychology*, 131(5), 477–480.

3. Mazur, J. E. (2016). *Learning & Behavior: Eighth Edition* (8th ed.). Routledge. https://doi.org/10.4324/9781315450285

4. McGreevy, P., & Boakes, R. (2011). *Carrots and Sticks: Principles of Animal Training*. Darlington Press.

5. Heath, S. (2018). Understanding feline emotions: . . . and their role in problem behaviours. *Journal of Feline Medicine and Surgery*, 20(5), 437–444.

6. Heath, S. (2020). Environment and feline health: at home and in the clinic. *Veterinary Clinics: Small Animal Practice*, 50(4), 663–693.

7. Taylor, S., St Denis, K., Collins, S., Dowgray, N., Ellis, S. L. H., Heath, S., Rodan, I., & Ryan, L. (2022). 2022 ISFM/AAFP cat friendly veterinary environment guidelines. *Journal of Feline Medicine and Surgery,* 24(11), 1133–1163.

8. Heath, S. (2022). Feline behavioural medicine–An important veterinary discipline. *Advances in Small Animal Care*, *3*(1), 13–22.

9. Rodan, I., Dowgray, N., Carney, H. C., Carozza, E., Ellis, S. L. H., Heath, S., Niel, L., St Denis, K., & Taylor, S. (2022). AAFP/ISFM cat friendly veterinary interaction guidelines: approach and handling techniques. *Journal of Feline Medicine and Surgery*, 24(11):1093–1132.

10. Tooley, C., & Heath, S. E. (2023). Emotional arousal impacts physical health in dogs: A review of factors influencing arousal, with exemplary case and framework. *Animals*, 13(3), 465.

11. Yin, S. A. (2009). *Low Stress Handling, Restraint, and Behavior Modification of Dogs and Cats*. CattleDog Publishing.

12. Troisi, A. (2002). Displacement activities as a behavioral measure of stress in nonhuman primates and human subjects. *Stress*, 5(1), 47–54.

13. Hargrave, C. (2015). Anxiety, fear, frustration and stress in cats and dogs—implications for the welfare of companion animals and practice finances. *Companion Animal*, 20(3), 136–141.

14. Hargrave, C. (2017). Canine stress in a nutshell—why does it occur, how can it be recognised, and what can be done to alleviate it? *The Veterinary Nurse*, 8(3), 140–147.

15. Hargrave, C. (2017). Feline stress in a nutshell—why does it occur, how can it be recognised, and what can be done to alleviate it? *The Veterinary Nurse*, 8(4), 192–199.

16. Siniscalchi, M., d'Ingeo, S., Minunno, M., & Quaranta, A. (2018). Communication in dogs. *Animals,* 8(8), 1–20. https://doi.org/10.3390/ani8080131

17. Friedman, S. G. (2009). Functional assessment: Hypothesizing predictors and purposes of problem behavior to improve behavior-change plans. *APDT Journal*, Sept. Based on a paper presented at the annual conference of the North American Veterinary Conference, Orlando, FL; January, 2009.

18. Moxley. (1996). The import of skinner's three-term contingency. *Behavior and Philosophy*, 24(2), 145–167.

19. Farhoody, P. (2012). A framework for solving behavior problems. *Veterinary Clinics: Exotic Animal Practice*, 15(3), 399–411.

20. Friedman S. G., Stringfield, C. E., & Desmarchelier, M. R. (2021). Animal behavior and learning: Support from applied behavior analysis. *The Veterinary Clinics of North America. Exotic Animal Practice*, *24*(1), 1–16. https://doi.org/10.1016/j.cvex.2020.08.002

21. Alberto, P., Troutman, A. C., & Axe, J. B. (2006). *Applied behavior analysis for teachers* (pp. 1–474). Upper Saddle River, NJ: Pearson Merrill Prentice Hall.

22. Brambell F. W. R. & Technical Committee to Enquire into the Welfare of Animals kept under intensive livestock husbandry systems. (1965). Report of the technical committee to enquire into the welfare of animals kept under intensive livestock husbandry systems. Her Majesty's Stationery Office.

23. Mellor, D. J. (2016). Updating animal welfare thinking: Moving beyond the "five freedoms" towards "a life worth living." *Animals* 6 (3): 21.

24. Arhant, C., Bubna-Littitz, H., Bartels, A., Futschik, A., & Troxler, J. (2010). Behaviour of smaller and larger dogs: effects of training methods, inconsistency of owner behaviour and level of engagement in activities with the dog. *Applied Animal Behaviour Science*, 123(3–4), 131–142.

25. De Castro, A. C. V., Araújo, Â., Fonseca, A., & Olsson, I. A. (2021). Improving dog training methods: Efficacy and efficiency of reward and mixed training methods. *PloS One*, 16(2), e0247321.

26. Deldalle, S., & Gaunet, F. (2014). Effects of 2 training methods on stress-related behaviors of the dog (Canis Familiaris) and on the dog–owner relationship. *Journal of Veterinary Behavior*, 9(2), 58–65.

27. Haverbeke, A., Laporte, B., Depiereux, E., Giffroy, J.-M., & Diederich, C. (2008). Training methods of military dog handlers and their effects on the team's performances. *Applied Animal Behaviour Science*, 113(1), 110–122.

28. Hiby, E. F., Rooney, N. J., & Bradshaw, J. W. S. (2004). Dog training methods: their use, effectiveness and interaction with behavior and welfare. *Animal welfare*, 13(1), 63–69.

29. Reisner, I. (2016). The learning dog: A discussion of training methods. In J. Serpell (Ed.), In: *The Domestic Dog: Its Evolution, Behavior and Interactions with People* (pp. 210–226). Cambridge: Cambridge University Press. doi:10.1017/9781139161800.011

30. Vieira De Castro, A. C., Barrett, J., De Sousa, L., & Olsson, I. A. S. (2019). Carrots versus Sticks: The relationship between training methods and dog-owner attachment. *Applied Animal Behaviour Science*, 219, 104831.

31. Ziv, G. (2017). The effects of using aversive training methods in dogs—a review. *Journal of Veterinary Behavior*, 19, 50–60.

32. De Castro, A. C. V., Fuchs, D., Morello, G. M., Pastur, S., De Sousa, L., & Olsson, I. A. S. (2020). Does training method matter? Evidencefor the negative impact of aversive-based methods on companion dog welfare. *PloS One*, 15(12), e0225023.

33. Guilherme Fernandes, J., Olsson, I. A. S., & De Castro, A. C. V. (2017). Do aversive-based training methods actually compromise dog welfare? A literature review. *Applied Animal Behaviour Science*, 196, 1–12.

34. Daniels, J. T., Busby, D., Chase-Topping, M., & Brown, S. M. (2023). A survey of dog behavior modification practice in the UK: Who is offering it? What methods are they using and how effective do their clients perceive practitioners to be? *Journal of Veterinary Behavior,* 59, 1–7.

35. Daniels, J. T., Busby, D., Chase-Topping, M., & Brown, S. M. (2023). I wish he'd listen: client-centered interviewing approaches are associated with higher compliance with behavioral modification advice in pet dog owners. *Journal of Veterinary Behavior*, 63, 22–30

36. Dinwoodie, I. R., Zottola, V., & Dodman, N. H. (2021). An Investigation into the effectiveness of various professionals and behavior modification programs, with or without medication, for the treatment of canine aggression. *Journal of Veterinary Behavior*, 43, 46–53.

37. Casey, R. A., Naj-Oleari, M., Campbell, S., Mendl, M., & Blackwell, E. J. (2021). Dogs are more pessimistic if their owners use two or more aversive training methods. *Scientific Reports*, 11(1), 19023.

38. Herron, M. E., Shofer, F. S., & Reisner, I. R. (2009). Survey of the use and outcome of confrontational and non-confrontational training methods in client-owned dogs showing undesired behaviors. *Applied Animal Behaviour Science*, 117(1), 47–54.

39. Masson, S., De La Vega, S., Gazzano, A., Mariti, C., Da Graça Pereira, G., Halsberghe, C., Leyvraz, A. M., McPeake, K., & Schoening, B. (2018). Electronic training devices: Discussion on the pros and cons of their use in dogs as a basis for the position statement of the European Society of Veterinary Clinical Ethology. *Journal of Veterinary Behavior*, 25, 71–75.

40. Schilder, M. B. H., & Van der Borg, J. A. M. (2004). Training dogs with the help of the shock collar: Short and long term behavioral effects. *Applied Animal Behaviour Science*, 85(3–4), 319–334.

41. Strickler, B. G. (2018). Helping pet owners change pet behaviors: an overview of the science. *Veterinary Clinics: Small Animal Practice*, 48(3), 419–431.

42. Siracusa, C., Provoost, L., & Reisner, I. R. (2017). Dog-and owner-related risk factors for consideration of euthanasia or rehoming before a referral behavioral consultation and for euthanizing or rehoming the dog after the consultation. *Journal of Veterinary Behavior*, 22, 46–56.

43. Horwitz, D. F., & Pike, A. L. (2014). Common sense behavior modification: A guide for practitioners. *The Veterinary Clinics of North America. Small Animal Practice*, 44(3), 401–426.

44. Stellato, A., Jajou, S., Dewey, C. E., Widowski, T. M., & Niel, L. (2019). Effect of a standardized four-week desensitization and counter-conditioning training program on pre-existing veterinary fear in companion dogs. *Animals*, 9(10), 767.

45. Bouton, M. E., Westbrook, R. F., Corcoran, K. A., & Maren, S. (2006). Contextual and temporal modulation of extinction: behavioral and biological mechanisms. *Biological psychiatry*, 60(4), 352–360.

46. Mech, L. D. (2012). *Wolf.* Doubleday.

47. Mech, L. D., & Boitani, L. (Eds.). (2019). *Wolves: Behavior, Ecology, and Conservation*. University of Chicago Press.

48. Schenkel, R. (1946). *Behavior Study of Wolves Observed in Captivity*. Canadian Wildlife Services.

49. Schenkel, R. (1947). Expression studies of wolves. *Behaviour*, 1, 81–129.

50. Schenkel, R. (1967). Submission: its features and function in the wolf and dog. *American Zoologist*, 7(2), 319–329.

51. Bradshaw, J. W. S., Blackwell, E.-J., & Casey, R. A. (2016). Dominance in domestic dogs—A response to Schilder Et al. (2014). *Journal of Veterinary Behavior*, 11, 102–108.

52. Bradshaw, J. W. S., Blackwell, E. J., & Casey, R. A. (2009). Dominance in domestic dogs—useful construct or bad habit? *Journal of Veterinary Behavior*, 4(3), 135–144.

53. Van Der Borg, J. A. M., Schilder, M. B. H., Vinke, C. M., De Vries, H., Geagskliniek, S., Animal Ecology, S. E. & E&C2, Ass. (2015). Dominance in domestic dogs: A quantitative analysis of Its behavioral measures. PloS One, 10(8), e0133978.

54. Leotti, L. A., Iyengar, S. S., & Ochsner, K. N. (2010). Born to choose: The origins and value of the need for control. *Trends in Cognitive Sciences*, 14(10), 457–463.

55. Jones, E. (2023). Cooperative care for companion dogs: emotional health and wellness. *Companion Animal*, 28(7), 1–6.

56. Jones, E. (2023). Preparing fearful dogs for vaccinations with cooperative care. *Animal Behaviour and Welfare Cases*.

57. Wess, L., Böhm, A., Schützinger, M., Riemer, S., Yee, J. R., Affenzeller, N., & Arhant, C. (2022). Effect of cooperative care training on physiological parameters and compliance in dogs undergoing a veterinary examination – A pilot study. *Applied Animal Behaviour Science*, 250, 105615.

Author: Sherrie Yuschak, RVT, VTS (Behavior), KPA-CTP

CHAPTER 5

Preventative Behavioral Health for Puppies

5.1 Introduction

Proper care of puppies is essential for their well-being and development, addressing both their physical and emotional health. This care includes providing proper nutrition, regular veterinary check-ups, socialization, and safe, engaging environments. These measures are needed to support both immediate health and long-term emotional development, helping to prevent future behavioral issues. Early education through environmental enrichment and training plays a key role in this process.

Veterinarians and their team members, often the first point of contact with new puppy caregivers, help educate them about puppy development, behavior, and the importance of meeting their basic needs. Introducing puppy kindergarten at this early stage provides caregivers with the knowledge to create a nurturing environment and navigate the formative behavioral developmental stages of their puppies. This guidance helps establish a strong, healthy relationship between puppies and caregivers, providing veterinarians with an opportunity to recommend evidence-based, ethical training resources and classes.

5.2 Sensitive Periods of Learning

Puppies progress through several developmental stages, from the neonatal phase to their senior years, which include transitional, socialization, juvenile, adolescence, and adulthood stages. Each stage presents its own set of physiological and behavioral milestones. For a puppy's well-rounded development, the complexity of their environment should offer appropriate stimuli and challenges to match their specific developmental needs. As caregivers guide their puppies through these stages, recognizing and understanding the unique requirements of each phase supports their physical and emotional growth.

Utilizing the Sensitive Period for Socialization

Behavioral development in puppies is influenced by several factors, including genetics, early weaning, maternal stress, and early life experiences, or lack thereof. The sensitive period of learning occurs between three and 12 weeks of age.[1,2] During this time frame, the goal is to introduce the puppy carefully, thoughtfully, and gradually to other animals, people, novel environments, noises, surfaces, handling, and husbandry. Missing these opportunities can lead to underdeveloped coping and social skills, significantly increasing the risk for behavioral problems later in life.[2,3] During the socialization process, puppies need to set the pace and caregivers should monitor the puppy's body language to ensure they are comfortable and not at risk for flooding and sensitization. The process of socialization should focus on positive experiences and interactions rather than merely "checking" items off a list.

Understanding Fear and Fear Periods

Starting around five weeks of age, puppies may begin to show fear responses towards people. However, with positive interactions, this fear often dissipates.[1] Puppies weaned before eight weeks are more prone to exhibiting fearful or anxious behaviors.[4,5] For this reason, it is important that they receive adequate and appropriate human interaction before reaching 14 weeks of age; otherwise, they may struggle to form appropriate social bonds with people.[2,6,7] Similarly, a lack of interaction with socially adept dogs can hinder a puppy's acquisition of necessary social skills, increasing the likelihood of fearfulness and aggression toward other dogs as they mature.[5]

Fear periods, during which puppies become more sensitive to external stimuli, typically occur between eight to 10 weeks and again at four to 11 months of age.[8–10] Negative experience during these periods can have long-lasting effects.[8] Given that many puppies experience transitions to new homes and their first veterinary visits during this timeframe, it is important to educate caregivers on how to facilitate smooth transition.

Transitioning into the New Home

The socialization period generally ends around 12 to 14 weeks, although it may vary from one puppy to another.[1,10,11] During this time, as the puppy's immune system develops, socialization is still necessary for their growth and development of social skills. Balancing the need to protect the puppy from diseases while meeting their socialization needs can be achieved by taking proper precautions to minimize the risk of disease.[12–15] The focus should be on preventing future behavioral issues, which are more likely to arise if the puppy is isolated during this important developmental stage.[13–15]

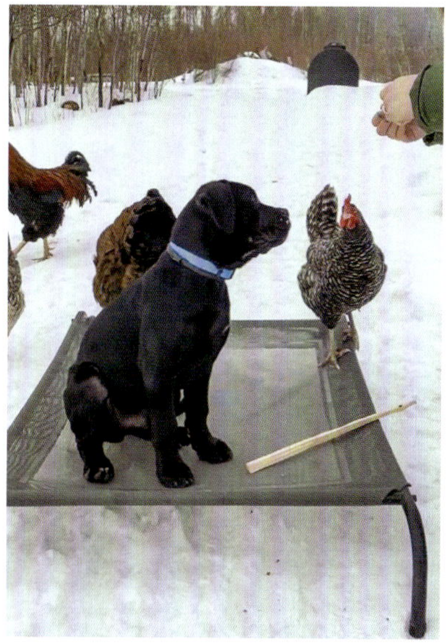

Fig. 5.2 A: Puppy and chicken getting treats for being near one another during a calm interaction. (Photo courtesy of Jessica Benoit)

Learning How to Live in the Human World

When learning how to live in a human world, providing opportunities for interactions with unfamiliar people, places, sounds, textures, animals, and objects helps to build new relationships and experiences. The more diversity experienced in a puppy's life from a young age, the more likely they are to be a behaviorally sound adult. This process should be gradual, giving the puppy a choice to engage or not. Rather than being forced into unfamiliar situations, it is best to let the puppy approach and retreat at their own pace. If a puppy shows signs of fear, such as panting, averting gaze, hiding, running away, or freezing, steps should be taken to improve their comfort and safety. Start by gently moving the puppy away from the fear source to a distance where they feel more comfortable, while offering them a tasty treat. This helps assess their comfort level and can aid in establishing positive associations with the

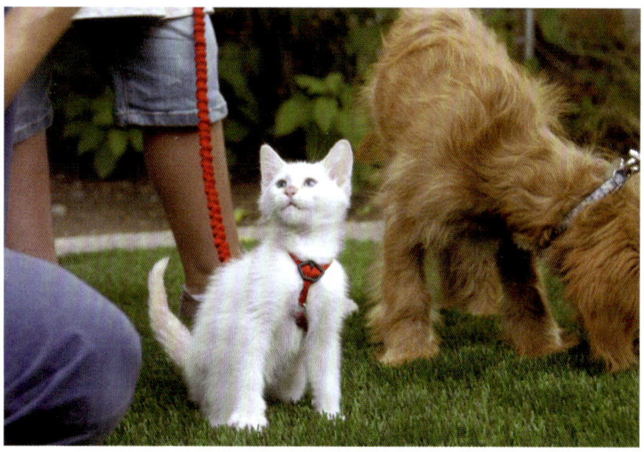

Fig. 5.2 B: Puppy and kitten getting treats together while supervised.

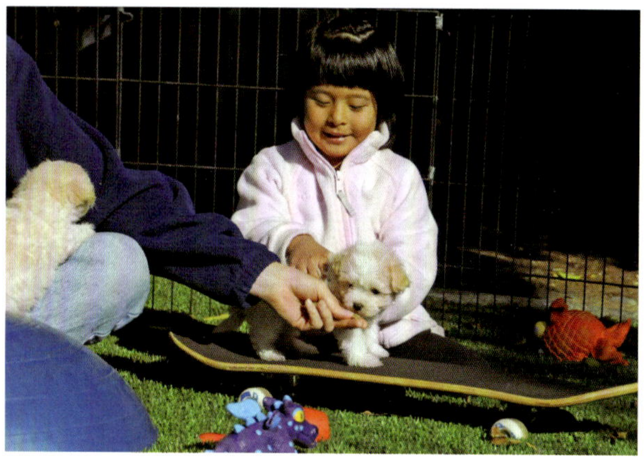

Fig. 5.2 C: Puppy enjoying treats while on a skateboard and interacting with a child.

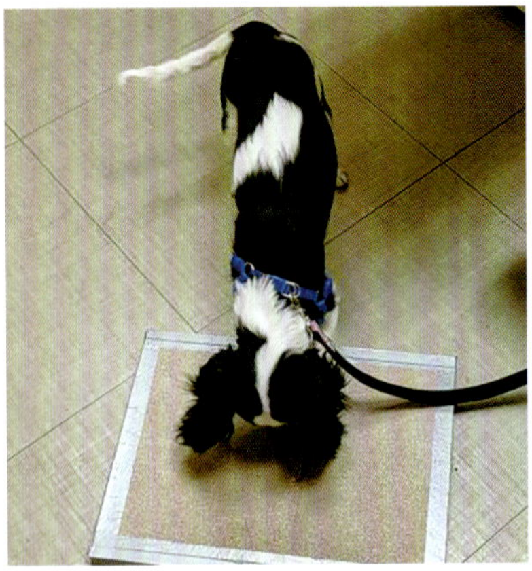

Fig. 5.2 D: Puppy getting treats on a new substrate (nail board). (Photo courtesy of Jessica Benoit)

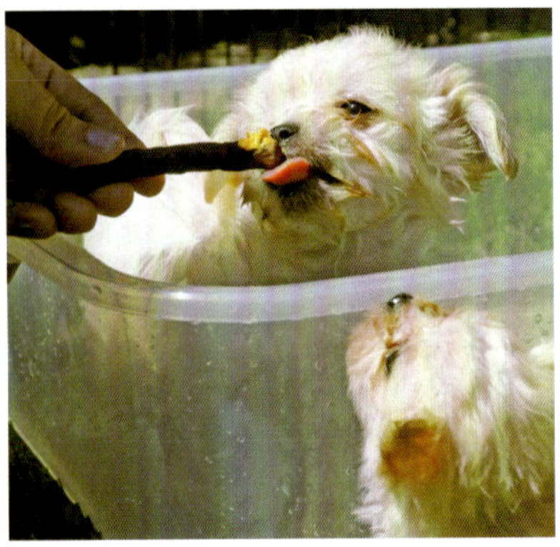

Fig. 5.2 E: Puppy being introduced to water while receiving treats.

situation. If these fear-related behaviors are consistent across various situations, consult with a board-certified veterinary behaviorist for further support and guidance.

A Caution About Flooding

During the process of socialization, be aware of the potential for flooding. This can inadvertently occur when attempting to desensitize a puppy. Flooding happens when a puppy is exposed to a feared stimulus at a high intensity, in an effort to reduce their fear or until they stop reacting (a state known as learned helplessness). Since the puppy is unable to move away, this restriction often leads to an increase in the fear response (sensitization), rather than the intended desensitization.[3,16]

Often, when flooding is used, it is not intended to overwhelm the puppy; rather, it stems from the misconception that the puppy will simply become accustomed to or "get over" their fear.[3] For instance, consider a puppy being physically restrained for a nail trim. Initially, they may tolerate it, but with successive attempts, their response may shift to active avoidance or even aggression. This principle also applies to other husbandry procedures, such as bathing, teeth brushing, or grooming. Flooding can commonly occur in various settings, including dog parks, doggie daycare, and while walking in large crowds or through big-box stores. It can also happen when the puppy meets large groups of people, is passed from person to person, held while children pet them, or during veterinary visits.

5.3 Normal Behaviors and Meeting Basic Needs

Understanding and managing typical puppy behavior cultivates a positive relationship between puppies and their caregivers, while also establishing realistic expectations. Common puppy behaviors, such as nipping, mouthing, biting, chewing, jumping, digging, and barking, can be effectively addressed through several approaches. These include meeting puppies' basic needs, providing suitable outlets for their behavior, teaching new behaviors using positive reinforcement training, and reinforcing alternative and incompatible behaviors. Meeting a puppy's basic needs in accordance with the *Five Domains Model of Animal Welfare*,

Table 5.3.1 The Five Domains Model

Domain	Description
Nutrition	Adequate access to a proper diet to maintain health.
Environment	Providing a suitable living environment free from stress.
Health	Ensuring the absence of disease or injury.
Behavior	Allowing for natural behaviors and mental stimulation.
Mental State	Freedom from suffering and distress.

a comprehensive framework designed to assess and enhance the well-being of animals across various environments is always the first step in this process.[17,18]

Safe Space

Access to a safe space is a fundamental need for all dogs. While a crate can provide this safe space and offers many benefits, it is not suitable for every dog. The belief that dogs prefer crates due to their den-like atmosphere has been challenged by studies of free-ranging dogs, which show a variety of den choices and preferences, ranging from open fields to smaller spaces, with only pregnant females typically seeking dens.[19] Unlike being confined to a crate, free-ranging dogs have the freedom to enter and exit their chosen dens as they please.[19]

Crates can be useful for travel, veterinary visits, post-surgery recovery, and dog sporting events. When introduced in a slow and positive manner, these and other confinement spaces can become a safe, in-home retreat for overwhelmed, fearful, anxious, or tired dogs and puppies.

When selecting a crate for a puppy, consider both the size and setup of the crate. The crate should be spacious enough to allow the puppy to move around, stand up, turn around, and lie down comfortably. It should also have enough room to accommodate water and safe toys. Metal crates are a practical option since they are easy to clean and can be adjusted to suit the growing needs

Addressing Animal Welfare

The ***Five Domains Model*** and the ***Five Freedoms*** are both frameworks designed to measure animal welfare, but they approach the concept from slightly different angles. The Five Freedoms focus on providing essential freedoms to animals and emphasizing the absence of negative experiences. These freedoms include freedom from hunger, discomfort, and fear.[17,18] In contrast, the Five Domains Model offers a more comprehensive approach by examining five key domains: nutrition, environment, health, behavior, and mental state.[18] It emphasizes not only the absence of negative experiences but also the promotion of positive aspects of animal well-being.[18] While the Five Freedoms offer a fundamental set of principles, the Five Domains Model offers a more detailed and multifaceted perspective on evaluating and enhancing the overall welfare of animals.[17,18]

of the puppy. Fabric crates can be a good choice while the puppy matures and is housetrained. Some puppies may prefer covered crates, as these can reduce visual stimuli, thereby enhancing opportunities for rest and relaxation.

The Crate Fairy Game

The crate fairy exercise, effective for crate training success, involves placing high value treats in the puppy's crate throughout the day while they are not watching. This way, when the puppy chooses to enter their crate, they will be surprised with delicious treats.

Exercise pens or gated rooms offer more space and can serve as alternative confinement areas. Placing a crate within an exercise pen allows for the door to be taken off so puppies have a choice to enter and exit the crate on their own terms. This helps to prevent negative associations with premature confinement. If used, the enclosed area should provide for the puppy's basic needs including an elimination area, feeding station, and toys.

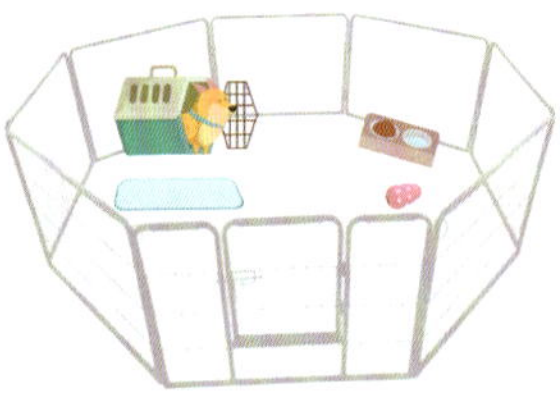

Fig. 5.3 A: Example of a confinement space set-up, including the crate, elimination area, food and water, and a food-storage toy. (Illustration courtesy of Jessica Benoit)

Initially, most puppies are uncomfortable with crates, especially overnight. As social sleepers, they are used to sleeping in piles with littermates.[1] Separation from their mother and littermates can cause undue stress for puppies and if they are immediately expected to sleep alone in a crate, a negative association may occur. To reduce stress, place the crate near the caregiver's bed, use a gated bathroom, or let the puppy sleep in the bed, ensuring they can safely get on and off. Caregivers should be prepared for nighttime elimination trips.

Crate training requires patience to build positive associations. Regularly offering food puzzle toys in the crate reinforces positive feelings and independence. The crate fairy exercise, which involves hiding treats in the crate when the puppy is not looking, fosters positive crate associations. The crate should never be used for punishment and should always be a safe, comfortable space.

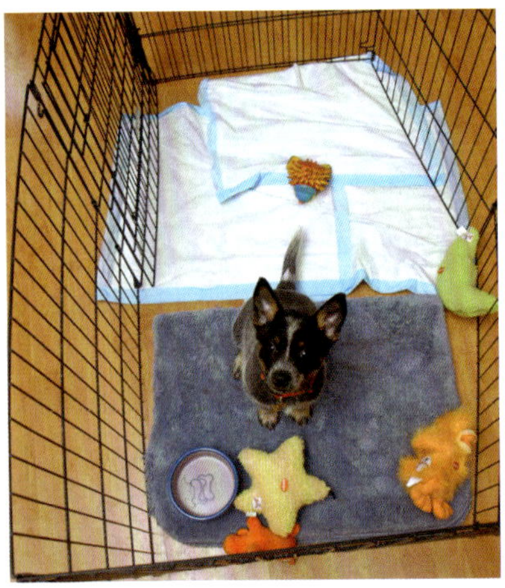

Fig. 5.3 B: Exercise pen set-up as a confinement space for a puppy.

For departures, offer a food puzzle in the safe space five to 10 minutes before leaving. This helps the puppy associate departures with positive experiences. Video recording departures can identify puppies uncomfortable with being left alone, signaling the need for early intervention.[20]

If a puppy shows distress upon departure, it is best to return and consider alternatives like a pet sitter or family member until a behavioral plan is in place. Comfortable puppies will typically engage with their toys and rest during the caregiver's absence.

Housetraining Puppies

Housetraining starts when puppies are just three weeks old. Around eight and a half weeks, they typically pick a specific spot for their bathroom needs.[21] Caregivers should identify the puppy's preferred substrate and location, guiding them there consistently.

Key to Success: Supervision

Direct supervision is key to housetraining success. It helps in the recognition of signs like sniffing, scratching, and circling, indicating the puppy's need to eliminate. With their small bladders, puppies need frequent bathroom breaks. They should be taken outside after waking, eating, playing, wandering away, or if they appear distracted during activities.

Initial Routine: Frequent Breaks

Keeping the puppy on a schedule (feeding, playing, napping, and sleeping) creates consistency and allows caregivers to better predict when the puppy needs to eliminate. Start by taking the puppy outside at least hourly. They need to go every one to two hours until about 12 weeks of age. As they mature, their bathroom schedule will become more predictable.[1] The more a puppy is rewarded for outdoor elimination, the fewer indoor accidents they will have.

Table 5.3.2 Outdoor Training Tips

Tip	Description
Use a leash for guidance and reward.	Guide the puppy to the chosen spot with a leash and reward them immediately after they eliminate.
Food or toy lures for leash-aversive puppies	For puppies that are uncomfortable with leashes, use food or toy lures to encourage them to go to the designated spot.
Small exercise pen or barrier	To minimize distractions for off-leash puppies, start with a small exercise pen or barrier in the elimination area.
Try again if the puppy does not eliminate as expected.	If the puppy does not eliminate when expected, bring them back inside, set a timer for ten minutes, then try again.
Indoor training	Follow the same steps for indoor training. Make sure the indoor area is clean and welcoming.

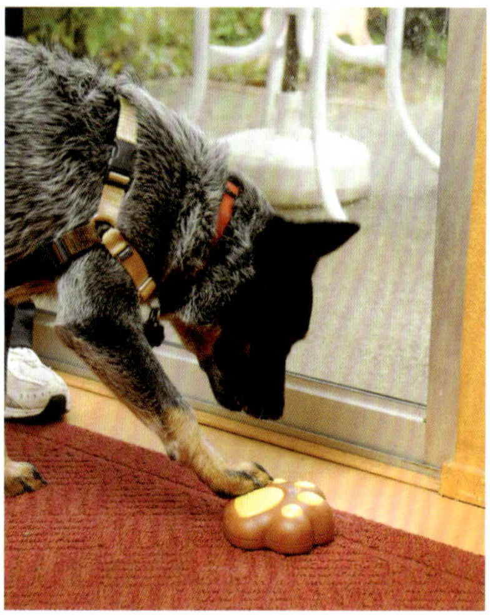

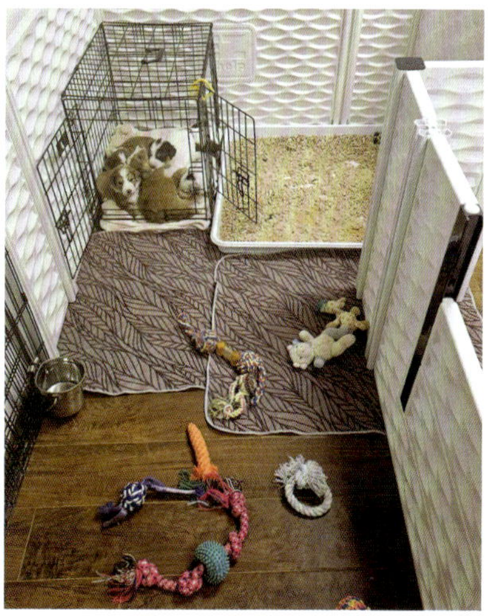

Figs. 5.3 C, D: Photo C, shows a puppy learning to press a button to signal a need for an outdoor bathroom break. Photo D, by Valerie Ayers, displays an indoor elimination area with an exercise pen and litter box.

Monitoring Confinement Comfort

Avoid using crates or exercise pens if the puppy is uncomfortable with them. Provide puppy toys and monitor for comfort.

Access to Water

Puppies should always have free access to water. Withholding water is never considered a humane or effective housetraining strategy.

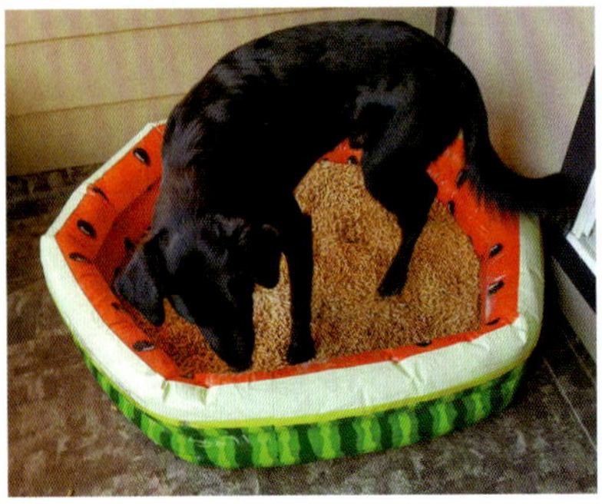

Fig. 5.3 E: Outdoor balcony elimination area with a children's pool and litter substrate, suitable for older puppies. (Photo courtesy of Jessica Benoit)

Patience with Housetraining

Housetraining takes time. Each puppy is an individual and this timeline depends on many factors such as size, age, temperament, and consistency with training.[22]

Mouthy Behaviors

Nipping, mouthing, and chewing are all biting behaviors, varying in intensity and frequency. Less intense behaviors can be precursors to more intense behavior, therefore recognition and early intervention is important.

Avoid Punishment

Never scold, hit, or push a puppy's face into their urine or feces if they have an accident. These outdated methods are ineffective and inhumane. Using this type of harsh punishment can make training take longer and cause the puppy to become fearful, anxious, and frustrated. This may lead to the puppy hiding when eliminating in an attempt to avoid unpleasant consequences.

Handling Accidents

In the event of an accident, calmly guide the puppy to their outdoor elimination area instead of resorting to scolding or punishment. The same approach should be applied if you use an indoor elimination area. Consistently encourage and positively reinforce the use of this specific spot. Regularly replace pads or litter substrate to keep the area clean. This indoor elimination area should always be easily accessible to the puppy.

Nipping, Mouthing, Biting, and Chewing

Puppy caregivers often encounter challenges with behaviors like nipping, mouthing, biting, and chewing, typically during play. Understanding that puppies use their mouths to explore is important. While these behaviors are normal among littermates, they require a different approach when directed at people, particularly in homes with young children. Caregivers need to identify and differentiate these behaviors, since what is normal for puppy interactions may not be suitable for human interaction.

Managing these behaviors involves meeting the puppy's basic needs, educating caregivers, and implementing strategies for safe and healthy development. Puppies experiencing teething discomfort, similar to human infants, can find relief through chewing. Providing safe toys, such as durable rubber toys filled with kibble or treats, can effectively redirect inappropriate chewing. Food dispensing and puzzle toys offer mental enrichment, and rotating these toys helps to keep interest. Techniques such as confinement strategies, using gates or exercise pens, and consistent positive human interactions can also effectively manage these behaviors.

Effective Management Strategies for Puppy Biting Behaviors

Understanding the differences between nipping, mouthing, biting, and chewing is important. Nipping and mouthing are less intense forms of biting, but if not addressed properly, can evolve into more severe behaviors. The first line of defense in managing any of these behaviors is to prevent the rehearsal of these behaviors through effective management strategies. Coupled with redirection and avoiding the use of punishment, this approach fosters positive relationships between puppies and their caregivers.

When a puppy engages in nipping, mouthing, or biting, caregivers should avoid initiating play with their hands or permitting puppies to chew or mouth them. Allowing such behaviors can confuse the puppy, making it challenging for them to distinguish between hands and toys. It may also lead to uncertainty about whether hands might be used for punishment, such as in discipline. The guiding principle should be that hands are for loving; toys are for biting and chewing.

Enrichment

When considering the basic needs of puppies and managing their normal behaviors, enrichment is an essential element. Enrichment involves creating experiences and environments that engage the five senses, enabling dogs to express normal species-specific behaviors.[23–26] Such enrichment opportunities are needed to meet the basic needs of puppies in alignment with the *Five Freedoms* and *Five Domains of Animal Welfare*.[17,18] The concept of enrichment is categorized into five distinct types:

1. **Occupational enrichment**: Providing dogs with jobs or tasks that fulfill instinctual behaviors.

Table 5.3.3: Pause, Take a Breath, and Redirect

Pause and take a breath.	If the puppy starts biting, pause for a moment, and take a breath. Puppy biting can be frustrating and can even be painful, so it is important to remain calm.
Redirection	Unlike simply ignoring the behavior, redirection reduces frustration and offers an opportunity to reinforce a positive alternative behavior. Setting up toys and treat stations in areas of the home where excitement is likely to occur can be an effective prevention strategy. For example, place a basket of toys near the front door where excitement and biting are most likely to happen.
Reinforce an alternative behavior.	Anything other than biting is a good place to start. For example, once the puppy has calmed down, capturing desirable behaviors such as moving their mouth away, four feet on the floor, or eye contact are good alternative behaviors. Using familiar cues, such as "touch" provides predictability, clear communication, and sets the puppy up for success.
Take a break	If family members become frustrated or need a break, this is a perfect opportunity to provide the puppy with a long-lasting chew or food dispensing toy in their safe haven. Place the puppy into their safe haven using a food or toy lure as needed to avoid a potentially aversive interaction such as picking them up, stern voices, chasing, or yelling.

2. **Physical enrichment**: Modifying a puppy's environment for new exploration opportunities and increasing complexity within the home, such as adding new comfy beds, new toys (or rotating toys), and exploring new environments.

3. **Social enrichment**: Fulfilling the need for interactions with other dogs, humans, and other species.

4. **Nutritional enrichment**: Commonly using food as motivation for foraging, problem-solving, and earning rewards.

5. **Sensory enrichment**: Engaging all five senses—smell, sight, taste, touch, and sound.[24]

Meeting Basic Needs

Canine instincts serve as reminders of needs that must be met. Often, an undesirable behavior is normal dog behavior that humans deem inappropriate or bad. For example, a dog digging up a flower bed in an attempt to find the source of an interesting scent. Digging is an instinctive behavior and if given a better outlet, such as a digging box filled with smelly treasures to find, the dog may be less likely to dig up the flower bed.

Understanding the types of enrichment and sensory experiences that are beneficial for puppies helps to create a complex and fulfilling environment that meets their basic needs. A study on the impact of environmental enrichment on shelter dogs supports this idea.[25] In this study, dogs received daily positive reinforcement training for desirable behaviors while in confinement and had access to food storage toys.[25] The results showed significant improvements in the dogs' overall welfare, evidenced by a decrease in unwanted behaviors like excessive vocalization and an increase in calm behaviors such as sitting and lying down.[25] This study highlights not only the effectiveness of positive reinforcement training and food storage toys as enrichment strategies but also their relevance for puppies in domestic settings.[25] While caregivers may not consider their puppies captive animals, the insights gained from learning about enrichment benefits in shelter or captive settings can be valuable when addressing the physical and mental needs of puppies in home environments.[18,24,26]

Guidelines for Enrichment Safety

During the use of all enrichment items and opportunities, safety should be a priority. Here are some guidelines to make these experiences both safe and enjoyable:

1. **Supervision**: Always monitor puppies during enrichment activities to prevent accidental ingestions or other injuries.

2. **Appropriate materials**: Be mindful with puppies prone

to ingesting non-food items. Avoid giving puppies access to shreddable materials like cardboard or wood if they show a tendency to ingest these substances.

3. **Low stress introduction**: Introduce new enrichment opportunities in a way that is fun and engaging.
4. **Manageable food puzzles**: Start with simple food puzzles and gradually increase the difficulty as the puppy successfully navigates the easier challenges. This prevents frustration and enhances the learning experience.
5. **Monitor arousal levels**: Pay attention to the puppy's level of excitement during activities like tug-of-war or playing with flirt poles. Flirt poles are large wand toys that encourage puppies to chase and grab. Since most puppies don't know a "drop it" cue, toss a few treats on the ground to encourage the puppy to release the flirt pole while redirecting them. The toy can then be picked up while the puppy is eating the treats. Restart the game once the puppy offers a calm, alternative behavior, such as all four paws on the floor, looking up at you, or a sit.
6. **Rotate enrichment activities**: Regularly change and introduce new enrichment toys and activities to keep a puppy's interest and prevent habituation. This keeps the environment dynamic and encourages ongoing learning and exploration.

Flirt Pole Safety

When engaging a puppy with a ***flirt pole***, to keep playtime safe and enjoyable, move the toy along the ground to reduce jumping, erratic movements, and potential for injury.

Sensory Enrichment

Appealing to a puppy's five senses through enrichment is important for their development and well-being. By engaging these senses, caregivers can create a diverse and stimulating environment that caters to the puppy's natural behaviors and instincts.

Olfactory

A dogs' olfactory function is far superior to that of a human. For example, bloodhounds have 300 million olfactory receptors compared to humans' five million.[27] This advanced olfactory ability is why activities such as foraging and scavenging for food are effective in enriching a puppy's environment. Long-line sniff walks or "sniffaris" enable puppies to follow scents, combining olfactory

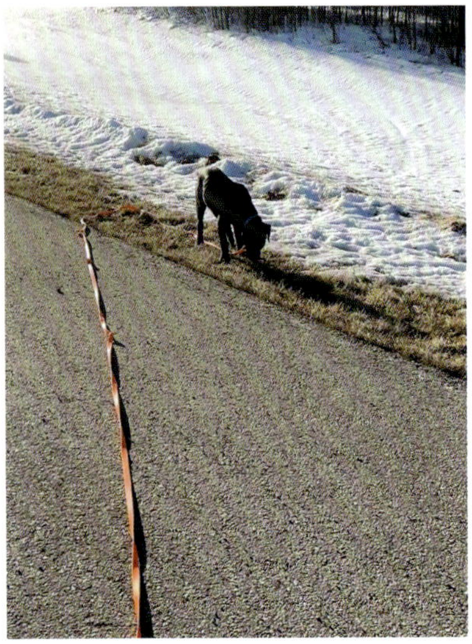

Fig. 5.3 F: Puppy on a long-line leash, sniffing, and exploring. (Photo courtesy of Jessica Benoit)

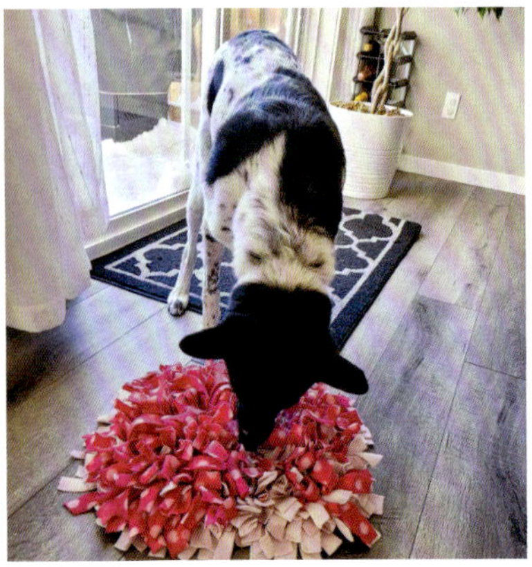

Fig. 5.3 G: Dog sniffing out hidden treats in a snuffle mat. (Photo courtesy of Jessica Benoit)

stimulation with physical exercise.[28] Introducing new scents of people or animals, scent swapping, and nose-work training also prove to be beneficial. Studies have shown that nose-work not only enhances a dog's sense of optimism but also improves their overall welfare.[29]

Gustatory

Gustatory enrichment, involving food toys and chewable items, is particularly satisfying due to its multisensory nature. Food puzzles and toys are useful during handling and medical procedures as they distract and help form positive associations. Start with simple food puzzles, gradually increasing complexity to prevent frustration in puppies. If the puzzle is too challenging, the puppy might give up or lose interest in problem-solving. This was observed in a small study that investigating the behavioral effects of feeding kenneled dogs with enrichment toys.[30] This study found that using suitably challenging food-storage toys like the Kong® motivated the dogs to seek food and solve problems, but also reduced barking while enhancing the dogs' overall welfare.[30] Therefore, starting with easily accessible food toys and progressively introducing more complex puzzles as the puppy develops can be an effective way to engage and foster their problem-solving abilities.

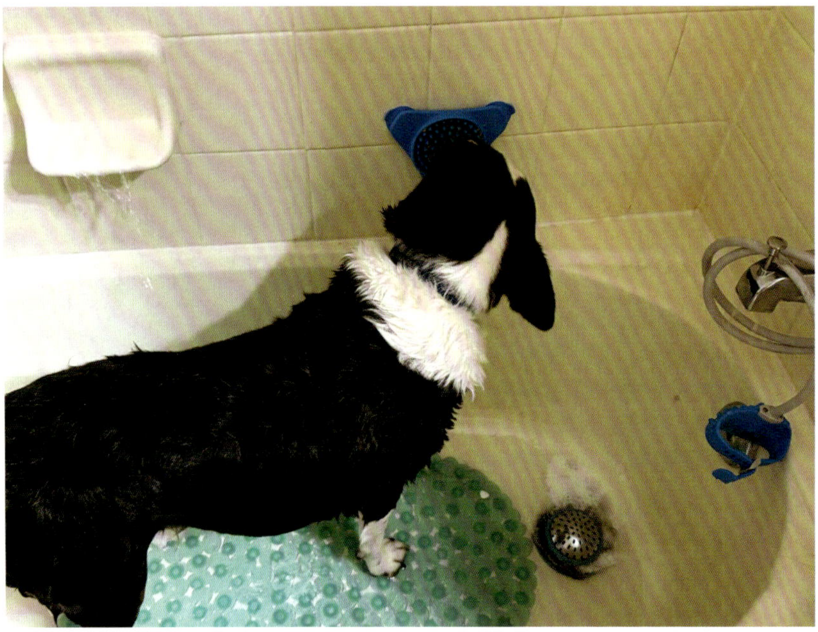

Fig. 6.3 H: A lickable mat can be used in the bath tub as an easy distraction. (photo courtesy of Reilley Calder)

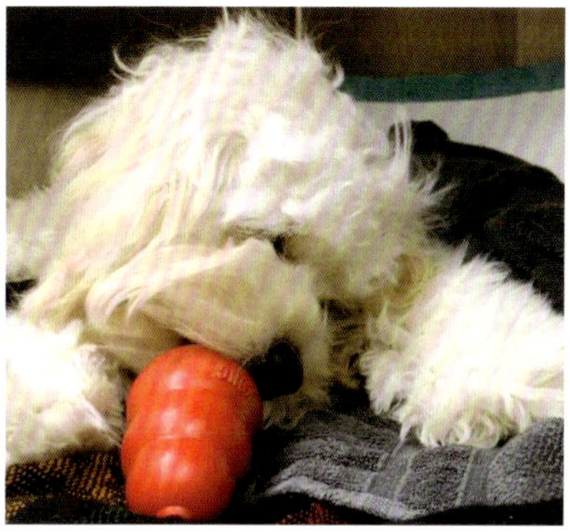

Fig. 5.3 I: Puppy enjoying a food-storage toy in his kennel postoperatively. (Photo courtesy of Jessica Benoit)

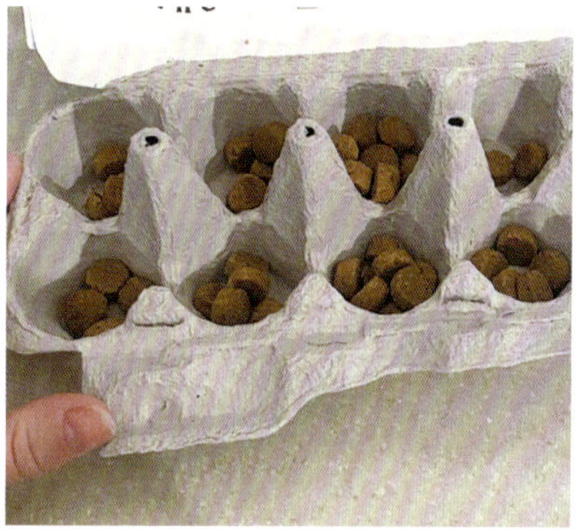

Fig. 5.3 J: Egg carton filled with kibble. (Photo courtesy of Jessica Benoit)

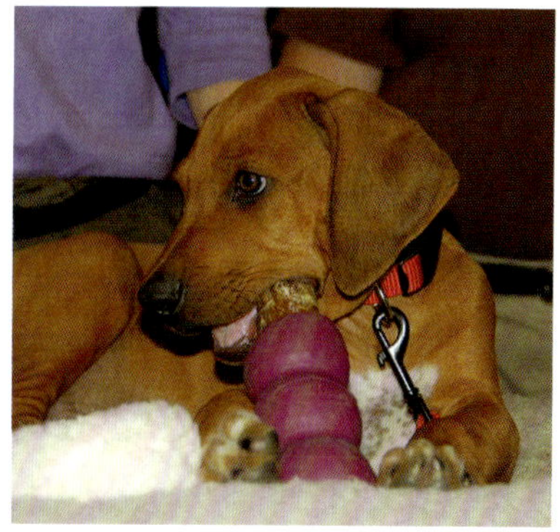

Fig. 5.3 K: Puppy enjoying a puzzle toy at puppy class.

Tactile

Dogs have various sensitive touch areas, including the paws, mouth, face, ears, tail, and genitals, and tactile enrichment should respect each dog's comfort level.[16] This can include activities like brushing, petting, and providing different textures for them to feel and chew.[31] It is essential to ensure these items are safe and to supervise puppies to prevent ingestion or dental injuries. Some dogs may enjoy brushing or experiencing certain textures under their paws, such as fleece blankets or sand.[31] Preference can often be observed in their choice of resting spots, as they might consistently choose one area over another when given various options.[31] By offering a range of surfaces, like different types of beds, blankets, and platforms, caregivers can learn more about what their puppy prefers.[18,31] These preferences can evolve as the puppy grows older, so regularly reassessing and adapting to their changing likes and dislikes is beneficial.[31]

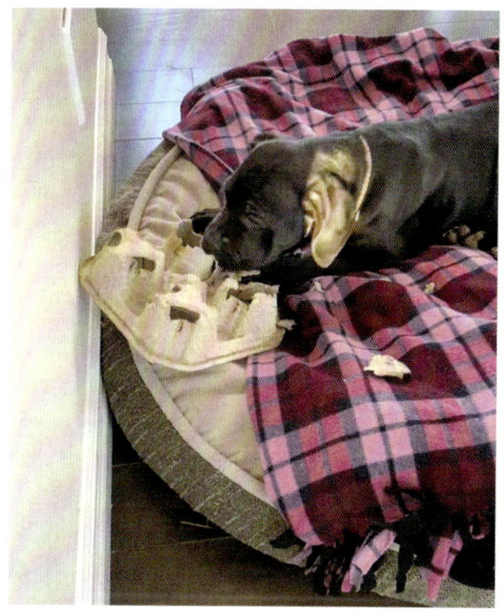

Fig. 5.3 L: Puppy shredding a cardboard drink tray as a form of tactile and gustatory enrichment. (Photo courtesy of Jessica Benoit)

Visual

Dogs possess dichromatic vision, making them particularly adept at detecting movement. They can see across the blue-violet and yellow-green spectrums and see objects clearly at close range. Consequently, toys like flirt poles and dynamic activities such as car rides and watching television can provide suitable visual stimulation for some dogs. However, these activities can be overly stimulating for others. In shelters, visual enrichment through dog-specific programming on

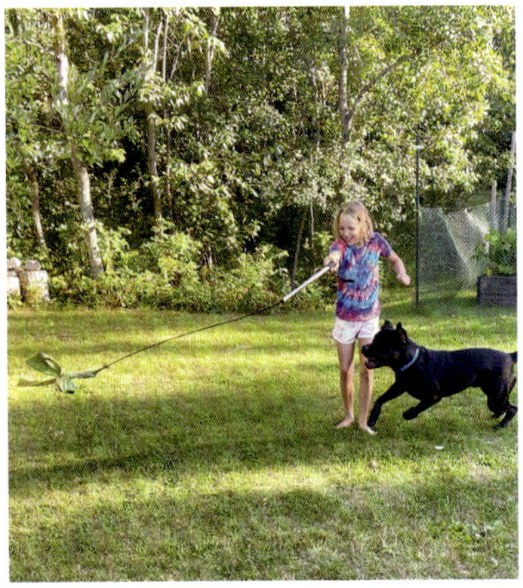

Fig. 5.3 M: Chasing a flirt pole provides visual enrichment for some dogs. (Photo courtesy of Jessica Benoit)

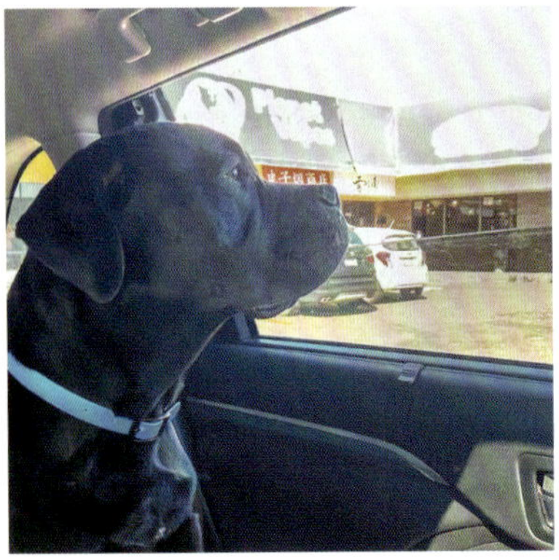

Fig. 5.3 N: Puppy observing the environment on a car ride. (Photo courtesy of Jessica Benoit)

video devices has been shown to decrease the time dogs spend at the back of the kennel and reduce stress behaviors, such as pacing.[32] This suggests that similar methods of visual enrichment could also be advantageous for puppies, particularly during periods when they are left alone or as part of their daily enrichment routines.

Auditory

Puppies' hearing starts to develop during the transitional phase of development, roughly between 11 to 21 days of age, as their ears begin to open.[11] As a species, dogs can detect frequencies much higher than humans, and are capable of hearing up to 65,000 Hz, surpassing the human range which caps at around 20,000 Hz.[11] Exposing puppies to a variety of sounds during this sensitive learning period can enrich their environment and reduce future noise sensitivities. Studies have consistently shown that classical music, particularly those with lower pitches and slower tempos, can have a soothing effect on dogs.[32–34] For example, one study found that playing such music for kenneled dogs led to better rest and reduced vocalization.[33] This means that playing classical music compilations could be beneficial for puppies during times of confinement or when undergoing home-alone training, helping them relax and enriching their auditory environment.[32–34]

Social Enrichment: Puppy Play

Play helps dogs learn social cues and practice their motor skills. During appropriate play, puppies take turns chasing and jumping on each other. Pawing, mouthing, and biting are also common play behaviors. Vocalization to solicit play, such as barking and growling, can be normal. Occasionally puppies yip, growl more forcefully, or show their teeth to tell another puppy that they are not comfortable with their play style.[35]

During play, frequent breaks should be provided to encourage appropriate social interactions. This gives puppies an opportunity to self-regulate and to reduce overarousal.[35] A "shake off" can be one indicator that arousal levels are too high and the puppy needs a break. If this is observed, a food lure or toy can be used to redirect and interrupt play. Puppies should not be left to sort it out on their own as play can quickly escalate.[36]

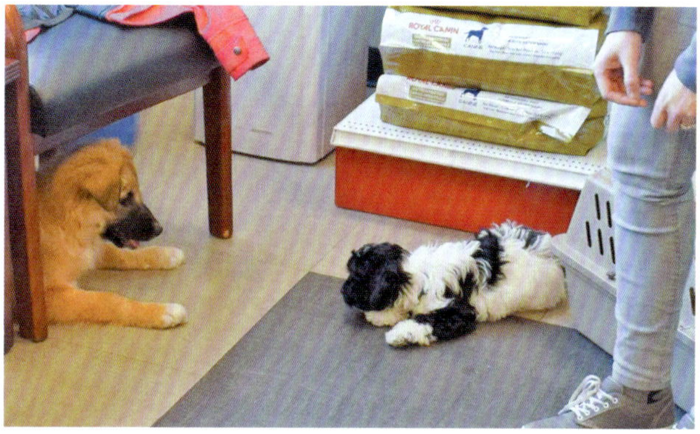

Fig. 5.3 O: Two puppies taking a break during play. Often, one puppy will use a chair or go behind a barrier when a break is needed. To provide choice, these options need to be available during puppy playtime. (Photo courtesy of Jessica Benoit)

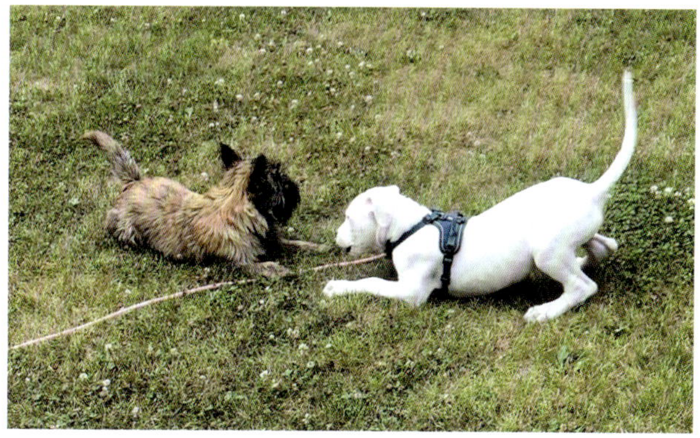

Fig. 5.3 P: The puppy on the right displays a play bow, with his forearms on the ground, keeping his hind end and tail in the air, to solicit play from the puppy on the left. (Photo courtesy of Jessica Benoit)

Recognizing Normal Play

Normal play behaviors can include play bows, chasing, biting, mouthing, vocalizations, and mounting. By understanding these behaviors, caregivers and trainers can ensure interactions remain safe and contribute positively to development. Recognizing abnormal play provides an opportunity for timely intervention.

Play Bows

This posture involves a dog placing their forelimbs on the ground while the hind legs remain standing, often accompanied by a raised, sometimes wagging, tail.[37] Play bows are typically used to initiate play or signal a desire to continue playing after a pause.[37–40] A play bow can also be a displacement or abnormal behavior depending on the body language of the other puppies.

Chasing

Puppies often chase each other during play. Healthy play is evident by the chase being reciprocal. If one puppy is constantly being pursed, avoiding, or hiding from the other puppies, then intervention is needed.

Play Biting and Mouthing

Biting is a common part of play, teaching puppies to regulate their bite pressure. Typically, the areas most often bitten include the legs, tail, back, and flanks. When a bite is too forceful, a sharp yip from the bitten puppy signals the need to reduce the intensity. However, this feedback might not occur during atypical play. While gentle bites on the neck are normal, persistent biting, especially if it causes pain or is accompanied by head shaking, is considered abnormal.

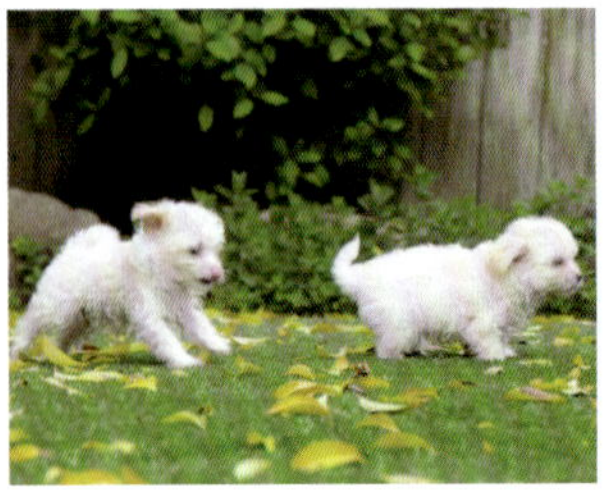

Fig. 5.3 Q: Puppies playing chase.

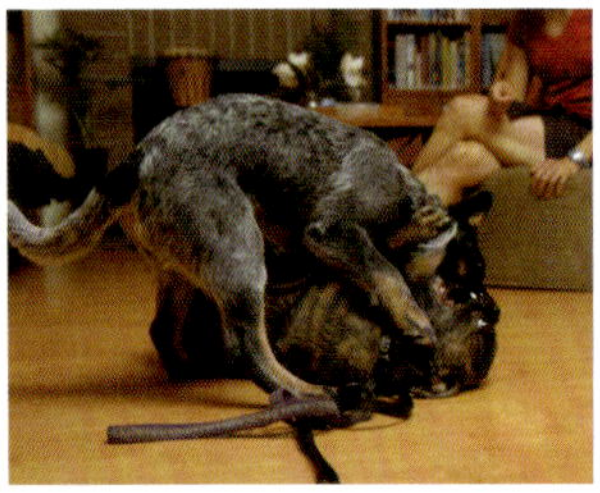

Fig. 5.3 R: Puppies wrestling with one another.

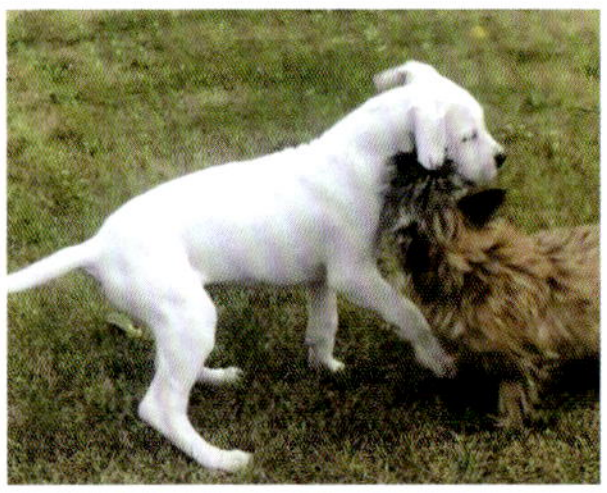

Fig. 5.3 S: The puppy on the right is biting the other puppy's neck during play. (Photo courtesy of Jessica Benoit)

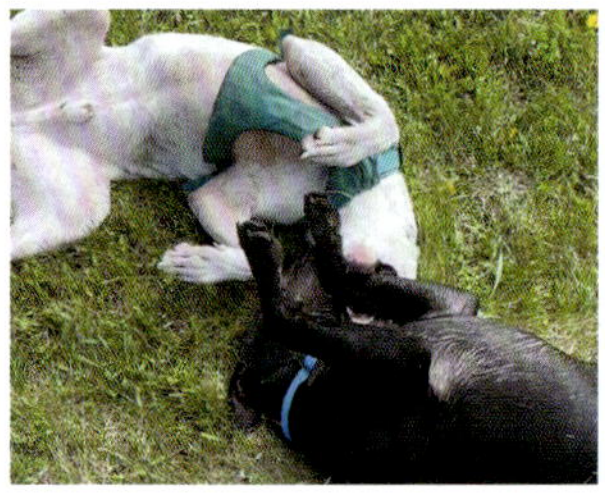

Fig. 5.3 T: The adolescent puppy on the left bites the other puppy's leg during a play session. (Photo courtesy of Jessica Benoit)

Vocalization

Barking and growling occur frequently during play. Barking can be used as an invitation for play; however, repetitive barking can indicate over-arousal and a need for intervention. Similarly, growling often occurs during play and typically features a higher frequency and pulsing rhythm compared to non-play growls.[41] Should growling escalate to air snapping or hard contact bites, play should be stopped. Low, throaty, sustained growls are warning growls, indicating that a puppy may be feeling stressed or defensive during play. These growls would be accompanied by body language indicating stress.[42]

Mounting

Mounting behavior in puppies, often misinterpreted as a sign of dominance, is actually a normal part of their behavior repertoire. This behavior can be triggered by various emotions, including excitement, conflict, anxiety, frustration, or over-arousal. Caregivers should recognize that this as normal behavior, although it may sometimes lead to stress or embarrassment. Reactions to mounting can vary among puppies; some tolerate it well, whereas others do not, and it does not always negatively impact their overall well-being. Intervention becomes necessary if the recipient of the mounting behavior is uncomfortable or signals that the behavior is unwelcome. Effective redirection techniques, such as cueing a touch, recall, or using a food or toy lure, can help reduce escalation.

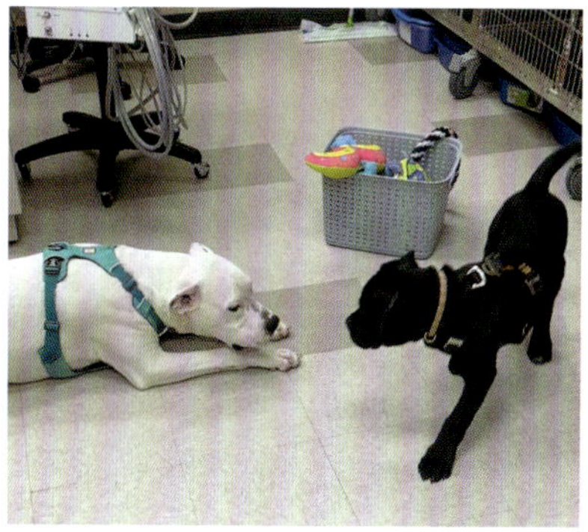

Fig. 5.3 U: Large adolescent puppy greets the 13-week-old puppy by lying down to make play easier between the two dogs. (Photo courtesy of Jessica Benoit)

Adaptive Play

When there is a size or age discrepancy between dogs, the larger or older dog may get down to the level of the puppy to make play easier. Interactions with older puppies and dogs should be calm and respectful. For example, an older dog that frequently needs to correct a puppy by growling or snapping does not provide a safe learning experience for the puppy and can also be stressful for the adult dog. The older dog should always have a safe space to retreat, and the puppy should be redirected when necessary.

Inappropriate Play

Inappropriate play in puppies is characterized by one puppy persistently chasing, jumping on, mouthing, snarling, growling, or biting another without role reciprocation, such as taking turns in chasing or wrestling. This lack of role-switching can suggest a puppy's inability to read and interpret social cues correctly. Signs of stress, such as averting gaze, freezing, lip licking, yawning, rolling onto their back, pulling ears back, tucking the tail, or exposing the belly indicate that play may not be appropriate or comfortable. If these signs are ignored, some puppies may respond defensively with growling, lip lifting, snarling, air snapping, or biting.

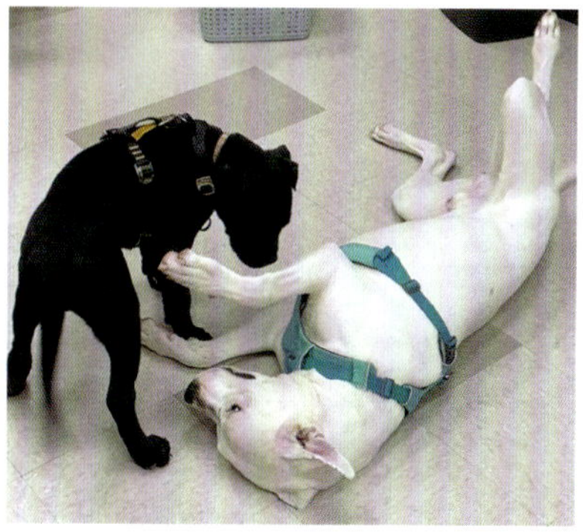

Fig. 5.3 V: To further encourage play, the adolescent dog lies on his side. (Photo courtesy of Jessica Benoit)

5.4 Puppy Kindergarten and Socialization Classes

Behavioral issues are a leading cause of dogs being euthanized, rehomed, or surrendered to shelters.[43–45] Puppy socialization classes significantly help reduce and prevent such problems, keeping dogs in their homes.[12–15,46] Despite concerns about disease risk before full vaccination, the safety and importance of early socialization are supported by studies and professional statements.[12,14] For instance, a 2013 study published in the Journal of the American Animal Hospital Association reported that none of the 279 puppies attending socialization classes contracted canine parvovirus

(CPV), demonstrating that participation in these classes does not increase the risk of CPV infection for vaccinated puppies.[14]

Furthermore, the American Veterinary Society of Animal Behavior (AVSAB) emphasizes the importance of socialization before full vaccination, particularly in the first three months, to help puppies adapt to new environments, people, and animals.[12] Research indicates that puppies in positive reinforcement-based classes are more likely to remain in their original homes, are easier to train, show less aggression towards familiar dogs, and have less situational fear.[13,47]

Puppy kindergarten and socialization classes are essential for puppies as young as seven to eight weeks old, and can be held at training facilities, veterinary hospitals, and shelters.[35,36] To minimize disease transmission, disinfectants that are both safe and effective such as accelerated hydrogen peroxide, can be used to clean the environment.[35,36] Puppies must have received vaccinations at least one week prior to attending, adhere to a recommended vaccination and deworming schedule, and have settled into their new homes for at least 10 days before joining.[35,36] Classes should be small, capped at six puppies, and led by qualified behavior trainers or veterinary technicians with the support of one assistant.[35]

5.5 Foundation Behaviors

Foundation behaviors help puppies develop appropriate social skills and adapt to life with humans. These skills, established early, serve as a basis for further development as the puppy grows. Training puppies requires an understanding of both the caregiver's and the puppy's lifestyles to establish realistic and appropriate training goals. For instance, certain breeds, such as bulldogs, may not be suited for activities like running. In such cases, alternative methods, such as teaching the dog to be comfortable in a stroller while the caregiver runs, can be explored.

Each puppy is unique. While some behaviors are essential for all puppies to learn, others should be tailored to the individual needs of the puppy and their caregiver's lifestyle. Giving puppies time to explore and become accustomed to leash-walking equipment, such as leashes, collars, and harnesses, helps minimize fear or discomfort associated with these items. Good observational skills enable caregivers to interpret body language, ensuring the puppy remains comfortable during the socialization process. By capturing and reinforcing desirable behaviors, caregivers encourage good habits in their puppies while refining their own training skills.

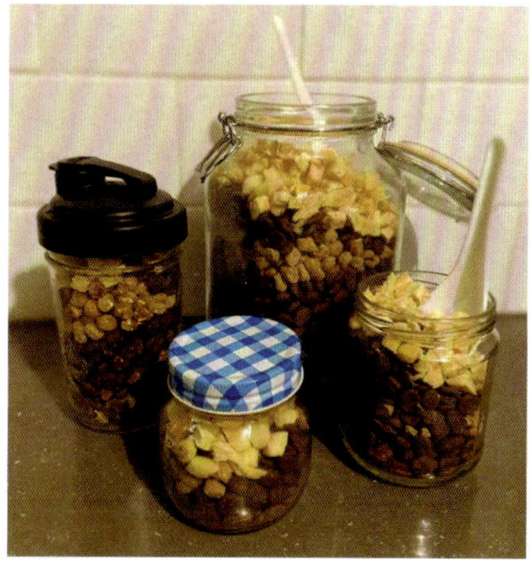

Fig. 5.5 A: Treat station jars filled with a combination of high and low value treats. These jars are placed around the home to reinforce desirable behaviors. (Photo courtesy of Alecia Muirhead of MUTTLIFE Dog Training and Behavior)

Capturing Desirable Behaviors

Capturing desirable behaviors is an effective game-like approach to building and changing behavior. It involves closely observing a pet and immediately rewarding naturally occurring desirable behaviors. Rather than forcing new behaviors, this technique reinforces the pet's natural actions, making learning instinctive and enjoyable. Not only does it build a repertoire of desirable behaviors, but it also strengthens the bond between humans and animals. Additionally, it enhances caregivers' skills in training and observation, particularly in timing and understanding reinforcement rates.

Touch

Touch training, a form of targeting where a puppy learns to touch their nose to a specific object such as a target stick or a hand, is an important technique in puppy training. Known as the touch cue, this behavior serves as a versatile tool in a puppy's training repertoire. It can be used during walks to keep the puppy close, redirect them from pulling, or aid in recall. Additionally, the touch cue is useful for guiding a puppy through various transitions, including entering or exiting vehicles, moving off the road, or stepping onto a scale at the veterinary office.

Incorporating touch training into a puppy's socialization process boosts their confidence and encourages interaction with new people, dogs, and objects in their environment. When shaped as a sustained target behavior, touch in the form of a chin rest or nose to hand can serve as a foundational behavior for cooperative care training.

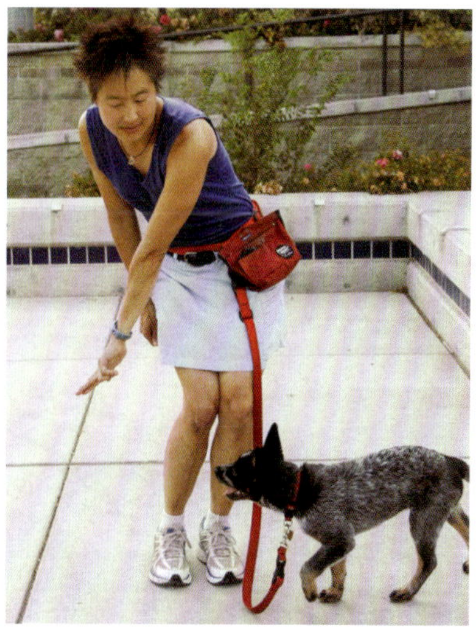

Fig. 5.5 B: The touch cue can help guide a puppy back to the caregiver's side to maintain a loose leash while walking.

Leash, Collar, and Harness Training

Socializing puppies involves safely introducing them to the world, starting with their walking gear such as leashes, collars, and harnesses. Classical conditioning introduces the gear in a non-threatening manner, creating a positive conditioned emotional response (+CER) by placing these items on the ground and scattering tasty treats around them. This encourages the puppy to sniff and scavenge near them. After one to two minutes, if the puppy appears relaxed—indicated by ears forward, a loosely wagging tail, and an eagerness to approach and interact with the equipment—it is time to move to the next step. Step two in this process involves placing the equipment on the dog to transfer the positive conditioned emotional response to wearing the gear, rather than just being in close proximity to it. This step is achieved by first fitting the equipment on the puppy and then offering a food puzzle toy. If the puppy moves away or shows signs of discomfort, the equipment should be immediately removed, and an alternative considered. However, if the puppy remains engaged and continues eating, the

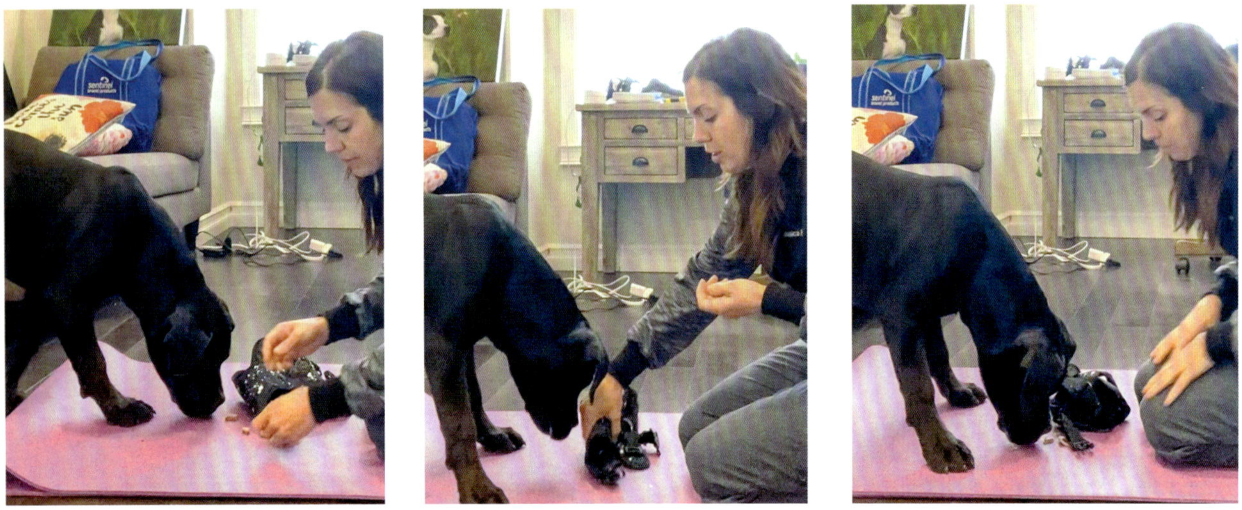

Figs. 5.5 C, D, E: Puppy eating treats near a harness on the ground. Once finished, pick up the harness and repeat. Observe comfort levels such as ears forward, tail wagging at midline, sniffing, or nudging the equipment. (Photos courtesy of Jessica Benoit)

equipment should stay on until they finish with their food toy. This gradual and positive introduction ensures that the puppy feels comfortable with the leash and walking gear, setting the stage for the next step: walking.

Monitor Body Language

If the puppy runs away, lowers their head, or otherwise avoids the equipment, go back to the previous step.

Loose Leash Walking

A loose leash enhances the walking experience for both the puppy and the caregiver, yet leash pulling is common due to puppies' enthusiasm for exploration. To tackle this and foster loose leash habits, start training in a low-distraction setting, such as indoors, initially without a leash. Encourage the puppy to stay close by rewarding them every few steps. As the puppy remains engaged, gradually make the training more complex by moving outdoors into a fenced yard or enclosed area. At this point, higher value treats may be necessary to keep the puppy focused and engaged around distractions such as other dogs and exciting scents in the environment.

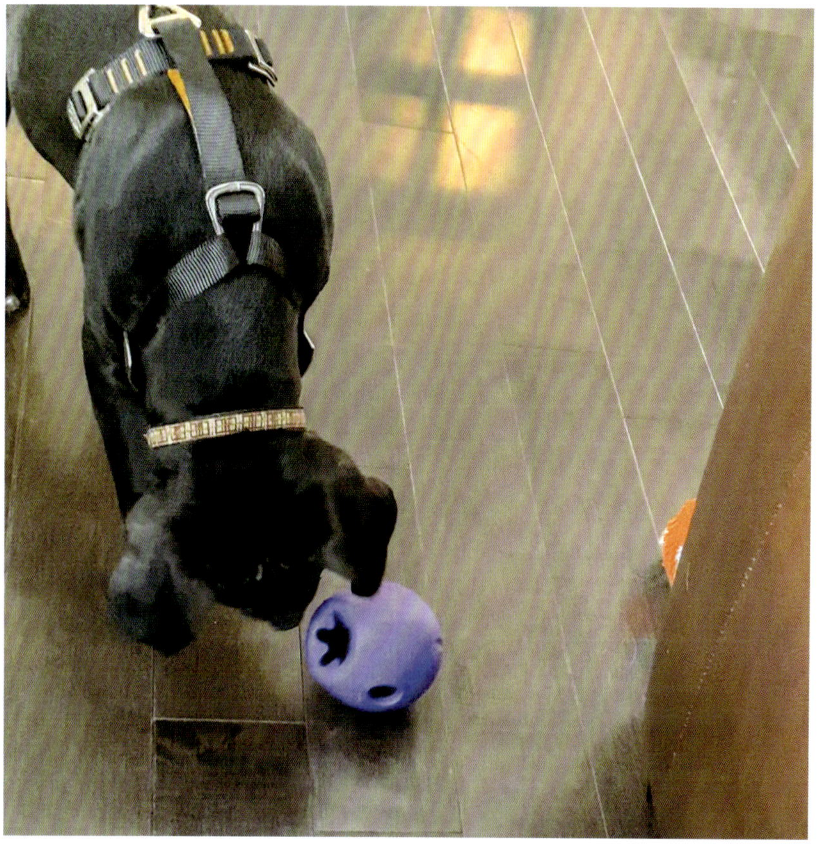

Fig. 5.5 F: Puppy enjoying a food toy while wearing his harness. (Photo courtesy of Jessica Benoit)

As loose leash training progresses, keep each session short and tailored to the puppy's attention span. Once the puppy remains engaged without a leash, introduce a long line. Avoid using short leashes during training and, whenever possible, as they can limit freedom, cause frustration, and put undue pressure on the puppy's collar or harness. Just like with the harness, when first introducing the leash, scatter treats on the ground while allowing the puppy to drag the leash. This approach helps the puppy get accustomed to the sensation of wearing the leash without feeling restrained. Once comfortable, caregivers can pick up the leash and hold it loosely, moving along with the puppy and continuing to offer treats.

At this stage, the primary goal is exploration, not teaching the puppy to walk in a straight line or maintain a specific position. As the puppy becomes more comfortable moving around while attached to a leash and harness, caregivers can start to introduce more structured loose leash walking and periodic check-ins.

Using a Waist Leash

A ***waist leash***, especially when using a clicker for loose leash-walking, frees up one hand for marking and treating. The waist leash should be at least eight feet long, to give the puppy enough space to sniff and take bathroom breaks.

Check-Ins

A check-in, or offered eye contact, occurs when a puppy looks at their caregiver without being prompted. This versatile behavior, applicable in many situations, can be taught both on and off the leash, helping to monitor the comfort level of the puppy and maintain engagement, especially in distracting environments. For

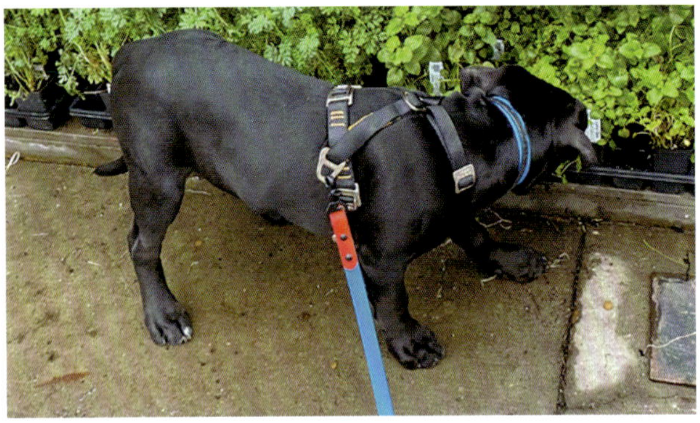

Fig. 5.5 G: Puppy exploring an outdoor environment with an attached harness and leash. (Photo courtesy of Jessica Benoit)

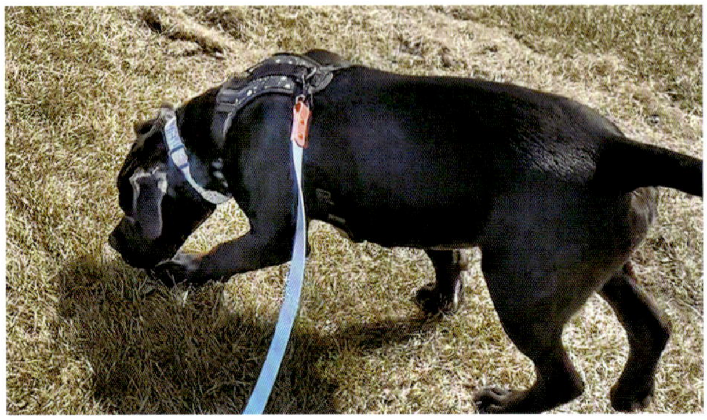

Fig. 5.5 H: A puppy on a sniff walk with a long line and harness. (Photo courtesy of Jessica Benoit)

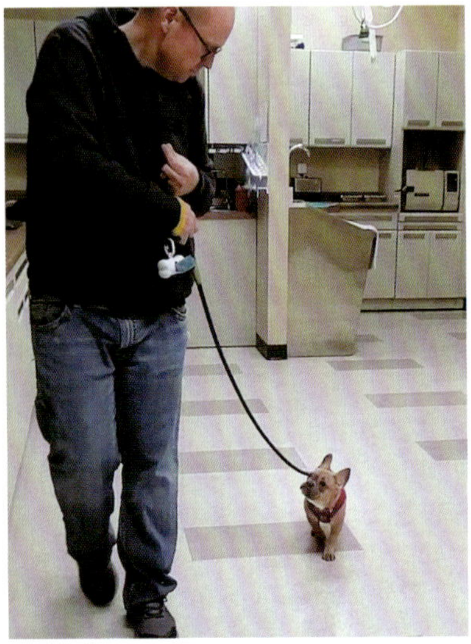

Fig. 5.5 I: Puppy practicing check-ins with the caregivers during a puppy class. Notice how the caregiver skillfully keeps the leash loose. (Photo courtesy of Jessica Benoit)

shy or fearful puppies, who may find direct eye contact intimidating, even a brief glance towards the caregiver should be rewarded.

Recall

An essential and potentially lifesaving behavior, the recall (come when called) serves as an effective means to redirect a puppy's attention when needed. A specific word, sound, or visual signal, this cue should consistently be associated with high-value treats to effectively encourage the puppy's response. and engagement. Punishment should never be used, even if the puppy does not immediately return or runs away, as this can damage the relationship and make the puppy less likely to return when called in the future.

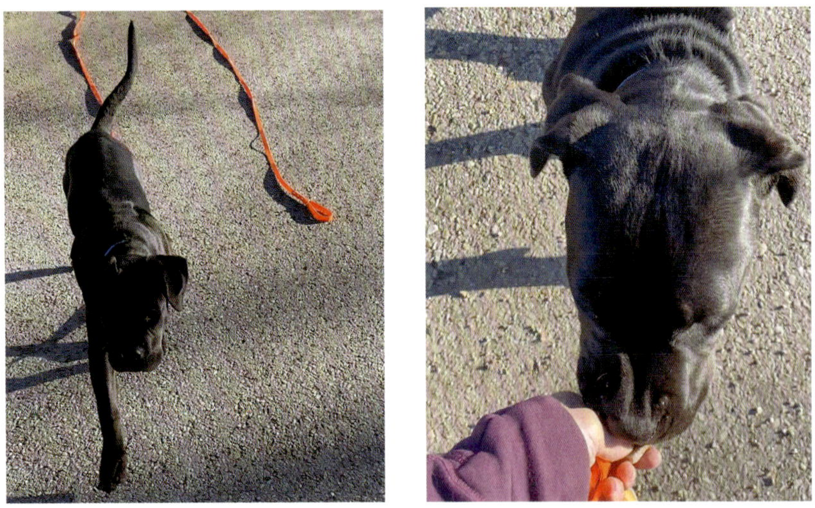

Figs. 5.5 J, K: Puppy practicing recall and being reinforced on a long line. (Photos courtesy of Jessica Benoit)

Mat Work

Learning how to stay out from underfoot, as well as developing independence and relaxation, can be challenging for some puppies. Mat work helps puppies form a positive association with a specific item, such as a mat, platform, or similar non-slip surface, and teaches them to stay in one place, a concept known as stationing. The portability of a mat adds versatility, allowing its use in various areas and environments. Suitable for both puppies and adult dogs, mat work is effective in everyday settings and in environments with more distractions.

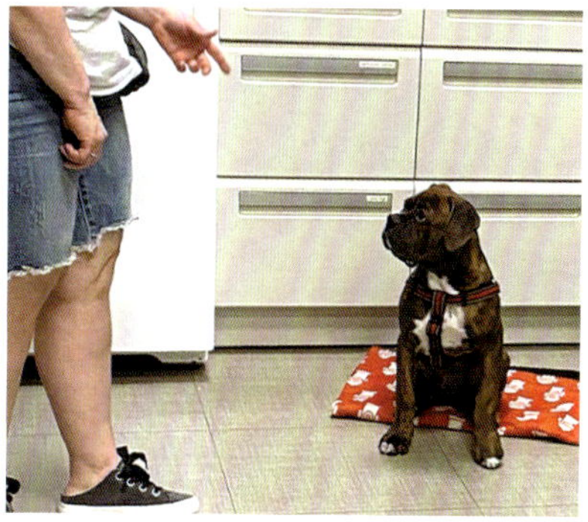

Fig. 5.5 L: In a training session, a caregiver teaches a puppy the "place" cue, guiding them to relax on a mat in response to a visual signal. Training starts with simpler tasks like sitting and lying down on the mat in low-distraction environments, such as at home. As the puppy becomes more proficient, the caregiver gradually transitions to practicing these behaviors in more distracting environments. (Photo courtesy of Jessica Benoit)

Key Application of Mat Work

Mat work is especially useful in teaching a puppy to stay stationed amidst various distractions, such as during meal preparation and eating, excitement at the front door, interactions with children, or in new places like a friend's or in-laws' home, veterinary clinics, and grooming parlors. This training encourages more desirable behaviors, such as sitting instead of jumping during greetings, and teaches valuable social skills and independence, such as knowing where to go to avoid being underfoot during high excitement times or when food is present. Common verbal cues for this behavior include "place" and "settle." A visual hand signal, such as pointing towards the mat, may also be used. Sometimes, the mat itself or its strategic placement within the environment naturally serves as a cue. For instance, during family dinner times or food preparation, the presence of food or the act of sitting down can prompt the puppy to go to the mat, reinforcing it as the preferred place instead of begging at the table or being underfoot.

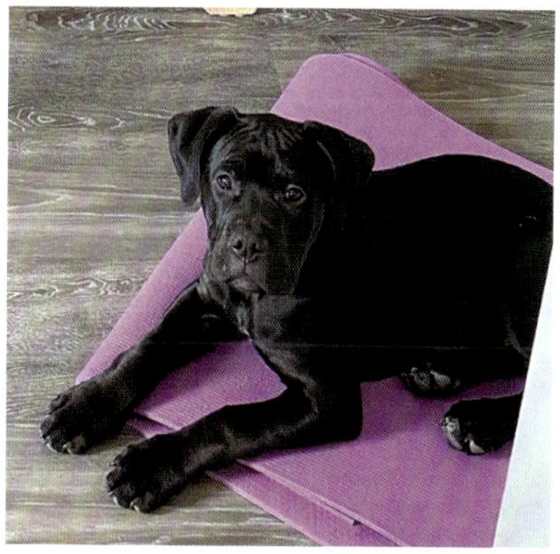

Fig. 5.5 M: Puppy practices mat work on the ground in the kitchen during mealtime. (Photo courtesy of Jessica Benoit)

Effective Mat Placement and Training Techniques

Begin by placing mats in high-traffic areas such as kitchens, living rooms, and near front doors to teach this behavior. Keep a variety of treats, mixing kibble with high and low-value treats, in containers near each mat or station for easy access. This setup allows you to capture opportunities when the puppy steps onto the mat and gradually settles. Puppies should be able to freely come and go from the mat. Initially, a reward may involve the puppy having all four feet on the mat, progressing to sitting or lying down as they get comfortable. It is important to distinguish between stationing and relaxation, which are often confused: stationing is staying in

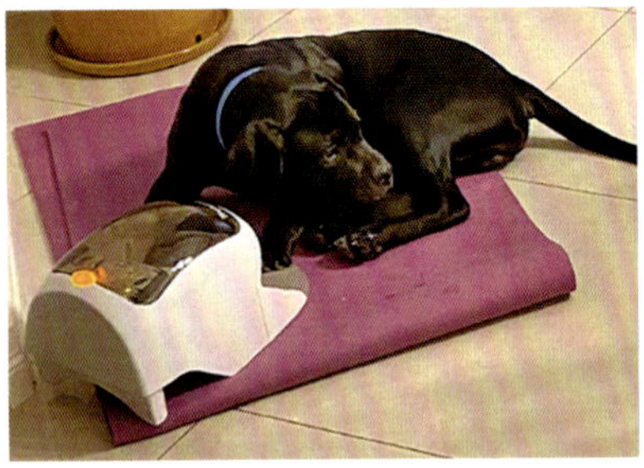

Fig. 5.5 N: Puppy is managed during dinner time using a Treat and Train® for mat training. (Photo courtesy of Jessica Benoit)

a designated spot briefly, while relaxation involves both physical and psychological calmness for an extended period. As the puppy becomes accustomed to the mat, encourage longer stays by using lickable mats or offering food-stuffed toys while they are on it. The "Relax on a Mat" technique focuses on shaping relaxed behaviors such as placing the head down on the mat, shifting the hips and extending out the hind legs, and deeper breathing. For extended durations, remote treat delivery systems like Treat and Train® are effective. Use the mat or platform exclusively during relaxation training and structured sessions to reinforce its significance.

5.6 Troubleshooting Common Puppy Behaviors

Training is a life-long commitment, that typically requires only minor adjustments as puppies mature. Puppies undergo significant brain development during their sensitive learning period from 12 to 16 weeks, transitioning into the juvenile and adolescence stages.[3,10,11] This phase, influences adult behavior and varies among breeds and size.[3] Common behaviors such as jumping, barking, counter-surfing, and digging are normal, stemming from a dog's instinct to scavenge, socialize, and explore. As dogs mature, however, these behaviors may become less acceptable, perceived as annoying or problematic. Consistently providing opportunities for dogs to express these natural behaviors, coupled with management and teaching alternative behaviors through positive reinforcement training methods, helps shape more appropriate and manageable behaviors for both dog and caregiver.

Using Stations

Strategically placed treat stations create opportunities to capture and shape desirable behaviors during both structured and passive training sessions. Set up these stations as small jars or cups, within easy reach for the human but out of the puppy's reach. For passive training, position these stations near all resting spots in the home. This setup allows for immediate marking and treat delivery when the puppy settles in these areas, and gradually encourages a more relaxed posture while on the mat.

Jumping

Jumping in puppies typically occurs when they are excited or over-aroused and is often reinforced by petting and attention. Such behavior might be tolerated or even encouraged in young puppies, human responses often become inconsistent as puppies grow, making the behavior hard to extinguish. This inconsistency can lead to fear, anxiety, and frustration due to mixed signals.

Prevention is key to stopping jumping behavior. Turning away or ignoring jumping behavior rarely stops it. Using barriers such as gates or exercise pens to confine the puppy before guests arrive can effectively prevent jumping. Instead of ignoring the behavior,

Adolescent Wellness Exams

Adolescent wellness exams offer an opportunity for early identification and management of behavioral issues, and help determine which dogs might benefit from a referral to a board-certified veterinary behaviorist.

encourage guests to squat to greet the puppy at their level and drop treats as the puppy approaches. Focus on teaching and reinforcing more desirable behaviors, such as keeping all four feet on the floor, stationing, or using a "touch" cue for greetings.

See note: https://cattledogpublishing.com/blog/jumping-up-how-to-help-your-pup/

Barking

Barking is a natural and common form of communication for dogs. They bark for various reasons, including fear, anxiety, frustration, alerting others to changes in their environment, or as an invitation to play.[40] Barking due to fear and anxiety can be particularly challenging to address. When dogs bark at external triggers or things such as people, animals, cars, or delivery trucks passing by their home, they often perceive this action as successful in making the perceived threat leave, inadvertently reinforcing the behavior. Managing this behavior largely depends on the dog's motivation. For barking triggered by unpredictable noises, using music or white noise to mask these sounds can be highly effective. Similarly, limiting a dog's ability to see external stimuli by closing blinds or applying window film, can also significantly reduce instances of barking.

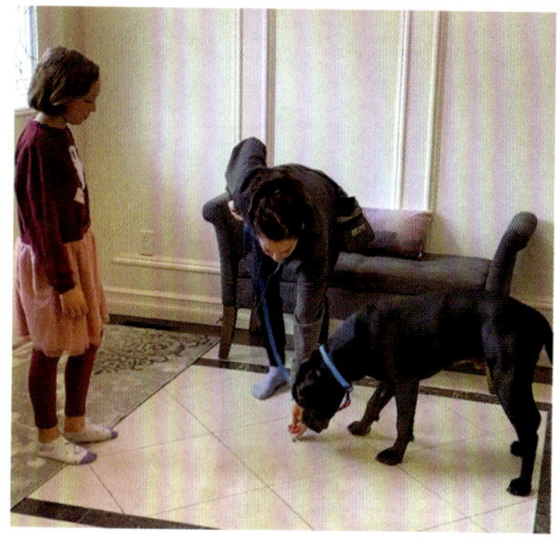

Fig. 5.6 A: Training session with a six-month-old puppy. The puppy is reinforced for all four feet on the floor. (Photo courtesy of Jessica Benoit)

Counter-Surfing

Counter-surfing often becomes more prevalent during a dog's adolescence, as puppies grow tall enough to reach food left on counters or tabletops. This behavior is highly self-rewarding, as the dog continues to find and access tasty food items when no one is around. The most effective management strategy for this behavior is to keep counters clear of food and to use a gate or exercise pen during meal preparation or whenever food is left unattended. Puppies can be positively reinforced for lying on a mat when food is present as an alternative behavior and long-term solution.

Leash Management for Jumping

If leashes are used, they should only be used during controlled training sessions. Caregivers should avoid using the leash to jerk or pull the puppy off a person, as these actions can lead to injury and create a negative association with people.

Teaching Alternative Behaviors

Capturing desirable behaviors gives an opportunity to reinforce quiet and calm behaviors, incompatible with or as an alternative to barking. Additional strategies to promote engagement to reduce barking, include Control Unleashed® Pattern Games, such as "Give Me A Break," "Up Down," and "1–2–3" Game.[48] Using "touch" can effectively interrupt the behavior and encourage a recall back to the caregiver for reinforcement. When called, the puppy should be continuously engaged with the caregiver until the stimulus is gone, otherwise an unwanted cycle may occur—bark, approach, get a treat, repeat.

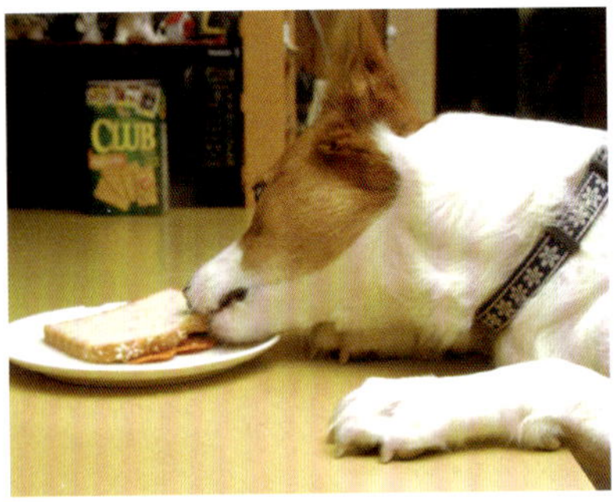

Fig. 5.6 B: To prevent counter surfing behavior, ensure that no food is left on the countertop, use a gate to restrict dogs' access to the kitchen or food prep areas, and teach alternative behaviors, like settling on a mat when food is present.

Addressing Stealing and Guarding Behaviors in Puppies

As natural scavengers, puppies often pick up non-food items such as sticks, mulch, and rocks in the yard and on walks, and they may even scavenge from countertops and trash cans. A common myth related to this behavior is that caregivers *should* be able to take food or other items from their dog's mouth. This belief system often leads to frustration and misinterpretation, resulting in the use of punishment, such as scolding, chasing, or forcefully removing the item, which may actually make the guarding behaviors worse.[49,50]

Effective Management of Stealing and Guarding Behavior

When addressing stealing and guarding behaviors, effective management strategies are key. This includes puppy-proofing to limit access to important, sentimental, expensive, or potentially dangerous items. Non-confrontational trade-offs reduce conflict and create positive associations when people approach while the puppy has a valued item. Offering higher-value food and toys encourages the puppy to voluntarily bring and exchange items, promoting cooperative behavior and reducing guarding or reluctance to relinquish items.

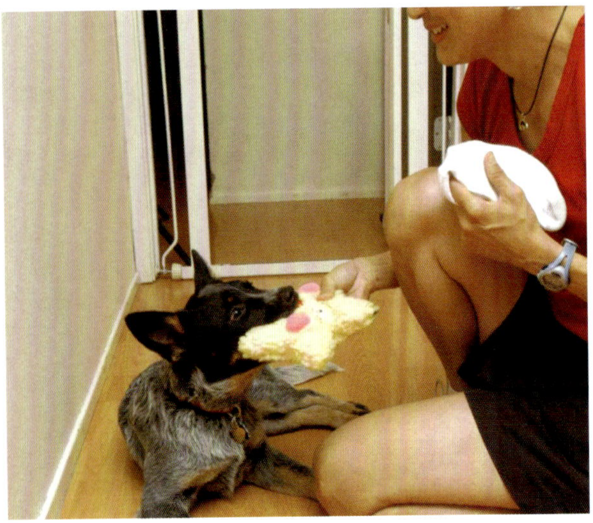

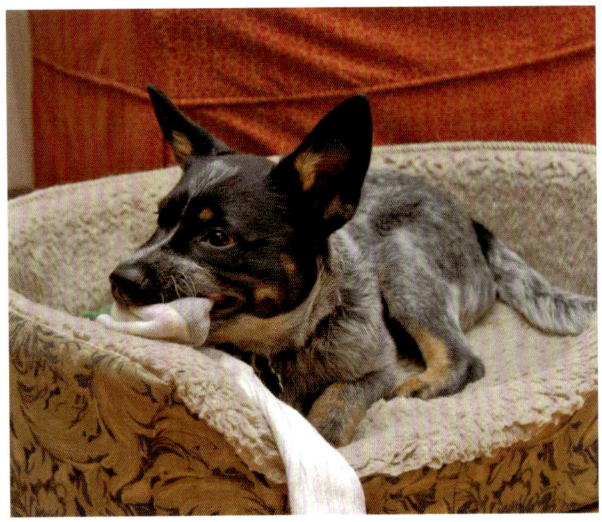

Figs. 5.6 C, D: Evaluate whether an item with a puppy is valuable or dangerous before removal. Not all items need to be taken; playful trade-ups can be used for items that are less critical.

Digging

Digging is a natural and common behavior in both puppies and adult dogs, driven by various motivations such as exploration, scent tracking, unearthing buried objects, cooling off, or seeking shelter.[3] To effectively manage this behavior, start by making sure the dog's basic needs are met, including providing adequate exercise, mental stimulation, and positive attention. Additionally, restrict access to preferred digging spots by using physical barriers and maintaining close supervision when the dog is outdoors.

An effective strategy to channel their digging instincts appropriately is to create a designated digging area. For example, a kiddie pool filled with play sand and pea gravel, or a sandbox, can provide an attractive alternative for dogs who love to dig. Enhance the appeal of these designated areas by, hiding treats and toys within them, encouraging digging in these desired locations over the undesirable ones.

Table 5.6.1 Non-confrontational strategies to remove an item from a puppy's mouth

Removing Items From A Puppy's Mouth	
Item is *not* Dangerous or Valuable **Goal:** Reduce conflict and help the puppy associate a person's approach with positive outcomes rather than losing their item.	**Item *is* Dangerous or Valuable** **Goal:** Must retrieve
Cheerful Approach Approach the dog with a friendly voice, asking, "Whatchya got?" Toss a treat when they look up, then walk away without immediately taking the item.	**Higher Value Trade** Offer a high-value item (food or toy) to distract them and lure to a safe location. Retrieve the original item after the puppy is safely contained elsewhere.
Reward Release If the dog drops the item, reward with multiple treats but do not take the item immediately. Give treats regardless of whether they drop the item before looking up.	**Avoid Conflict** Distract or lure the puppy from the area and away from the item without picking them up or grabbing their collar. Use a toy, treat, the sound of a doorbell, or offer an opportunity to go outside, an invitation for a walk, or car ride.

5.7 Preparing for the Future

At some point in their lives, puppies will need to be handled, examined, or need medications for their health. Incorporating handling exercises into a puppy's daily routine and interactions can help them become more comfortable with physical touch and routine husbandry procedures. Using lickable mats or other food-based distractions can make this process more enjoyable and less stressful for the puppy with minimal conditioning. Preparing puppies to willingly take medications simplifies the administration process, reduces conflict, and successful administration of medications in the future.

Handling Exercises

Handling exercises help caregivers learn how to gently interact with their puppies, building a positive conditioned emotional response (+CER). These exercises are designed to acclimate puppies to common types of touch and handling they will encounter throughout their lives, such as veterinary examinations and regular husbandry activities like brushing, bathing, and grooming. Familiarizing puppies with these interactions from a young age makes routine care activities more comfortable and less stressful for both the puppy and their caregiver.

Body Handling

If the puppy displays any signs of stress, ***stop***. Go back a step, then end the session on a positive note. For future sessions, consider breaking the steps down further and advancing more slowly.

Starting Handling Exercises

Begin handling exercises in a comfortable and relaxed environment for the puppy. Offer high-value treats while briefly touching less sensitive areas of their body, like the back, neck, and shoulders. If they are comfortable, transition to a "touch then feed" technique: touch their back, stop touching then offer a food reward. Gradually move from the less sensitive areas to the more sensitive ones, such as their mouth, paws, tails, and abdomen. During the session, toss treats away to give the puppy a break and the opportunity to choose to re-engage. Repeat this process several times a week for one to two minutes, focusing on different body parts as appropriate while letting the puppy set the pace.

Predictor Cues

During handling exercises, ***predictor cues***, such as naming the body part to be touched, can be added to make the handling process even more predictable for the puppy.

Preparing for Routine Care

The purpose of these exercises is to gradually accustom puppies to gentle handling and restraint, focusing particularly on areas frequently examined, such as the eyes, ears, teeth, and abdomen for palpation. Additional focus areas include parting fur for skin checks, inspecting genitals and anus, assessing lymph nodes, handling feet, and preparing for procedures like venipuncture. By gradually familiarizing puppies with a variety of touches, these interactions become predictable, helping them become comfortable with different types of handling. This makes veterinary examinations, procedures, and routine husbandry more manageable and less stressful for them in the future.

Preparing Puppies for Medication Administration

As part of preventative care and husbandry training, teaching puppies to willingly accept oral medications helps minimize stress and improve the success rate of medication administration when treatments are required in the future. There are a variety of techniques that can be used to make the process as smooth and low stress as possible for both the puppy and their caregiver. By focusing on

Table 5.7.1 Low Stress Handling® Medication Administration Strategies

Method	Description
Food ball method	Start by creating a consistent routine using small creamy food balls as rewards. Introduce a piece of kibble or a gelatin capsule hidden inside these treats to familiarize puppies with taking something unusual but still in a familiar form (the food ball).
Syringe training	Begin by smearing some creamy food on the syringe and encouraging the puppy to lick it off. Progress to attaching a food ball to the end of the syringe, allowing the puppy to take it off. Gradually, introduce the syringe into the puppy's mouth, initially without administering any liquid, and then slowly incorporate liquid medication.
Liquid medication	Start administering small amounts of a tasty liquid, like meat broth, using the syringe. Over time, increase the amount and switch up the flavors to keep the puppy engaged and comfortable with the process.
Lickable treat mat	Place medicated food balls on a lickable treat mat. This encourages the puppy to consume medication in a fun and non-threatening way.
Additional tips	• Encapsulate bitter pills to reduce taste aversion. • Use peanut butter or similar substances to disguise the texture of pills. • Practice with commercially available treat pouches for easy administration. • Administer medication as a treat to reinforce a cued behavior, as part of a game, or in an unsuspecting location such as on a walk.

creating a positive experience for the puppy any discomfort or fear associated with the medication process can be reduced.

5.8 Children and Dogs

Navigating the dynamics between puppies and children can present challenges to families. Following specific guidelines for safety and comfort aids in building positive relationships. It is not uncommon to hear people say, "My dog is so great with the kids" or "The children can do anything to the dog, and they don't react." Although it is commonly believed that dogs are generally tolerant of children, research indicates that many dog bite incidents involve familiar dogs biting children in their homes. These incidents particularly

Active Supervision

This is ***focused attention*** and ***intentional observation***. Distractions such as cooking, cleaning, reading, watching television, talking, or texting on the phone require the puppy and children to be separated because it only takes one second for an animal to become overwhelmed and bite a child.

affect younger children with bites usually occurring on the face and head.[51] This highlights the importance of bite prevention education, as advocated by veterinarians and other experts.

For safety, direct supervision of all interactions between children and dogs or puppies is essential. This involves actively observing their interactions and understanding body language that indicates fear and distress. These observations should be shared with children to teach them how to interpret the various signals a dog uses to communicate. By explaining this body language to children, they can understand and respond appropriately when the puppy is "talking" to them, fostering safe and positive interactions for everyone.

Young children often engage in activities like running, screaming, or speaking in high-pitched, excited tones, which can make it challenging for puppies to resist chasing and playfully nipping. It is therefore important to teach children how to remain calm and respectful around puppies. Involving children in the training process is beneficial, though the approach depends on the child's age and the puppy's temperament. One effective method is protected contact, where the puppy and child are separated by a barrier such as a baby gate or exercise pen. This approach helps children understand how their behavior influences the dog's emotional responses. It teaches them when to give the dog space and when to remove themselves from a situation, promoting safety and respect between the child and the dog.

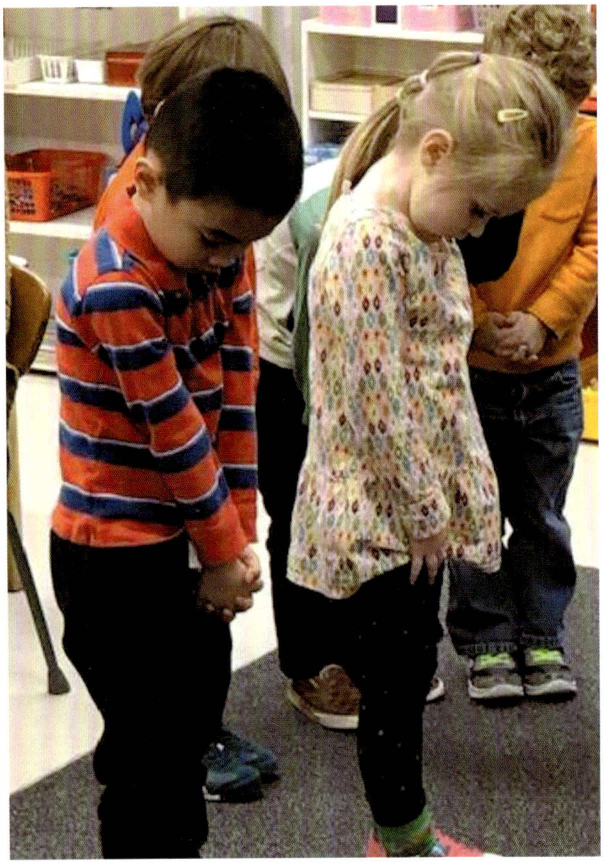

Fig. 5.8 A: Children learning to "be a tree" during an in-class school presentation. (Photo courtesy of Jessica Benoit)

Educational programs like Family Paws® and Doggone Safe (The Pet Professional Guild) offer animal professionals the chance to become licensed educators, assisting families with young children and dogs.[52,53] These programs provide valuable resources for teaching children about canine body language and safe interaction with both familiar and unfamiliar dogs. The Be a Tree™ program, for instance, instructs children to stand still, fold their arms, and lower their heads when around excited puppies and dogs. By removing attention and standing still, an overexcited dog's behavior should escalate quickly, giving the parents an opportunity to intervene.[52]

Helping puppies feel comfortable around children is just as important as it is to teach children how to interact with puppies. Puppies should always have the option to choose whether to interact with a child and should never be forced to interact. Teaching a puppy to hand target or "touch" is a great way to establish a positive relationship and have fun, while allowing the puppy to make choices. Additionally, to encourage calm behavior and familiarize the puppy with a child's touch, supervised gentle petting by a child can be combined with an adult giving treats to the puppy. When petting the puppy, pause frequently to assess body language.

Using barriers like baby gates and crates helps create safe spaces and manage interactions between children and dogs securely. When a baby or toddler is on the floor, it is safer to have the puppy

Additional Resources Available for Families and Expectant Parents

- familypaws.com
- poochparenting.net
- doggonesafe.com
- thebluedog.org
- dogmeetsbaby.expert
- colleenpelar.com
- thefamilydog.com

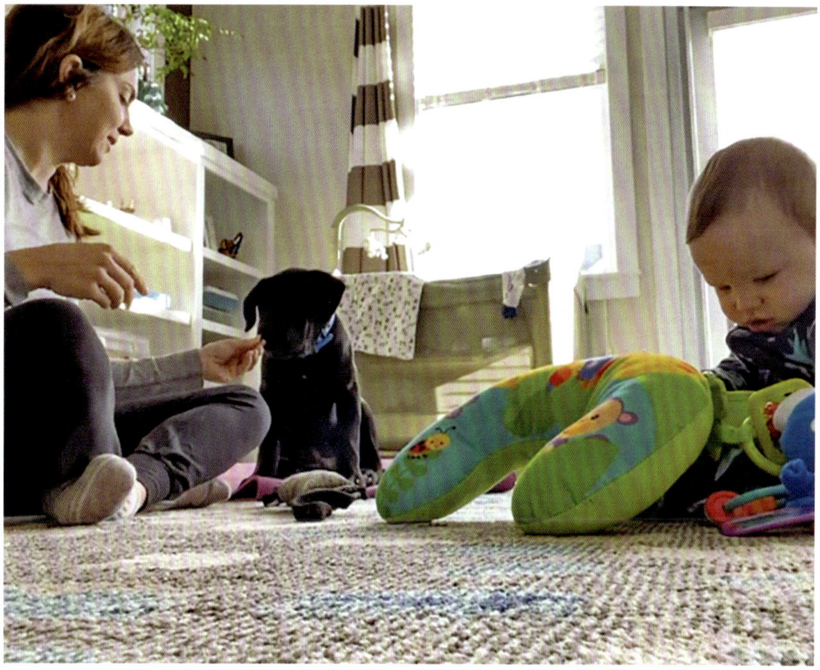

Fig. 5.8 B: An adult is on the floor with the baby while reinforcing the puppy for remaining on the mat. (Photo courtesy of Jessica Benoit)

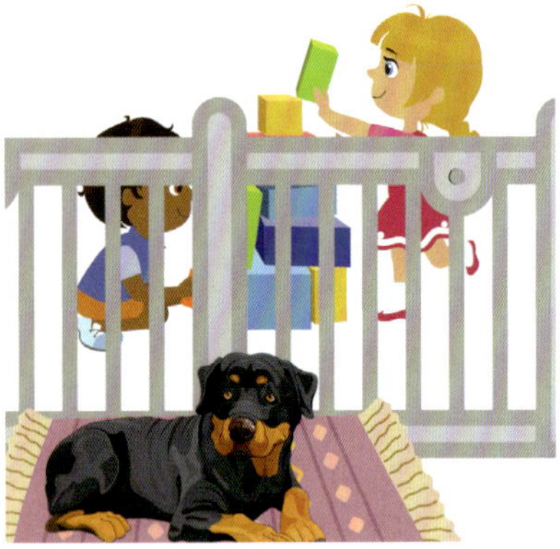

Fig. 5.8 C: Children playing with toys while the puppy is behind a baby gate. (Illustration courtesy of Jessica Benoit)

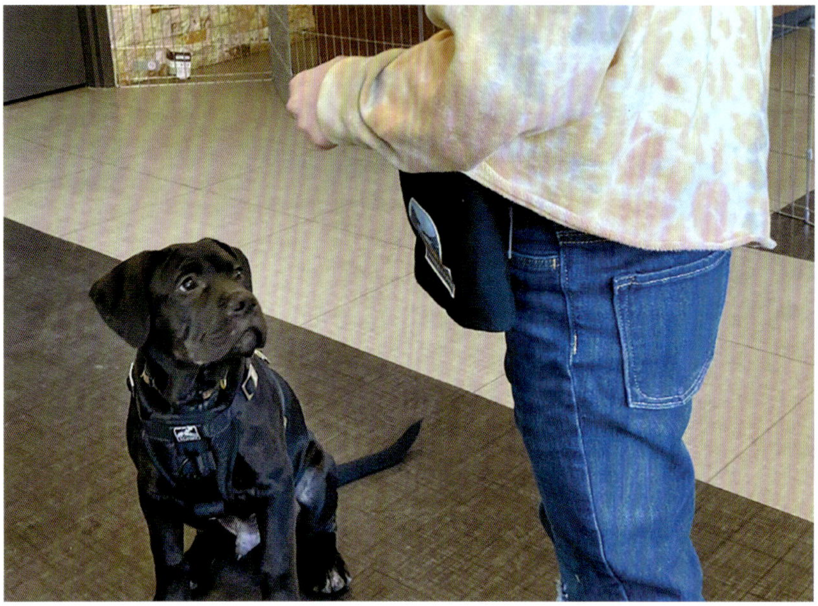

Fig. 5.8 D: When teaching children how to use a clicker for training, it is often easier to start with a stationary behavior such as sit rather than an active one like touch. Initially, children should focus on capturing the behavior (for example, clicking when they notice the puppy sitting naturally) instead of prompting the behavior with a cue. Once they achieve consistent timing with a verbal marker like "yes" or a clicker, they can then introduce the cue. An adult should have already taught a sit cue in a separate training session. (Photo courtesy of Jessica Benoit)

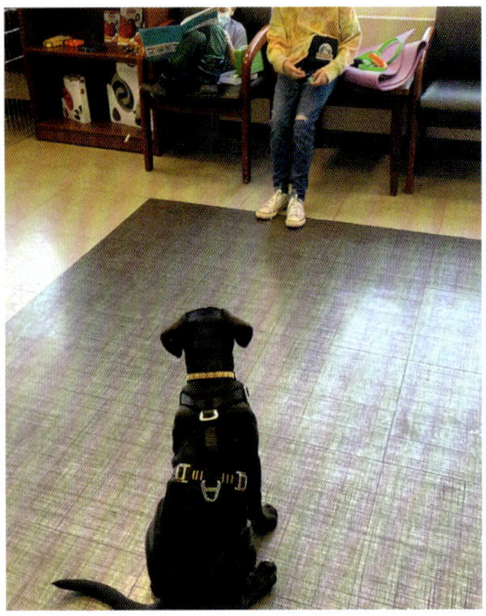

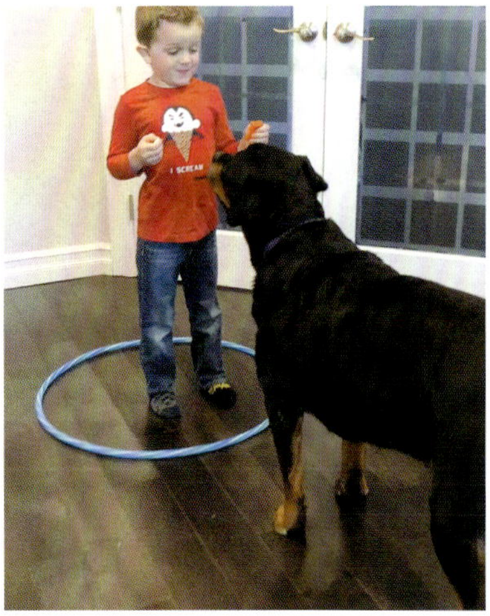

Figs. 5.8 E, F: Children should sit or stand while training. The more children move, the more difficult it can be for the puppy to pay attention. Some children do well if given a visual station like a hula hoop to stand in. (Photos courtesy of Jessica Benoit)

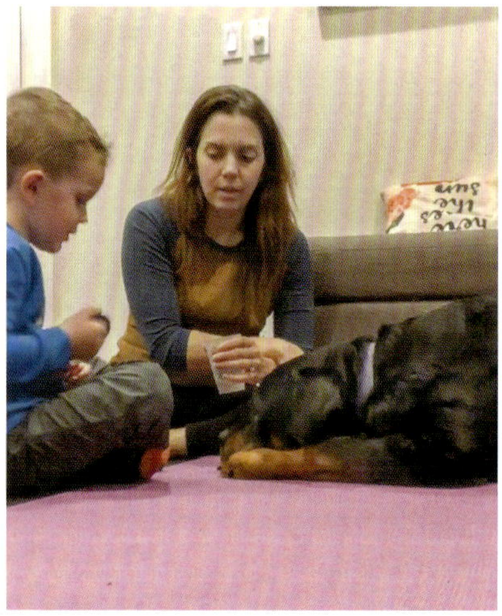

Fig. 5.8 G: Break up the task. Have a child oversee either clicking or tossing the treat, but not both. Children six years of age and older can often click and treat on their own. (Photo courtesy of Jessica Benoit)

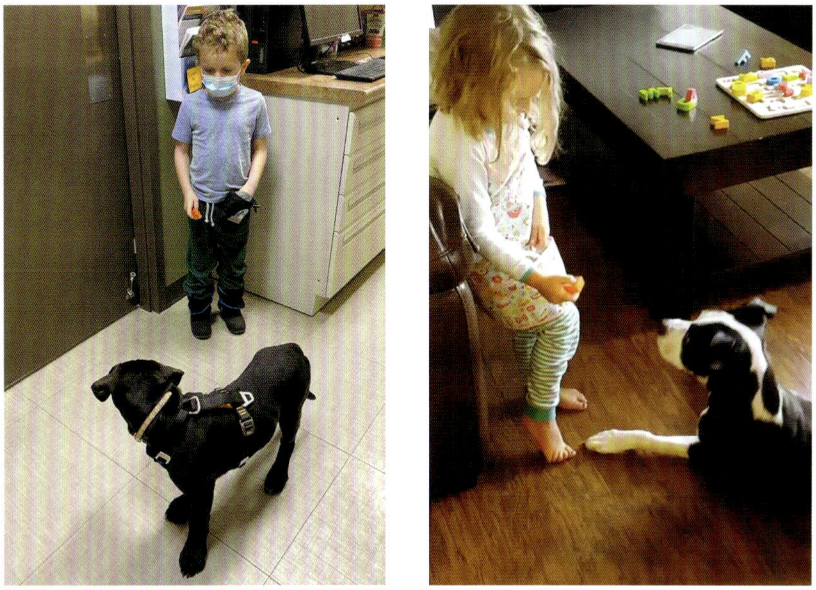

Figs. 5.8 H, I: Having treats in a treat pouch or apron can help make treat delivery easier for the child. (Photos courtesy of Jessica Benoit)

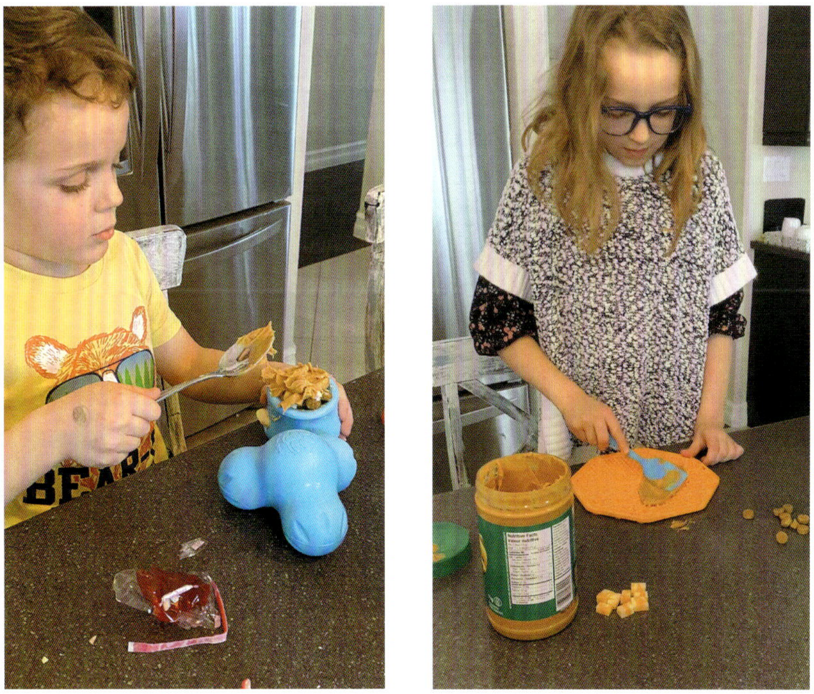

Figs. 5.8 J, K: In addition to training, involving children in the daily care of a puppy can be highly beneficial. One excellent activity for children is preparing food puzzle toys! (Photos courtesy of Jessica Benoit)

behind a visual barrier, either engaged with a food toy or simply resting. Relaxation exercises, such as having the puppy relax on a mat in their safe space, are also an integral part of this process.

5.9 Conclusion

In a world largely influenced by human actions, puppies need to be provided with opportunities to make choices and to create environments that support their natural canine instincts. Training puppies using positive reinforcement and establishing an environment suitable for their needs actively engages them in their own learning journey. Educating and supporting clients is key in maintaining the human-animal bond, establishing relationships based on trust, and promoting empathy and understanding. This method also gives caregivers a foundational skill set that can be enhanced and adapted as the puppy matures.

5.10 References

1. Scott, J. P., & Fuller, J. L. (1965). *Genetics and the social behaviour of the dog* (1st ed.). The University of Chicago Press.
2. Freedman, D. G., King, J. A., & Elliot, O. (1961). Critical periods in the social development of the dog. *Science*, 133, 1016–1017.
3. Overall, K. (2013). *Manual of Clinical Behavioral Medicine for Dogs and Cats*. Elsevier.
4. Pierantoni, L., Albertini, M., & Pirrone, F. (2011). Prevalence of owner-reported behaviours in dogs separated from the litter at two different ages. *Veterinary Record*, 169(18), 468. https://doi.org/10.1136/vr.d4967
5. Fox, M., & Stelzner, D. (1967). The effects of early experience on the development of inter and intraspecies social relationships in the dog. *Animal Behaviour*, 15(2–3), 377–386. https://doi.org/10.1016/0003–3472(67)90024–3
6. Scott, J., & Marston, M. V. (1950). Critical periods affecting the development of normal and mal-adjustive social behavior of puppies. *The Pedagogical Seminary and Journal of Genetic Psychology*, *77*(1), 25–60.
7. Feddersen-Petersen, D. (1994). Some interactive aspects between dogs and their owners: Are there reciprocal influences between both intra- and interspecific communication? *Applied Animal Behaviour Science*, 40, 78.

8. Fox, M. W., & Stelzner, D. (1966). Behavioral effects of differential early experience in the dog. *Animal Behaviour*, 14, 273–281.

9. Fox, M. (1971). *Behaviour of Wolves, Dogs, and Related Canids*. Dogwise Publishing.

10. Luescher, A. U. (2014). Canine behavior and development. In: *Canine and Feline Behavior for Veterinary Technicians and Nurses*, 30–50. John Wiley & Sons.

11. Radosta, L. (2023). Canine behavior and development. In: *Canine and Feline Behavior for Veterinary Technicians and Nurses*, 34–58. John Wiley & Sons.

12. American Veterinary Society of Animal Behavior. (2008). AVSAB position statement on puppy socialization. https://avsab.org/resources/position-statements/

13. Duxbury, M. M., Jackson, J. A., Line, S. W., & Anderson, R. K. (2003). Evaluation of association between retention in the home and attendance at puppy socialization classes. *Journal of the American Veterinary Medical Association*, 223(1), 61–66. https://doi.org/10.2460/javma.2003.223.61

14. Stepita, M. E., Bain, M. J., & Kass, P. H. (2013). Frequency of CPV infection in vaccinated puppies that attended puppy socialization classes. *Journal of the American Animal Hospital Association*, 49(2), 95–100. https://doi.org/10.5326/JAAHA-MS-5825

15. Hammerle, M., Horst, C., Levine, E., Overall, K., Radosta, L., Rafter-Ritchie, M., & Yin, S. (2015). 2015 AAHA canine and feline behavior management guidelines. *Journal of the American Animal Hospital Association*, 51(4), 205–221. DOI: 10.5326/JAAHA-MS-6527.

16. Howell, A., & Feyrecilde, M. (2018). *Cooperative Veterinary Care (1st ed.)*. Wiley-Blackwell.

17. Mellor, D. J., Beausoleil, N. J., Littlewood, K. E., McLean, A. N., McGreevy, P. D., Jones, B., & Wilkins, C. (2020). The 2020 five domains model: Including human–animal interactions in assessments of animal welfare. *Animals*, 10(10), 1870.

18. Littlewood, K. E., Heslop, M. V., & Cobb, M. L. The agency domain and behavioural interactions: Assessing positive animal welfare using the Five Domains Model. *Frontiers in Veterinary Science*, 10, 1284869.

19. Sen Majumder, S., Paul, M., Sau, S., & Bhadra, A. (2016). Denning habits of free-ranging dogs reveal preference for human proximity. *Scientific Reports*, 6(1). https://doi.org/10.1038/srep32014

20. Frank, D., Minero, M., Cannas, S., & Palestrini, C. (2007). Puppy behaviours when left home alone: a pilot study. *Applied Animal Behaviour Science*, 104(1–2), 61–70.

21. Ross, S. (1950). Some observations on the lair dwelling behavior of dogs. *Behavior*, 2, 144–162.

22. Learn, A., Radosta, L., & Pike, A. (2020). Preliminary assessment of differences in completeness of house-training between dogs based on size. *Journal of Veterinary Behavior*, *35*, 19–26.

23. Taylor, K. D., & Mills, D. S. (2007). The effect of the kennel environment on canine welfare: A critical review of experimental studies. *Animal welfare*, 16(4), 435–447.

24. Young, R. J. (2013). *Environmental Enrichment for Captive Animals.* Blackwell Publishing.

25. Herron, M. E., Kirby-Madden, T. M., & Lord, L. K. (2014). Effects of environmental enrichment on the behavior of shelter dogs. *Journal of the American Veterinary Medical Association*, 244(6), 687–692. https://doi.org/10.2460/javma.244.6.687

26. Hubrecht, R. C. (1995). Enrichment in puppyhood and its effects on later behavior of dogs. *Laboratory Animal Science*, *45*(1), 70–75.

27. Horowitz, A. (2015, February 2). How do dogs "see" with their noses? [Video]. YouTube. https://www.youtube.com/watch?v=p7fXa2Occ_U&t=70s

28. Stremming, S. (Host). (2018, Jan 9). Decompression walks [Audio Podcast Episode]. COG DOG Radio. *The Cognitive Canine*. https://thecognitivecanine.com/blog/a-decompression-walk-chat/

29. Duranton, C., & Horowitz, A. (2019). Let me sniff! Nosework induces positive judgment bias in pet dogs. *Applied Animal Behaviour Science*, 211, 61–66. https://doi.org/10.1016/j.applanim.2018.12.009

30. Schipper, L. L., Vinke, C. M., Schilder, M. B., & Spruijt, B. M. (2008). The effect of feeding enrichment toys on the behavior of kennelled dogs (Canis familiaris). *Applied Animal Behaviour Science*, 114(1–2), 182–195. https://doi.org/10.1016/j.applanim.2008.01.001.

31. Bender, A., & Strong, E. (2019). *Canine Enrichment for the Real World Workbook*. Dogwise Publishing.

32. Epstein, J., Dowling-Guyer, S., McCobb, E., Glotzer, C., & Dodman, N. H. (2021). Addressing stress in dogs in shelters through a novel visual and auditory enrichment device. *Applied Animal Behaviour Science*, 236, 105–215. https://doi.org/10.1016/j.applanim.2021.105215

33. Kogan, L. R., Schoenfeld-Tacher, R., & Simon, A. A. (2012). Behavioral effects of auditory stimulation on kenneled dogs. *Journal of Veterinary Behavior*, 7(5), 268–275. https://doi.org/10.1016/j.jveb.2011.11.002.

34. Bowman, A., Scottish SPCA, Dowell, F., & Evans, N. (2015). 'Four Seasons' in an animal rescue centre: Classical music reduces environmental stress in kennelled dogs. *Physiology & Behavior,* 143, 70–82. https://doi.org/10.1016/j.physbeh.2015.02.035.

35. Shaw, J., & Martin, D. (2023). *Canine and Feline Behavior for Veterinary Technicians and Nurses (2nd ed.).* John Wiley & Sons

36. Martin, D., & Martin, D. (2011). *Puppy Start Right: Foundation Training for the Companion Dog.* Karen Pryor Clickertraining.

37. Bekoff, M. (1977). Social communication in canids: Evidence for the evolution of a stereotyped mammalian display. *Science,* 197(4308), 1097–1099. https://doi.org/10.1126/science.197.4308.1097

38. Bekoff, M. (1995). Play signals as punctuation: The structure of social play in canids. *Behaviour,* 132(5–6), 419–429. https://doi.org/10.1163/156853995x00649

39. Maglieri, V., Zanoli, A., Mastrandrea, F., & Palagi, E. (2023). Don't stop me now, I'm having such a good time! Czechoslovakian wolfdogs renovate the motivation to play with a bow. *Current Zoology,* 69(1), 50–58.

40. Yin, S., & McCowan, B. (2004). Barking in domestic dogs: context specificity and individual identification. *Animal Behaviour,* 68(2), 343–355.

41. Faragó, T., Pongrácz, P., Range, F., Virányi, Z., & Miklósi, Á. (2010). 'The bone is mine': Affective and referential aspects of dog growls. *Animal Behaviour,* 79(4), 917–925. https://doi.org/10.1016/j.anbehav.2010.01.005

42. Landsberg, G. M., Hunthausen, W. L., & Ackerman, L. J. (2013). *Handbook of Behavior Problems of the Dog and Cat.* Saunders Elsevier.

43. New, J. C., Jr., Salman, M. D., King, M., Scarlett, J. M., Kass, P. H., & Hutchison, J. M. (2000). Characteristics of shelter-relinquished animals and their owners compared with animals and their owners in U.S. pet-owning households. *Journal of Applied Animal Welfare Science,* 3, 179–201. https://doi.org/10.1207/S15327604JAWS0303_1

44. Patronek, G. J., Glickman, L. T., Beck, A. M., McCabe, G. P., & Ecker, C. (1996). Risk factors for relinquishment of dogs to an animal shelter. *Journal of the American Veterinary Medical Association,* 209, 572–581.

45. Salman, M. D., Hutchison, J., Ruch-Gallie, R., Kogan, L., New, J. C., Kass, P. H., & Scarlett, J. M. (2000). Behavioral reasons for relinquishment of dogs and cats to 12 shelters. *Journal of Applied Animal Welfare Science,* 3(2), 93–106. https://doi.org/10.1207/s15327604jaws0302_2

46. González-Martínez, N., Martínez, M. F., Rosado, B., Luño, I., Santamarina, G., Suárez, M. L., Camino, F., de la Cruz, L. F., & Diéguez, F. J. (2019). Association between puppy classes and adulthood behavior of the dog. *Journal of Veterinary Behavior*, 32, 36–41. https://doi.org/10.1016/j.jveb.2019.04.011

47. Schulkey, R., & DePorter, T. (2017, August). Evaluation of the association between attendance at veterinary hospital-based puppy socialisation classes and long-term retention in the home. In *Proceedings of the 11th International Veterinary Behaviour Meeting*, 14–16th September 2017, Samorin, Slovakia (pp. 100–101). CABI.

48. McDevitt, L. (2019). *Control Unleashed: Reactive to relaxed.* South Hadley, MA: Clean Run Productions LLC.

49. Jacobs, J. A., Coe, J. B., Pearl, D. L., Widowski, T. M., & Niel, L. (2018). Factors associated with canine resource guarding behaviour in the presence of dogs: A cross-sectional survey of dog owners. *Preventive Veterinary Medicine, 161*, 134–142. https://doi.org/10.1016/j.prevetmed.2017.02.004.

50. Mohan-Gibbons, H., Weiss, E., & Slater, M. (2012). Preliminary investigation of food guarding behavior in shelter dogs in the United States. *Animals, 2*(3), 331–346. https://doi.org/10.3390/ani2030331.

51. Fein, J., Bogumil, D., Upperman, J. S., & Burke, R. V. (2018). Pediatric dog bites: A population-based profile. *Injury Prevention*, 25(4), 290–294. https://doi.org/10.1136/injuryprev-2017–042621.

52. Doggone Safe. (2018). About Us. https://www.doggonesafe.com/About

53. Family Paws. (2002). About Us. https://www.familypaws.com/about-family-paws/

Author
Jessica Benoit RVT, VTS (Behavior), KPA-CTP, CPDT-KA

Enrichment Benefits

All forms of enrichment offer important benefits. This chart outlines different types of enrichment and the sensory system they target.

	Occupational	Physical	Social	Sensory	Nutritional
Visual	Flirt poles Fetch Group training classes Agility Herding Lure coursing Dock diving Disc dogs Flyball	Agility and obstacle courses Explore surfaces & objects (bridges, tunnels, etc.) Exploration with new or favorite toys Walks	Group training classes Learning a new trick or behavior Tug/fetch Walks to new areas Dog parks Visiting friends at another house Introduction to veterinary professionals	Access to a window Walks to new areas Car rides TV programs	Chews Frozen food treats Snuffle mats for feeding LickiMat® Treat and Train®
Auditory	Clicker training Tracking Herding Canine freestyle	Explore children's toys that make sounds Dog toys that produce different sounds (crinkling) Different surfaces Walks in urban and rural environments (beaches, natural reserves, parking lots)	Walks to new areas Playgrounds Sounds of children, adults, animals, & birds	TV programs Classical music Use of sound apps (doorbell, door knock) New environments Car rides	Remote treat dispensers Clicker training

Enrichment Benefits *(continued)*

All forms of enrichment offer important benefits. This chart outlines different types of enrichment and the sensory system they target.

	Occupational	Physical	Social	Sensory	Nutritional
Olfactory	Scent detection sports (e.g. trailing, barn hunt, field trials, retrieving)	Finding treats in digging boxes Long-line walks dedicated to sniffing and exploring	Scent swapping Visiting dog friendly indoor/ outdoor establishments Intra-species and conspecific interactions	Long-line walks dedicated to sniffing and exploring Adding dog-safe essential oils to toys/objects Hide & seek with treats or people Bringing outdoor smells inside (leaves, grass, hay) Scent swapping (clothes or blankets rubbed on other canines or animals)	Snuffle mats for feeding Hide & seek with treats Forage for food using various commercial or DIY food toys or scattering kibble in snow, grass, or leaves
Gustatory	Forage for food in natural substrates (snow, grass, leaves) Snuffle mats for feeding Hide & seek with smelly treats	Forage for food by scattering kibble in snow, grass, or leaves		Introduce new foods Try freezing food toys	LickiMat® New foods to explore Food puzzle toys
Tactile	Flirt poles Digging boxes Agility & obstacle courses Swimming in a lake or pool	Comfortable bed Toys in a variety of textures Digging boxes Swimming in a lake or pool Explore surfaces & objects (metal, ladders, etc.)	Petting & massage Brushing	Shredding cardboard or other substrates Playing with toys of various textures	Chews Frozen treats Treats of various textures

Preventative Behavioral Health for Kittens

CHAPTER 6

6.1 Introduction

As both a predator and prey species, cats have many basic needs to stay physically and mentally healthy. Setting kittens up for success in the home environment and understanding the sensitive periods of learning is critical for their emotional health. Kitty kindergarten provides an opportunity for new caregivers to learn about fundamental needs of cats and how to set up their living environment. This knowledge, along with environmental enrichment, and training, is key for early intervention and prevention of future behavioral problems.

6.2 Sensitive Period of Learning

The sensitive period of learning in kittens is from two weeks to approximately seven weeks of age.[1–3] During this stage, kittens are most open to new experiences while they are still learning about what is safe or unsafe in life. It is important to give kittens plenty of positive experiences with a variety of stimuli during this time frame since experiences at this age influence how sociable or outgoing they will be later in life.

Utilizing the Sensitive Period for Socialization

Early gentle handling on a daily basis from birth to nine weeks increases friendliness towards humans.[1,4,5] Most kittens are not placed in homes until they are past this age, but some studies have shown that continuing daily gentle handling until 14 weeks still provides benefits.[1,6] It is impossible for kittens to experience every possible situation they will encounter as adult cats. Therefore, caregivers should focus on creating positive experiences with anything novel to best prepare them for the future.[1,7,8]

Quality, Not Quantity

A misconception about socialization is that it is solely about exposing kittens to a number of people, places, things, and environments (quantity). However, it is the quality of these experiences, rather than mere exposure, that is far more important.[9] Using food is the easiest way to create a positive association with each experience. Play is another. If a kitten refuses food or play, then the situation may be too stressful for them. During interactions, avoid overwhelming the kitten with forced interactions and always make sure to give an opportunities for breaks. Neglecting to do so could have repercussions and result in an increase in fear, anxiety, or frustration.[9]

Table 6.2.1: Table of Do's and Don'ts for Kitten Socialization

Do	Don't
Use food and distance	Use punishment for any reason
Allow kittens to explore at their own pace	Force kittens to explore new things or meet new people
Monitor kittens' body language closely	Ignore a kitten's emotional state

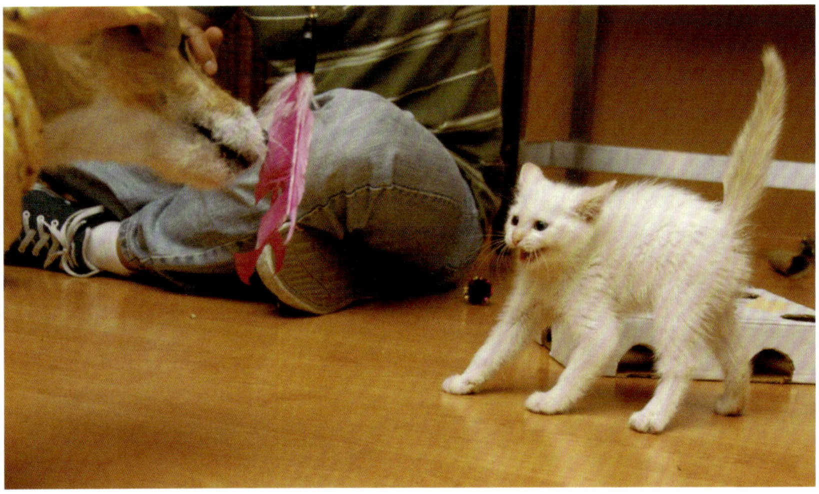

Fig. 6.2 A: This dog has come too close to this kitten, which has resulted in a fearful response. This is an example of flooding, one of the most common errors made during socialization. To prevent flooding, consider how the kitten may react to something new, including whether the intensity can be decreased and how to make it a positive experience for the kitten. Introducing novel and potentially intense stimuli from a greater distance and pairing those stimuli with food are common methods to enhance the experience.

Developmental Stage of Adolescence

Adolescence in cats spans from sexual maturity, around five to six months of age, to social maturity, which can extend up to two to four years.[1–12] During this period, there may be an increase in activity and the development of new, undesirable behaviors. Behaviors that were considered a minor issue during kittenhood can become more problematic.

The good news is that with their new physical prowess, there are more opportunities for reinforcement, for better or for worse. Continue applying the "Do's and Don'ts of Socialization" outlined in table 6.2.1 to provide a social and enriching environment to meet each cat's basic needs.

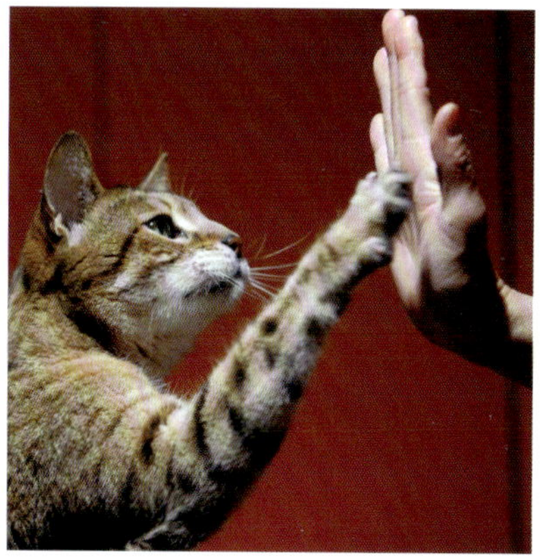

Fig. 6.2 B: High five is an easy trick to teach cats since they regularly make pawing motions.

6.3 Providing an Optimal Feline Environment

Cats are commonly thought to be easy keepers and low-maintenance pets. However, like all animals, they have specific needs that if not met, can lead to a variety of behavior problems such as aggression, elimination disorders, destructive scratching, and excessive vocalization.

The Five Pillars

Understanding and catering to their species-specific needs helps provide an ideal environment for cats. These requirements are recognized as the Five Pillars of a Healthy Feline Environment by the American Association of Feline Practitioners (AAFP) and the International Society of Feline Medicine (ISFM) and include:

Pillar 1. A safe space.

Pillar 2. Multiple and separate resources: food, water, toileting areas, scratching areas, play areas, and resting or sleeping areas.

Pillar 3. Opportunity for play and predatory behavior.

Pillar 4. An environment stimulating to the five senses (touch, smell, sound, sight, taste).

Pillar 5. Positive, consistent, and predictable human-cat social interaction.

Safe Space

Cats possess duel roles as both predator and prey, making them skilled hunters who are always alert to danger. Because they are also hunted, cats need to feel safe and secure. Therefore, safe spaces such as tall perches, cat carriers, and tunnels should be available in every room of the home. Cats particularly appreciate access to vertical spaces, which not only offer refuge but also enable them to observe their surroundings.

Resources

In a multi-cat household, provide approximately the number of resources equal to the number of cats plus one. Place these resources strategically using visual barriers such as solid pieces of furniture to separate them.

Multiple and Separate Resources

Cats need their resources to be readily available in multiple, separate locations, including choice areas for elimination, resting, eating and drinking. Multiple feeding stations should be available and separated from elimination areas. For those cats that prefer drinking out of the faucet, offer a water fountain in addition to a bowl.

Litterboxes

The litterbox set-up and elimination area are important resources for indoor-only cats. Most commercial litterboxes are too small; therefore, finding the ideal sized litterbox requires some creativity and compromise. Cats require a box that is at least 1.5 times their length from nose to tail tip. They should be able to turn around without touching the sides. Large plastic storage bins or under the bed containers can meet these needs. Having evolved from desert-dwelling ancestors, cats typically prefer fine, sand-like substrate in their litterboxes. Unscented, clumping, clay-based litter is preferred over other options such as wood, paper, corn pellets. Litter should be deep enough (approximately two to three inches) to encourage digging, an important part of their elimination ritual.

Litterboxes should be in quiet and easily accessible spaces. As prey species, cats monitor for signs of danger, especially, when they

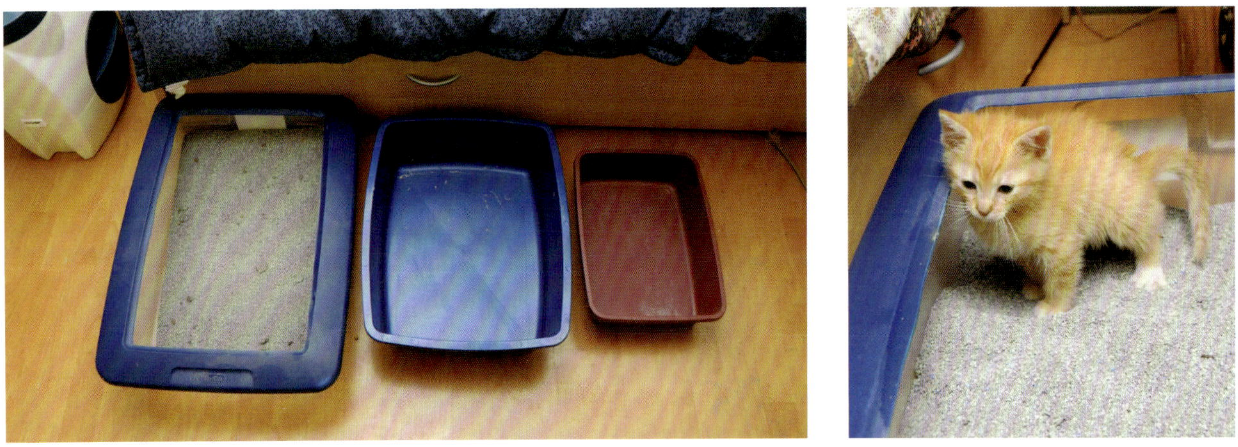

Figs. 6.3 A, B: Boxes should be large enough for a cat to turn around without touching the sides. Lower sided boxes are better for kittens and cats with arthritis.

feel vulnerable. This makes covered litterboxes less appealing. Also of importance, cats should not have to jump into their litterbox by way of one hole on the top. This would be uncomfortable for anyone with an urgency to eliminate and is especially difficult for older cats with arthritis.

Never place litterboxes in areas that may be periodically inaccessible or near loud appliances (e.g., washing machines, dryers, furnaces, etc.). Ideally, multiple entry and exit points should be available so that the cat can always easily escape if something scares them or blocks their exit. This often occurs in multi-cat homes where one cat blocks access or escape from the litterbox area. A screen in front of the litterbox is preferred to a cover. The screen should be placed several inches away but in front of the litterbox to allow easy access to enter and exit.

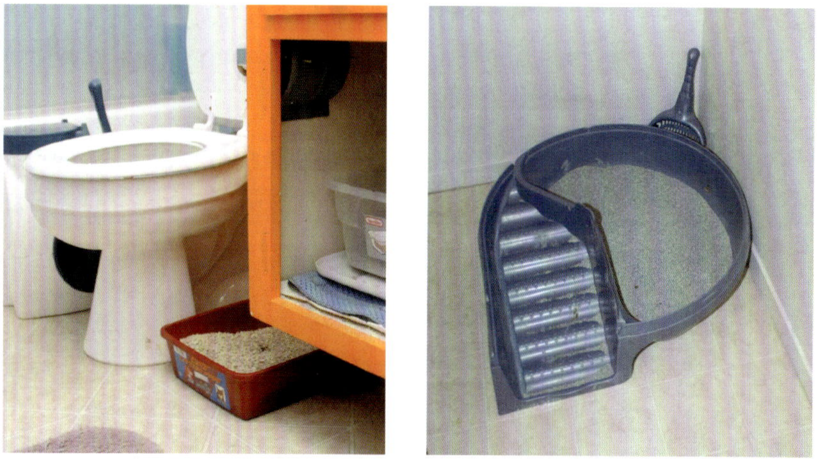

Figs. 6.3 C, D: Some cats prefer hooded boxes vs. open litter boxes.

Litterbox Accessibility

Arthritic cats may need a much lower entry to litterboxes.

When it comes to the number of litterboxes, a general rule is to provide one more litterbox than the number of cats in the home (e.g., three cats in the home = four litterboxes), and a box should be available on every level of the home. If litterboxes are placed side by side, cats will consider them as one elimination area or one litterbox.

Litter substrate needs to be scooped at least daily, if not more often. Litterboxes should be emptied and cleaned weekly. Plastic litterboxes should be replaced yearly because of urine buildup on a microscopic level. A litterbox liner is not recommended.

Scratching Behavior

Scratching is a normal behavior in cats. It keeps their nails sharp, removes the dead outer layer of the nail, deposits pheromones, and visually marks their territory. Typically, cats will scratch in socially prominent locations and near resting areas while stretching. Providing vertical and horizontal scratching surfaces near these locations helps to minimize damage. Vertical posts must have a sturdy base and be tall enough for the cat's entire body to stretch as they extend their front paws over their head. Rope is the preferred substrate, although individuals may enjoy carpet, cardboard, or wood posts.[13]

Hunting for Food

Cats should hunt for all their food using food puzzles. Providing food in small, frequent meals through a variety of puzzle toys encourages natural hunting behaviors, stimulates their minds, and helps keep them physically active.

Opportunity for Play and Predatory Behavior

Cats are solitary hunters that stalk and ambush their prey. In the wild, cats hunt multiple times a day, eating small, frequent meals. Although hunting provides sustenance, cats also benefit from the pleasure of hunting, which is an opportunity to learn and solve problems.

Domestic cats require opportunities to practice hunting in the home to satisfy their hunting instincts. Hunting opportunities should replicate a typical predatory sequence as much as possible (e.g., stalking, pouncing, killing, then consuming). Certain cat toys can mimic the types of prey they would typically hunt, such as small rodents, birds, and other small wildlife. Products that encourage predatory and hunting behavior include food puzzles and wand toys. Playing with a cat using interactive toys should always end with a food find to stop the hunting sequence. Regularly rotate toys to keep the cat's interest.[14] Hunting and play are forms of enrichment, improving quality of life and providing them with an opportunity to express normal, species-specific behaviors.[15]

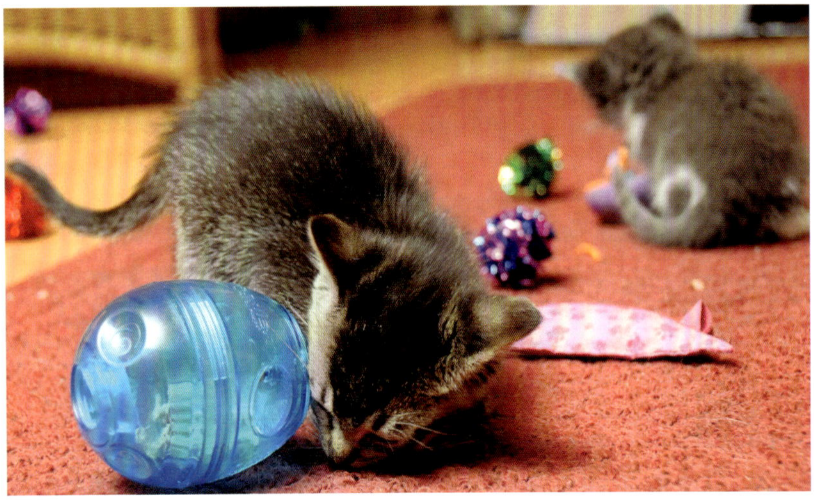

Fig. 6.3 E: Cats need opportunities to hunt. Food puzzles can help meet this need.

Enrichment and Meeting the Basic Needs of Cats

Cats, despite their domestication, retain many instincts from their wild ancestors. Enrichment should cater to these instinctive behaviors, meeting not only their basic needs but also an opportunity for mental stimulation and physical exercise.

Table 6.3.1 Enrichment Options

Toys	Interactive and structured playtime with humans helps to stimulate natural hunting instincts, provide physical exercise, and build relationships with humans and other animals.	Wand toys Laser lights/pointers Puzzle toys Fuzzy balls and mice Pipe cleaners
Puzzle Feeders	Food delivery to mimic the cat's natural feeding strategy: hunt, chase, grab, bat, or pounce to obtain multiple small meals. Should be difficult enough but not too difficult.	Open-ended or perforated tubes of different lengths Ice cube trays with wet food Freeze canned food in empty bottle caps or halve plastic Easter Eggs Commercial options are available too. See foodpuzzleforcats.com for additional ideas.
Vertical Spaces	Cats love to climb and explore their surroundings. Vertical spaces give opportunities for cats to climb, rest, jump, and observe their environment from different heights.	Cat trees Shelves Wall-mounted perches Catwalks
Hiding Areas	Cats are prey animals. Hiding spaces are important to keep them feeling safe.	Boxes Covered beds Towel over half the cage or enclosure (veterinary hospital and shelter)
Hide and Seek (Taste)	Hide toys or treats around the house for cats to find. This encourages normal hunting and foraging behaviors.	Scattering food in towels or blankets, or hidden around the house Creating a scent trail with tuna juice to a hidden meal
Scratching Posts	Cats need to scratch to stretch their muscles and maintain their claws.	Vertical posts Horizontal posts Curved posts- "S" shaped Cardboard posts
Window Perches	Position a post near the window for cats to observe the outside world.	Cat tree, window perch, bird feeder, hammock, window box
Outdoor time	Outdoor time provides an opportunity for cats to explore their environment. They can sniff, pounce, explore, and watch the world.	Catio Leash walks

Table 6.3.2 Sensory Needs

Scent	Cats use scent to communicate with other cats and to create a sense of security for themselves. Cats will spread their own pheromones throughout their home by rubbing their face on or scratching items.	Catnip, silvervine, and valerian root Cinnamon Lavender Peppermint Vanilla Pheromones Familiar bedding ** do not use essential oils**
Sound	Cats have very sensitive hearing. The absence of sound (i.e., dogs barking) is just as important as calming music especially in the shelter environment.	White noise machine Cat-specific music, classical, jazz, soft music, or audiobooks Soundtracks targeted toward cats
Sight	Cats see best in low light; however, movement catches their attention. Therefore, enrichment items that focus on movement help to keep them engaged.	Bubble machine Television playing a video targeted for cats Cat friendly apps for tablets and phones
Touch	Some cats enjoy touch, other cats do not. Monitor body language closely and do not force these interactions.	Petting, brushing, sitting next to or on laps (by their own choice)
Training	Positive reinforcement training provides mental enrichment and physical exercise. It also helps to build relationships and establish clear communication between cats and their caretakers. Training for handling, husbandry, and veterinary procedures can be part of this process.	Targeting Go to a mat Come when called (recall) Voluntary eye contact Pattern Games (Control Unleashed® by Leslie McDevitt)

Enrichment Considerations:

1. Species-specific needs: Cats have unique enrichment requirements distinct from other pets. Enrichment should reflect their natural behaviors, like hunting, scratching, and climbing.
2. Vary enrichment options: Just as individuals tire of the same puzzle and benefit from variety, cats also benefit from regularly switching out toys, scents, and other enrichment options.
3. Prioritize safety: Always guarantee the safety of new enrichment items or activities. Avoid small parts that could be ingested and provide initial supervision for new activities.

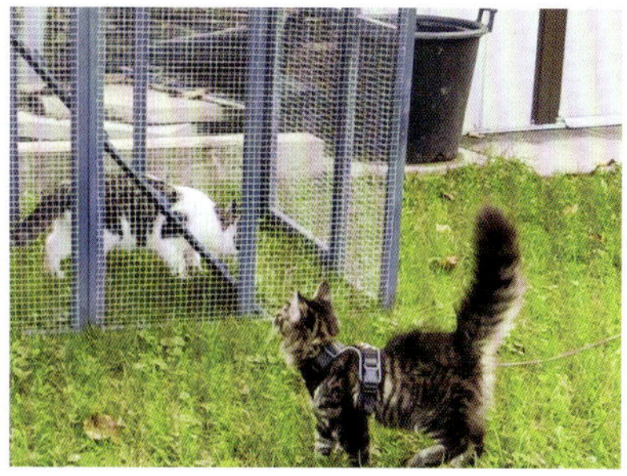

Fig. 6.3 F: Excursions outside, either on a leash or in a catio, provide a variety of enrichment for cats that they would not normally experience inside the home. (Photo courtesy of Danika Lamadeleine)

Food Dispensing and Puzzle Toys for Cats

Food dispensing and puzzle toys are innovative devices that stimulate a cat's mental and physical abilities. They are designed to challenge a cat to think and move in order to access their food or treats. These toys can range from simple to complex, offering cats of all ages and abilities a chance to engage their natural instincts and behaviors.

Why are Puzzle Toys Important?

Puzzle toys are important for cats for several reasons. They provide essential mental stimulation, much like the way humans benefit from mental challenges and puzzles. These toys require cats to strategize and problem-solve.

Many domestic cats lead sedentary lives. Puzzle toys serve as motivators, encouraging cats to move, play, and exercise, which can help prevent and reduce obesity. In the wild, cats spend a significant amount of time hunting for food. Puzzle toys simulate a cat's natural hunting behavior, allowing them to satisfy their instincts, both mentally and physically. For cats that tend to eat too quickly, puzzle toys can slow down their eating pace, potentially reducing digestive issues.

How to Use Puzzle Toys

To use puzzle toys effectively, several key strategies are recommended. Starting with a simple design helps cats become familiar with the concept and gives them an opportunity to get the hang of it. Using tasty motivators such as their favorite treats or kibble to fill the toy can encourage a cat to engage with it. Supervising a cat during their initial interactions with a puzzle toy is essential to prevent potential frustration or any attempts to break or ingest the toy. Over time, introducing different puzzle toys can help maintain a cat's interest. Toys need to be cleaned regularly especially when wet food is used.

Table 6.3.3: Puzzle Toys for Cats

Specific Examples	Description
Ball dispensers	Balls that dispense kibble or treats when moved in a certain way
Maze feeders	Require cats to navigate the maze to push food to an exit point
Mat feeders	Silicone mats with multiple compartments for hiding treats or food
Interactive puzzle boards	Feature different compartments and moving pieces to hide treats
Automated puzzle toys	Battery-operated toys that move or dispense food intermittently

Food Puzzles for Cats

For more information, detailed reviews, and further insights into food puzzles and how they benefit cats, visit **www.food-puzzlesforcats.com**.

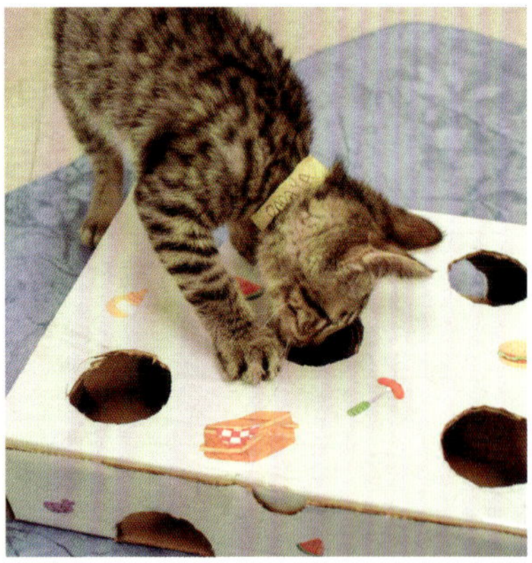

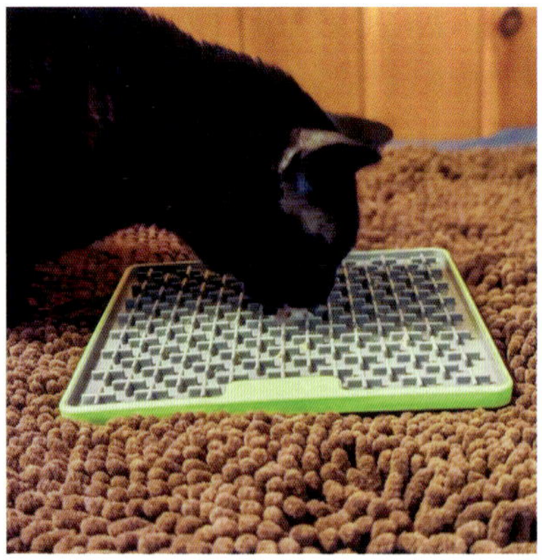

Figs. 6.3 G, H: Examples of a two food puzzle toys: a maze and lickable mat.

Consistency and a Predictable Environment

Social interaction is another form of enrichment. It involves spending time with humans or other pets. Meeting these social needs through these interactions provides an opportunity to create positive experiences and a predictable environment. Understanding feline body language helps to ensure this time spent with others is enjoyable from the cat's perspective.

6.4 Why Play is Important

Play mimics a cat's natural behavior, replicating the instinctive hunting cycle of stalking, pouncing, and catching prey. It offers an opportunity for physical exercise, promoting weight maintenance while enhancing strength, agility, and coordination. Play provides necessary mental stimulation through interactive toys and puzzles serving a social purpose through the strengthening of bonds with littermates, other pets, and human companions. Regular play sessions help to reduce stress, prevent, and manage undesirable behaviors.

Play and Developmental Milestones

Play is a critical part of a cat's development, evolving through distinct stages. It starts with gentle pawing from two to seven weeks, progressing to active play with littermates that enhances coordination, social skills, and bite inhibition. Between eight and twelve weeks, play intensifies with hunting behaviors such as stalking, chasing, and pouncing, making it an ideal time for interactive play with humans. From three to six months, kittens explore more, climbing and scratching. this is when to introduce climbing structures and scratching posts. Although the frequency of object play may decline after six months, it usually persists into adulthood, supporting the cat's emotional and physical health.

Playing with Cats

Engaging cats in play can be a rewarding experience; however, it is important to maintain their engagement with interactive toys like those that simulate flying insects or birds and encourage both jumping and pouncing behaviors. Laser pointers can be enjoyable, but to avoid frustration provide a food find for them to capture

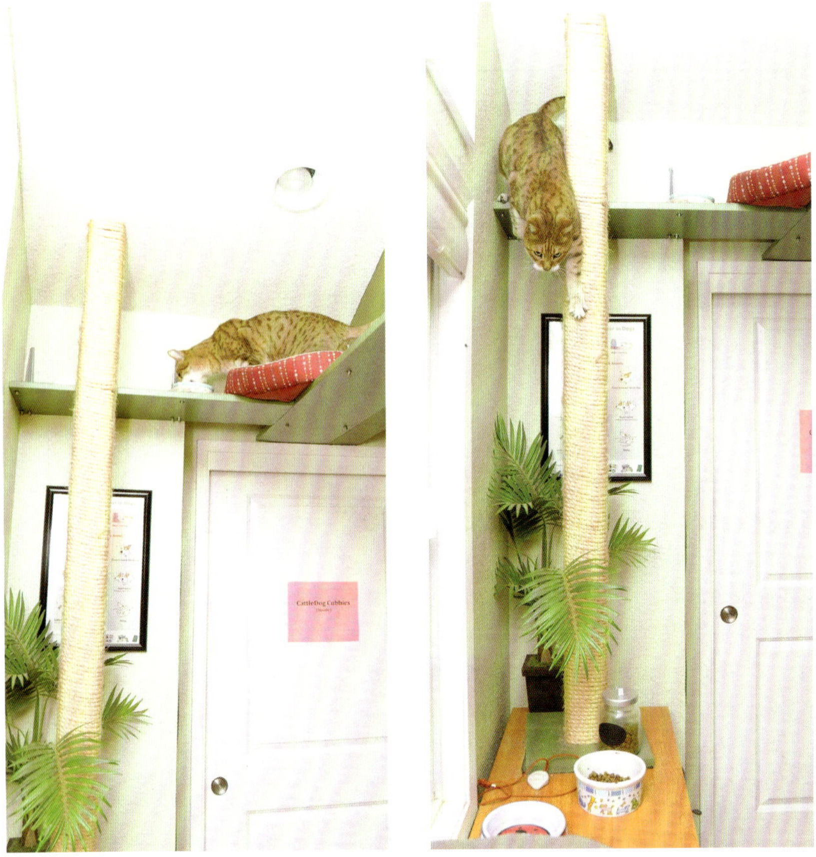

Figs. 6.4 A, B: Enrichment of the environment includes vertical spaces, resting areas, and separate feeding stations.

at the end of every play session. For solo play, consider using balls and mice that cats can bat around, or opt for catnip toys. Puzzle toys, such as those involving food puzzles, encourage problem-solving skills and mental stimulation. Structured play sessions lasting 10–15 minutes daily, designed to follow the hunt-catch-rest cycle, can keep a cat entertained fulfilling a basic need. Climbing structures such as cat trees and wall shelves, as well as, tunnels and paper bags (without handles), encourage stalking and pouncing type play.

6.5 Kitten Class Set-Up and Expectations

Kitty kindergarten provides a socialization opportunity for kittens to learn important social skills.[11] Often an under-utilized tool, these classes can be offered at both shelters and the veterinary hospital. Goals for kitten class include:

- Education about normal feline behavior and the unique needs of cats
- Early recognition and prevention of behavioral issues
- Opportunities to form positive associations with the veterinary hospital
- Acquiring social skills and learning new behaviors
- Socialization opportunities include handling and experiences with people, objects, sounds, smells, and other animals

Kitten Requirements

Kittens should be at least seven weeks of age and no more than 14 weeks by the end of class. After 14 weeks, they are less likely to interact with other kittens and may be more fearful.[10–13,16] Caregivers of older kittens can still benefit from attending class without their kitten, or virtual attendance could be considered.

Kittens should be in the home for at least seven days prior to the start of class to monitor for any health issues (e.g., diarrhea, vomiting, sneezing, eye or nasal discharge, etc.). Before starting class, kittens must be examined by a veterinarian and given their first vaccination at least 10 days before the start of class. They should be retrovirus negative and free of internal and external parasites, including a negative fecal test.[12,16–18] Instructors should examine each kitten as they arrive to ensure that they are bright, alert, and appear healthy. Unhealthy kittens should not attend class; however, caregivers can be encouraged to participate without their kitten or virtually from home.[12,16]

Classroom and Equipment

Kitten class requires a room large enough to accommodate the number of kittens and their caregivers. When there are more than three to four kittens in a class, an assistant may be needed. Provide seating for all human participants and a playpen for each kitten.

During class, each kitten should have access to a litter pan, toys, a scratching surface, water, and a hiding spot. Provide examples of specific resources to meet each cat's basic needs, such as food puzzle toys, vertical and horizontal scratching surfaces, ideal litter pans and substrates for kittens and adult cats, interactive and solo toys, carriers, harnesses, and grooming supplies (e.g., nail trimmers, scissors, electric clippers). Exploration items should also be available, such as climbing structures, objects for hiding (e.g., tunnels, cardboard boxes, step stools), veterinary tools (e.g., baby scales, exam tables, medical supplies, stethoscope, pen lights, otoscopes), household items (e.g., vacuum cleaner, fan, broom, umbrella, floor/carpet tiles), and outdoor objects (e.g. branches, leaves). Be creative and think about items that will provide novel sights, sounds, smells, tastes, and textures.

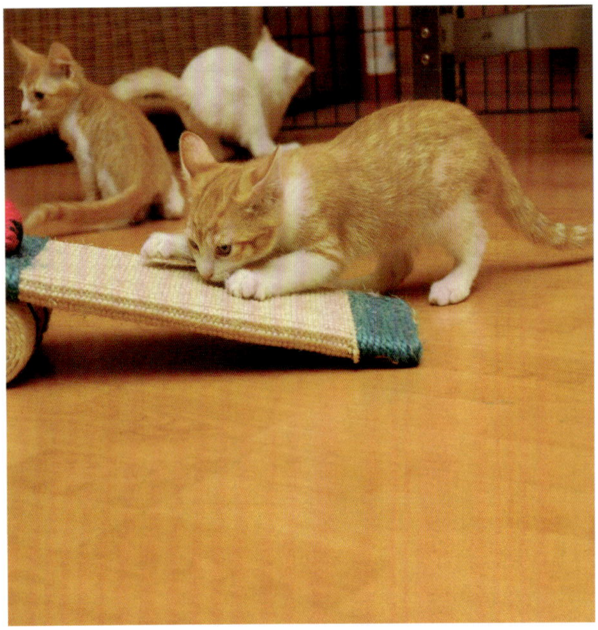

Fig. 6.5 A: Provide various types of scratching surfaces, including vertical, horizontal, sisal rope, cardboard, etc. This scratching post size is adequate for kittens but would be quite small for an adult cat.

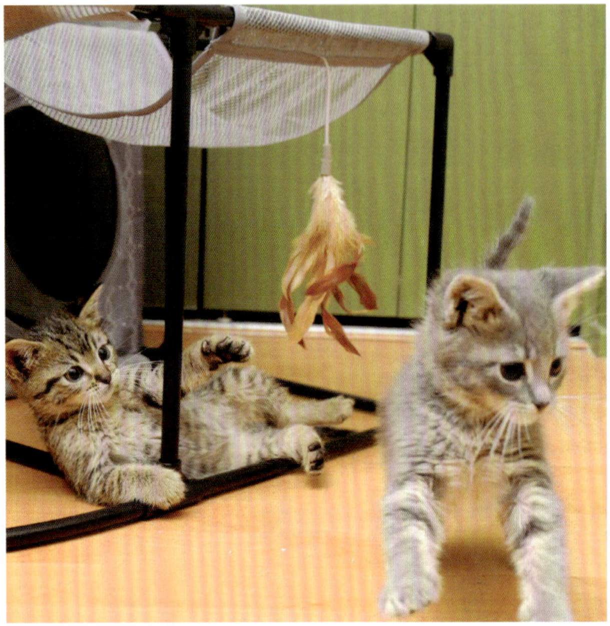

Fig. 6.5 B: Provide hiding spaces along with a variety of toys.

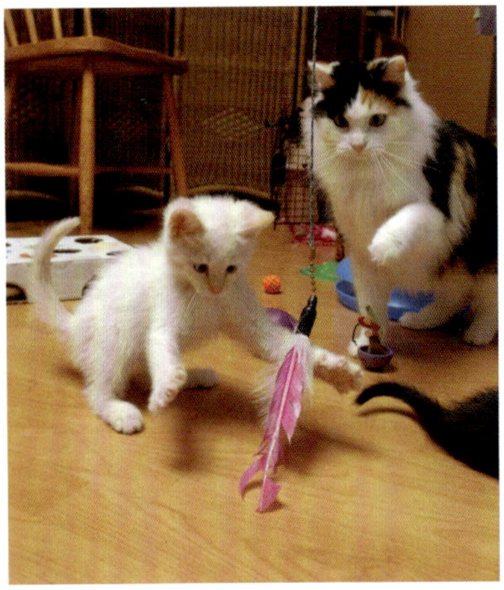

Fig. 6.5 C: Normal play among kittens does not typically include vocalization.

Kitten Play

If kitten play is allowed in class, monitor body language closely to ensure all kittens are having a positive experience. If some kittens are too fearful to play, allow them to stay in their carrier or playpen with a blanket blocking the view of other kittens.

Normal kitten play is usually a mix of wrestling, chasing, and mutual object play. Each kitten should take turns being on the top and bottom while wrestling, chasing, or being chased.[7,19] If a kitten shows a lack of interest in play or engages in inappropriate play (e.g., always chasing), separate and engage them in solo play or with an interactive toy.

Exploration

Kitten class provides an opportunity to learn about novel stimuli that will be encountered throughout their lives. In class, offer a variety of items for kittens to explore following the socialization guidelines above. These items should target the five senses: sight, sound, touch, scent, and taste.

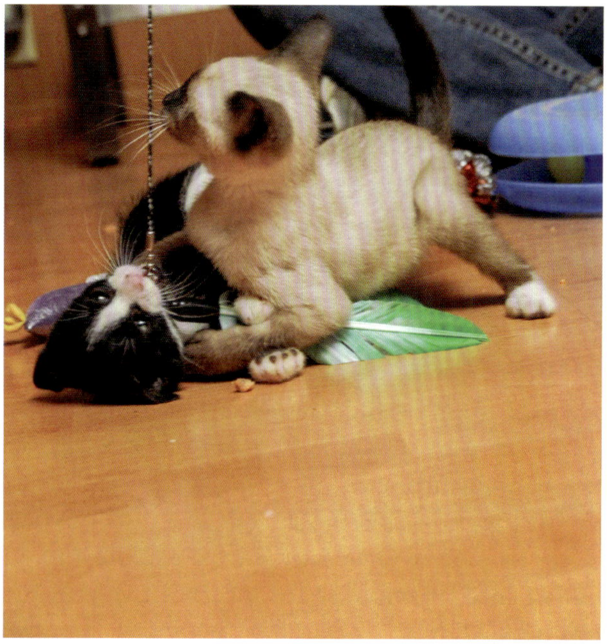

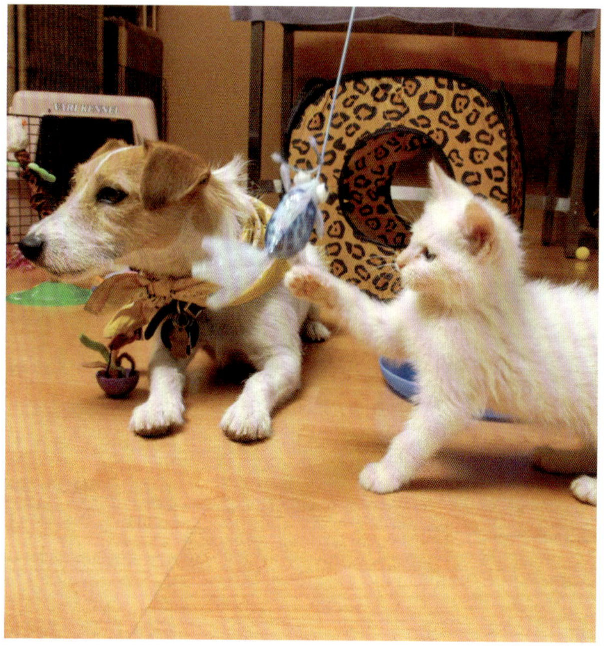

Figs. 6.5 D, E: Kitten play may appear rough to humans, but this type of play is normal between kittens.

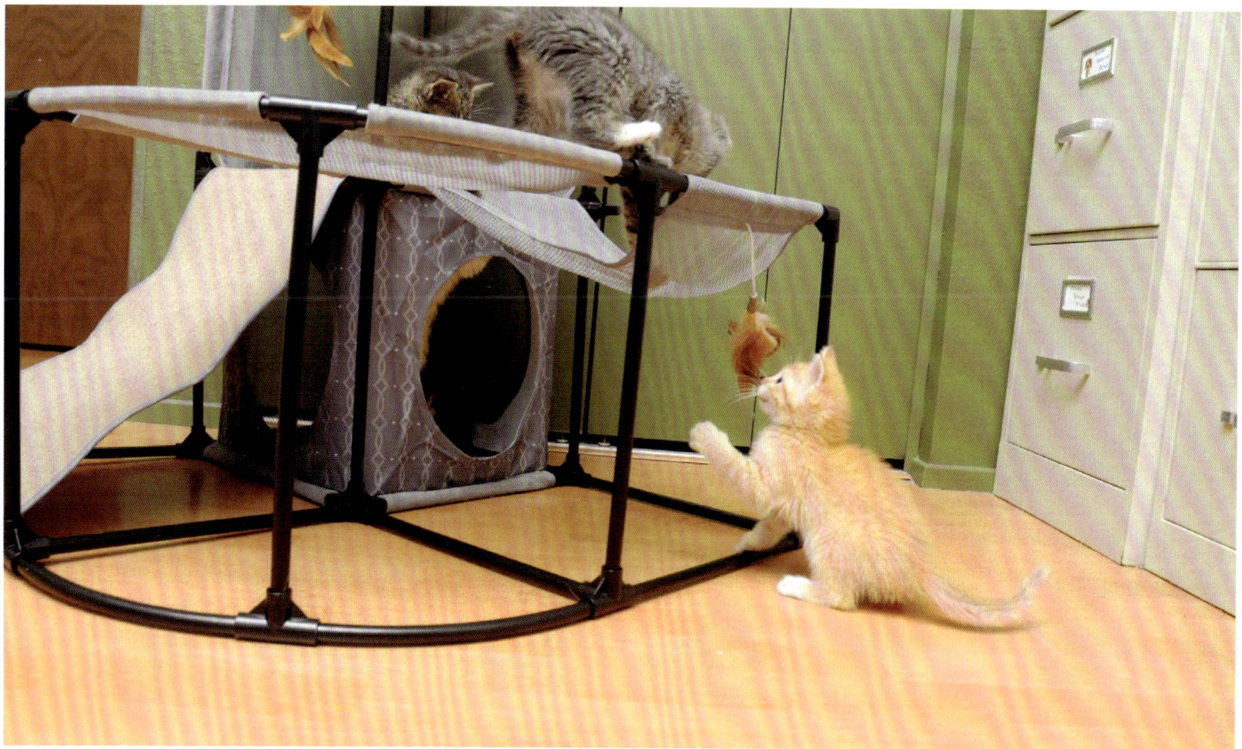

Fig. 6.5 F: Provide kittens with a variety of items that stimulate various senses.

Client Education

During class, handouts on topics to educate caregivers on the unique needs and normal behavior of cats should be available. Topics covered in class can include reading feline body language, health and veterinary care, providing a healthy feline environment, litterbox requirements and care, preventing scratching in undesirable locations, and appropriate play methods.

Additional Resources

- Veterinary Partner: veterinarypartner.vin.com
- CattleDog Publishing: cattledogpublishing.com

6.6 Foundation Behaviors

Positive reinforcement training establishes a common language and builds positive relationships with people. Methods such as luring, targeting, capturing, and shaping are preferred to provide an opportunity for choice and a sense of control. Molding (e.g., physically manipulating into position), a form of positive punishment, is never recommended.

Foundation behaviors such as sit, recall (come), targeting (touch), and stationing serve as building blocks for more advanced training in the future. These behaviors develop social skills and prepare kittens for various situations. By teaching these basics, it becomes easier to maintain engagement, redirect their attention and prevent unwanted behaviors.

Sit

"Sit" is an easy, versatile behavior to teach. This can be used as a building block for other behaviors, such as sitting for brushing teeth administering medications, performing, examinations, or venipuncture.

Luring is an effective method for teaching this behavior. To use this technique, hold a treat at the level of the kitten's nose and then arc it back over their head. As the kitten follows the treat with their eyes and head, their hind end should naturally lower into a sit position. As soon as the kitten sits, mark the behavior and give a treat. Alternative methods for teaching this behavior include capturing, which involves waiting for the behavior to occur naturally, and shaping, which rewards incremental approximations of the behavior.

Targeting

Targeting teaches a kitten to touch an object with a specific part of their body, such as their nose or paw touching a finger or target stick. This foundational skill is useful for teaching new behaviors, including positioning for veterinary visits, carrier training, and greeting new people. In shelters, teaching cats to target to the front of their enclosure has been shown to increase adoption rates.[20,21]

Most kittens naturally investigate nearby objects by sniffing them. An effective first step in targeting is to present a finger or target stick close to the kitten. When they sniff it, mark the behavior with a click or a verbal cue, and reward them with a treat. Once the kitten performs this behavior reliably—more than 80% of the time—introduce a verbal cue before marking and rewarding. Once learned, increase the challenge by placing the finger or target object a few inches away, allowing the kitten to choose to approach and touch it. Continue to gradually increase the distance as long as the kitten continues to target successfully.

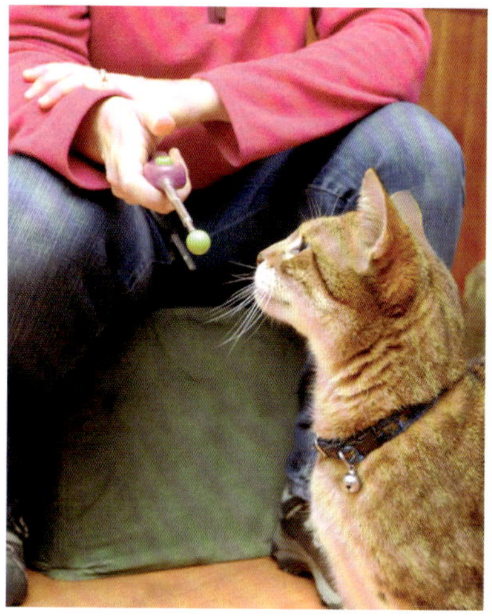

Fig. 6.6 A: Targeting using a target stick.

Recall

Teaching a kitten to recall (come) is one of the easiest behaviors to teach. Often, kittens naturally learn this behavior if they respond to the sound of food being poured into a bowl, a can of wet food opening, or shaking a treat bag. Cues like "come" can be useful to redirect kittens from unwanted behaviors or dangerous situations. To ensure success, always offer high value rewards each time the kitten comes when called.

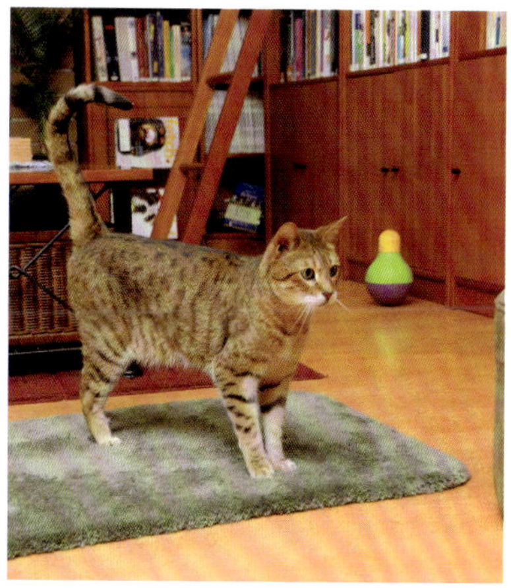

Fig. 6.6 B: Teaching a cat to station on a mat can be used in a variety of scenarios.

Stationing

Teaching kittens to go to a mat or station is a valuable technique for preventing them from running out the door, building consent for husbandry or medical procedures, and redirecting unwanted behaviors. The best methods for teaching stationing are capturing, shaping, and targeting. When the kitten is on the mat, allow them to choose the most comfortable position. The objective is not to require a specific sit or down behavior, but rather to target their body onto the mat.

6.7 Prevention Exercises

Carrier Training for Emergencies

During emergencies such as tornadoes, hurricanes, fires, or earthquakes, it is important to teach cats to seek out their carrier. Placing the carrier in a specific spot, like a bedroom closet, makes it easier to direct emergency personnel to where the cat may be hiding allowing for a swift retrieval. Quickly closing the door can lead to a successful rescue. Additionally, cats in carriers are typically accepted in national disaster shelters.

The following exercises provide a foundation for creating positive associations with various procedures and experiences that kittens will encounter throughout their lives. Always allow the kitten time to investigate and make a positive association with any tool being used.

Carrier Training

All kittens should feel comfortable in their carriers, viewing them as safe spaces rather than sources of anxiety or fear. To train a kitten to use a carrier, start by placing it in an area where the kitten frequently spends time. If the kitten is hesitant to enter, you can make the space more inviting by removing the top and door. Once the kitten is comfortable in the bottom half, gradually reintroduce the top and then the door. Enhance the appeal of the carrier by placing a soft blanket sprayed with pheromones inside, creating a cozy resting spot. Additionally, hide treats inside the carrier for the kitten to discover periodically throughout the day. Feeding wet food inside or near the carrier also helps build positive associations and encourages the kitten to explore the carrier.

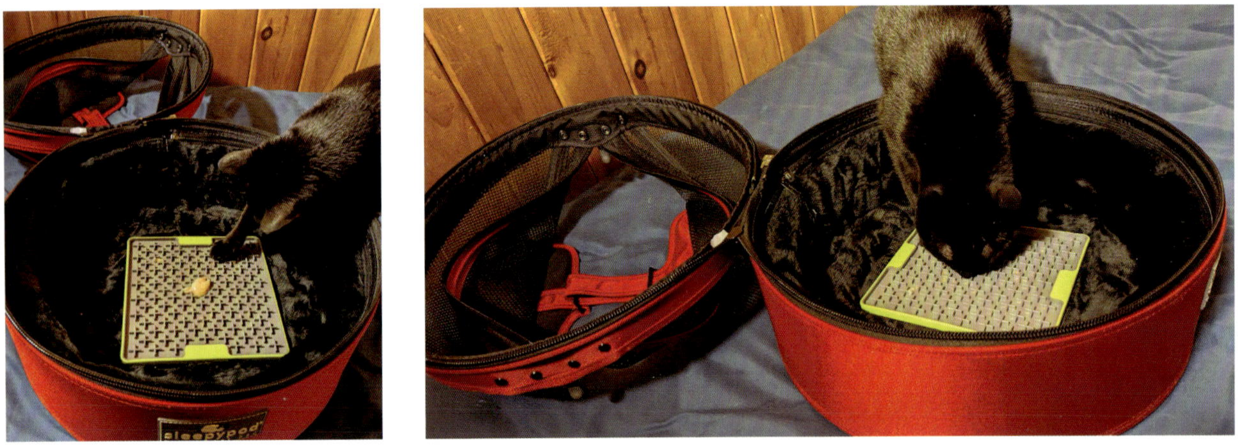

Figs. 6.7 A, B: Carrier training starts by leaving it in a location where the cat is comfortable and placing food in it to encourage exploration and positive associations.

Harness Training

Acclimating kittens to wearing a harness opens up numerous opportunities for safe enrichment. There are various types of harnesses available, including H harnesses, tiny puppy harnesses, or vests that cover more of the kitten's body. It is practical to begin with a harness that is easily available for initial training, and then invest in a larger harness as the kitten grows.

Initial Conditioning Steps

To condition a kitten to wear a harness, start by offering a treat syringe (or a favorite toy like a wand toy) through the head loop towards the kitten. Initially, do not move the syringe to lure the kitten's head through the loop.

Progressing the Training

Remove the treat and harness simultaneously and repeat this step three to five times before moving on to the next phase. Reposition the loop with the syringe closer to the head loop and repeat three

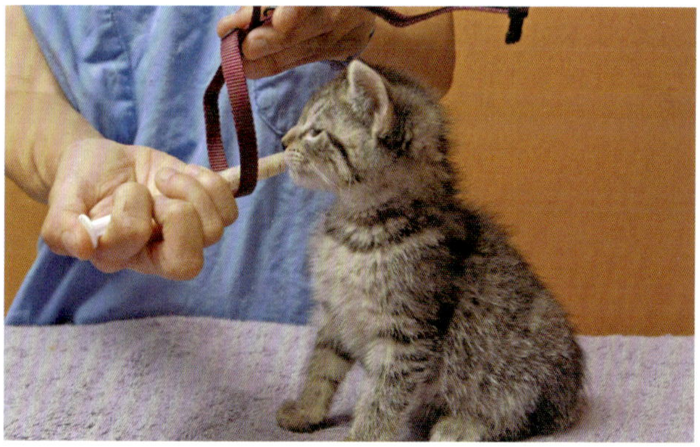

Figs. 6.7 C: Using a treat syringe helps keep harness training a positive experience.

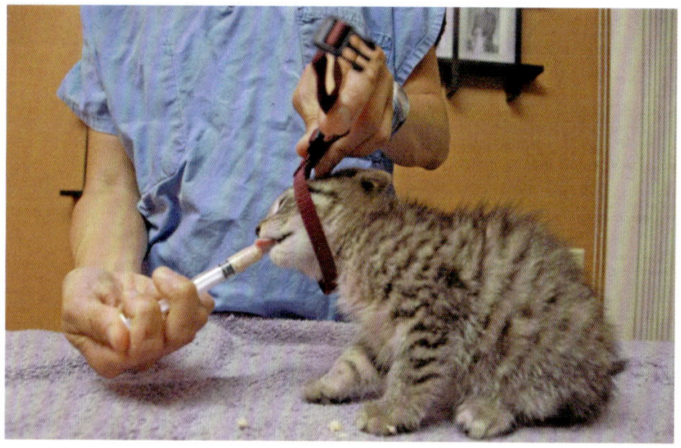

Fig. 6.7 D: The kitten should choose to place their head through the harness loop voluntarily.

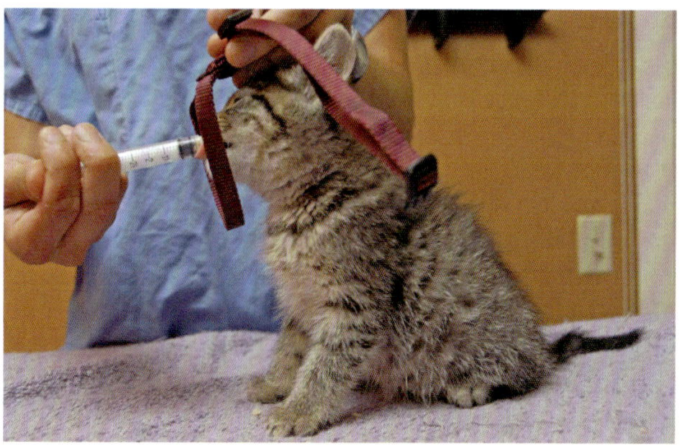

Fig. 6.7 E: As the harness is removed, continue to encourage them to eat.

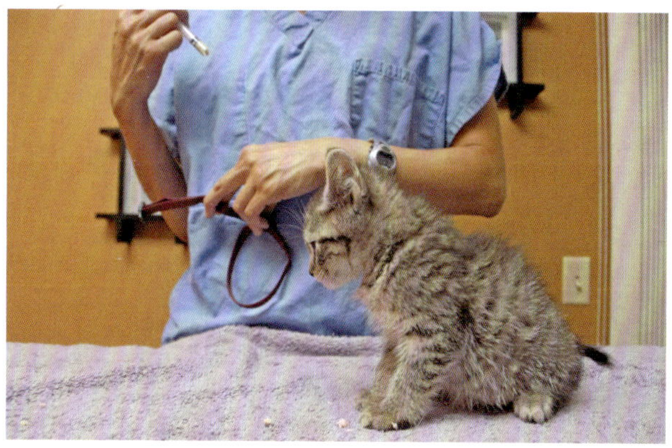

Fig. 6.7 F: Once the harness is removed, take away the treat as well.

to five times. Gradually present the syringe further away from the kitten until they voluntarily push their head through the loop. This step can be challenging, so patience is key. Once the kitten comfortably puts their head through the head loop, proceed cautiously towards clipping the body strap in place. Distraction with a lickable treat can be helpful while clipping the strap. Practice clipping the harness near the kitten with a treat, helping them acclimate to the sound before placing the harness on their body.

Finalizing Harness Training

Once the harness is clipped on, create a trail of treats to encourage movement. You can also use the "1-2-3 Game" to build the duration and to encourage walking. Start by having the kitten wear the harness for a short period of time, gradually increasing the duration as long as the kitten remains relaxed and comfortable.

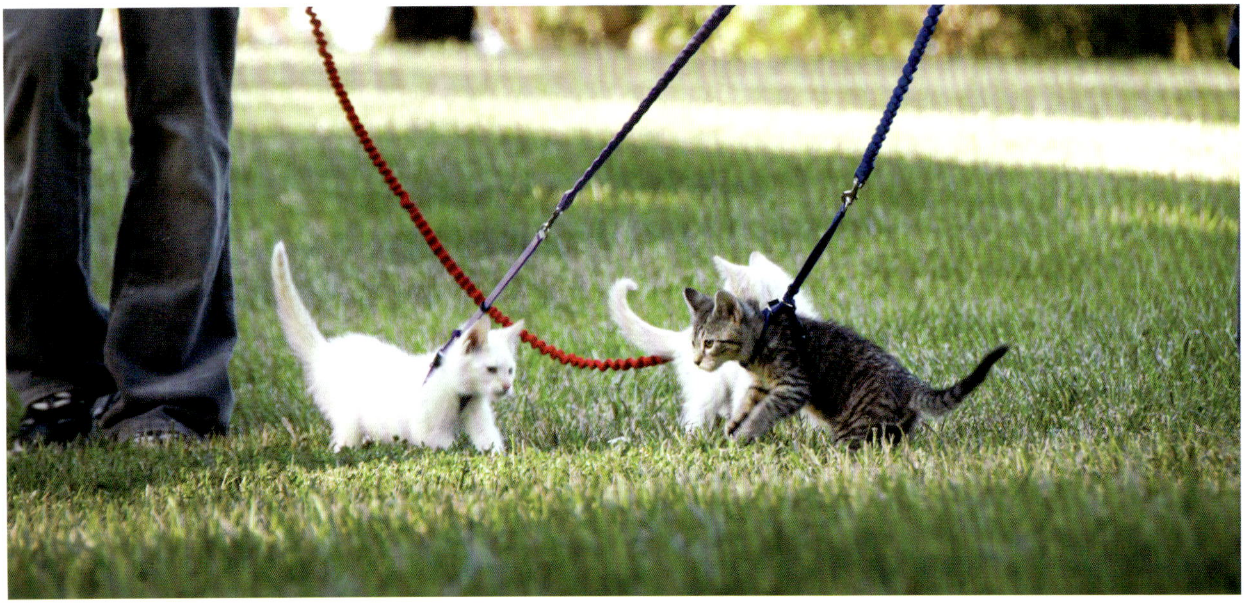

Fig. 6.7 G: Kittens that have learned to enjoy wearing a harness can go for walks and spend time outside.

Handling

Handling exercises help caregivers learn how to gently interact with their kittens, building a positive conditioned emotional response (+CER) to handling. These exercises are specifically designed to help kittens become comfortable with the kinds of touch and handling they will commonly experience throughout their lives, including physical examinations by veterinarians and regular husbandry activities such as grooming and being picked up. Familiarizing kittens with these interactions from a young age helps make routine care activities more comfortable and less stressful for both the kitten and their caregiver.

Start with Comfortable Petting

Forming a positive emotional response to handling begins in an environment where the kitten feels most comfortable and is relaxed. Offer high-value treats to the kitten while briefly petting the kittens in areas where they are comfortable, such as around their chin and face, for two to three seconds. As long as they are comfortable, transition to a "touch then feed" technique. Begin by touching the top of head, stop touching, and then offer a food reward. Continue with this technique, moving from the least sensitive part of their body to the most sensitive parts, such as their mouth, paws, back, and tail. Always toss treats away during the session to give the kitten a break and the chance to choose to re-engage in the session. Repeat this process several times a week for one to two minutes. Remember that not all parts of the body need to be handled in every training session; move at the kitten's pace.

Monitoring Body Language

If kittens display discomfort or become distracted during petting, reduce the petting interval and return to the location where they were most at ease.

Gradually Increasing Handling Complexity

Continue the training by gradually increasing the difficulty, such as the amount and length of petting, different locations on the kitten's body, and the pressure applied during petting. The goal is to work towards areas that are commonly involved in physical examinations or hygiene care, teaching the kitten to happily accept being touched in these ways. Examples include holding the head to look at the eyes, ears, and teeth; abdominal palpation with gentle pressure; parting fur to check the skin; lifting the tail for examination; assessing lymph nodes; and gentle preparation for procedures like venipuncture.[22]

Safety Between Kittens and Children

Kittens should always be supervised when interacting with children and other pets. Modeling and coaching how to gently handle kittens reduces rough handling and gives an opportunity for intervention when needed. Improperly holding kittens, pulling parts of their body, and preventing escape should never be allowed and can lead to protective emotions and defensive behaviors.

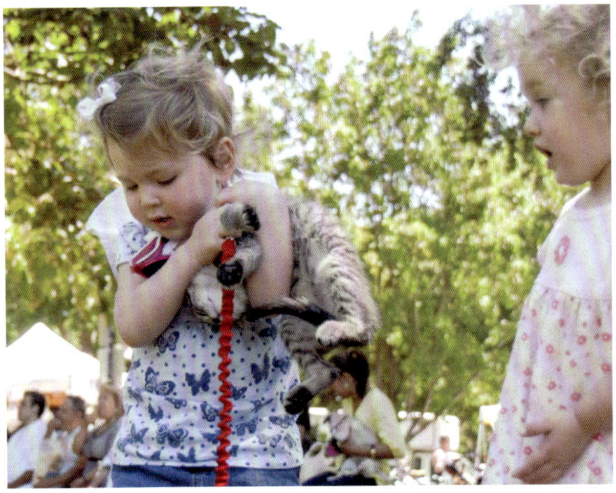

Fig. 6.7 H: Rough handling by children can result in fear and defensive behaviors.

Fear at the Veterinary Clinic

Low Stress Handling® and early intervention reduces fear and anxiety in the veterinary setting.

The use of distractions, cueing, luring, and play opportunities allow the cat choice and control over their space, examination location, and interactions.[22] Cooperative care training provides more opportunities to form positive experiences with handling.[22]

Nail Trims

Teaching kittens to be comfortable with nail trims is important since regular nail trimming will be needed for the life of the cat. Regular nail trimming prevents scratching of furniture or people and is important for their health. Long nails can cause pain, difficulty walking, and other medical issues. Introducing the nail trimming process to kittens improves their comfort level with this type of handling as they grow.

For each handling session, allow the kitten to choose their own position and have treats ready. Touch each foot and gently squeeze each toe to extend the nail while providing a steady stream of treats. A lickable mat or squeezable treats work well for this. Once the kitten is relaxed, introduce the nail clippers, and give an opportunity for the kitten to investigate. Feed treats while touching each toe with the trimmers without clipping. If comfortable, start trimming one nail at a time; choose the easiest nail first. As the kitten continues to eat, trim the nail quickly but carefully. Eventually, transition to clipping each nail then rewarding the kitten with a treat after each clip.

As the kitten becomes more comfortable with the process, more than one nail can be trimmed in a single session. Alternatively, teaching start signal behaviors, such as stationing to a mat, before starting the nail trim gives the kitten predictability, choice, and control.

Brushing Teeth

Cats should have their teeth brushed daily.[23] One way to teach kittens to hold their heads still for oral care is to use a syringe filled with something tasty. While supporting the kitten's chin, provide a reward whenever handling the head. Once the kitten is comfortable with chin touches, repeat the process and gently lift the lip. Next, touch a tooth with your finger and offer a taste of pet-friendly toothpaste. When the kitten is ready, introduce a toothbrush, starting with one or two teeth and gradually covering the rest of the mouth.

Oral Medications

All caregivers should be comfortable giving their cat medications and they should regularly practice delivering oral medications (e.g., without using real medication) to maintain a positive association and a practiced interaction.

Three Treat Trick

Prepare three treats using something soft like a pill pocket, squeeze cheese, or wet food. Test out different treats to find which one the kitten likes best. When adding medication, the first treat should be blank (e.g., no pill in it), the second treat contains the pill, and the third treat is another blank. Give in rapid succession to motivate the kitten to eat them quickly.

Using a Pill Gun

Place a treat in the pill gun and let the kitten eat it. They may be more willing to investigate the pill gun if it is placed on the ground. Offer the pill gun several times, allowing the kitten an opportunity to eat before gently depressing the plunger while pushing the treat into the kitten's mouth. Follow up quickly with plenty of treats to encourage the kitten to swallow without chewing.

When it is time to add medication, cover the pill with something tasty, keeping the size small. If using a pill gun, always follow up with treats and never forcefully hold their head or body. The reward should be exceptionally positive to outweigh any negative association.

Taking Liquid Medication from a Syringe

Prepare a syringe with puree, wet food slurry, or paste made for cats. Allow the kitten to lick the contents of the syringe. Next, gently dispense a small amount of the contents into the kitten's mouth. Move through the steps slowly to keep the kitten comfortable and to create a positive experience with the syringe.

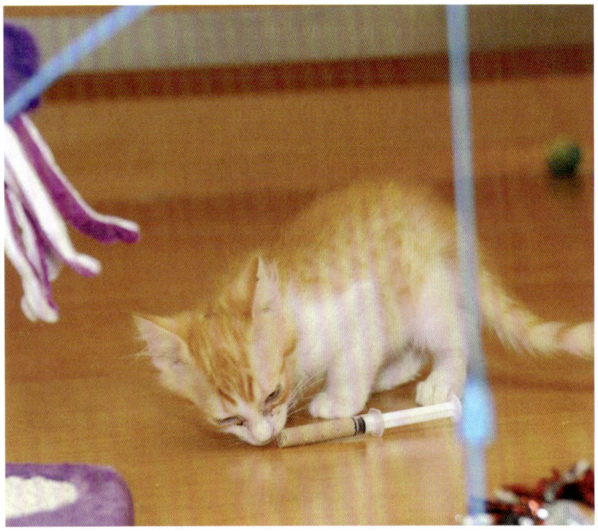

Fig. 6.7 I: Syringes with the tips cut off and filled with tasty wet food serve as a first introduction to liquid medications. This kitten is learning that syringes are not scary and contain tasty treats.

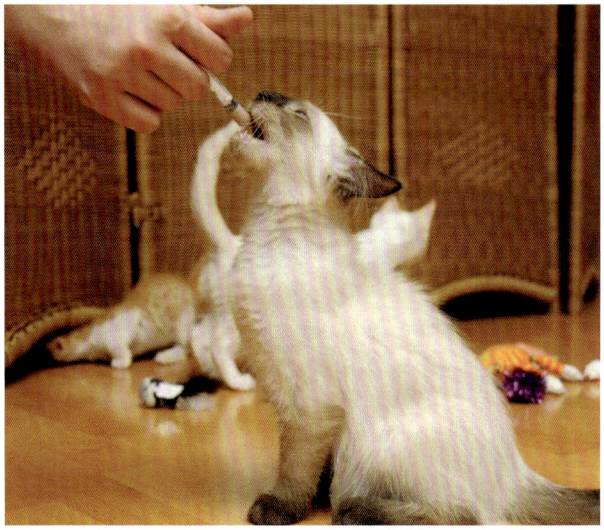

Fig. 6.7 J: Kittens can learn to accept food from a syringe, which can help make liquid medication delivery easier in the future.

6.8 Common Feline Behavior Concerns and Strategies

Behavior problems are common in cats. Some of these behaviors are normal (e.g., scratching, hunting, urine marking). Being able to recognize normal behaviors and educate pet caregivers about their cat's basic needs, the importance of enrichment, and how to provide outlets for their natural instincts can improve everyone's quality of life. When abnormal behaviors are present, medical causes should always be considered first.

ABCs of Behavior

Behaviors are best understood using the three-term contingency or ABC model. All behaviors have a purpose and follow a predictable pattern: antecedent (A), behavior (B), consequence (C). Antecedents prompt or precede the behavior. Consequences either increase or decrease the likelihood that a behavior will be repeated.

Externally influencing antecedents and consequences can alter behavior. For example, if a cat scratches the couch (B), by providing acceptable scratching surfaces near the couch (A), the scratching on the couch should decrease (C). Since scratching is a normal behavior in cats, punishment is not likely to decrease or stop it. When offered appropriate alternatives, cats are more likely to choose these scratching surfaces instead.

Inappropriate Play

Kittens that scratch and bite are typically doing so in play. Use toys and avoid using hands or feet when playing with kittens. When playing with people, object play ensures kittens are learning to play and use their claws in appropriate ways. Handling kittens roughly only teaches them to use their claws to avoid the unpleasant experience. Learning to handle kittens gently and observe body language reduces the kitten's need for defensive scratching.

Inappropriate Scratching

Kittens need access to appropriate scratching materials. Most cats prefer scratching posts made of rope; however, individual preferences will occur. Offer a variety of substrates, along with vertical and horizontal scratching surfaces. Vertical scratching surfaces should be tall enough for kittens to fully stretch and extend their bodies when scratching.

Place scratching surfaces in a variety of locations, especially in areas where the kitten is more likely to scratch. If scratching furniture, a plastic cover can be used to make it less appealing. One purpose of scratching is to deposit pheromones from the interdigital space between their toes as a form of communication; using a synthetic pheromone in these areas helps to decrease this type of marking behavior. Scat mats, compressed air, and snap traps are all positive punishments and not recommended as deterrents. Instead, use toys, treats, or catnip to redirect kittens away from furniture and encourage them to use the appropriate scratching surface.

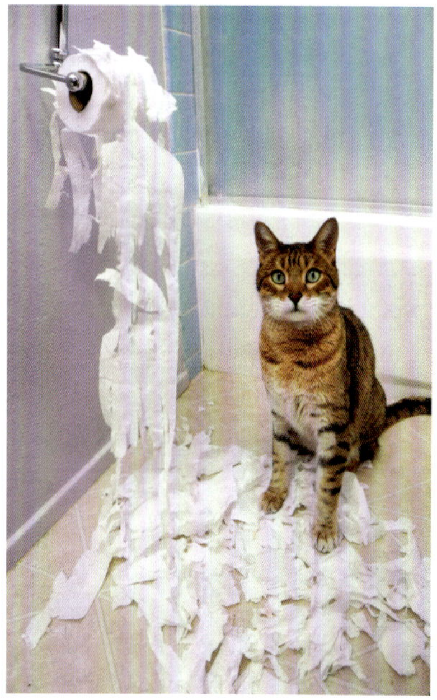

Fig. 6.8 A: If a cat's basic needs are not met, they will find a way to meet their own needs. This often occurs in ways that are undesirable.

House Soiling

Most kittens are easily trained to use a litterbox and do not require much assistance. Make sure the litterbox is easily accessible, especially for young kittens who may have trouble climbing into larger litterboxes or going up and down stairs if the box is in the basement. Use low-sided containers in easy and accessible locations when kittens are very young. A medical condition should always be investigated first when a cat or kitten starts to eliminate outside of the box. A dirty litterbox, location, substrate preference or aversion are other common causes for this behavior.[7] Cats should have litterboxes that meet their needs and individual preferences.

Climbing on Undesirable Surfaces

Since cats are natural climbers, having access to vertical spaces such as tall perches, shelves, and windowsills, provides enrichment, keeping them off counters. Cats can be encouraged to use appropriate perches by offering toys, treats, or catnip in these areas. If possible, prevent access to undesired areas, or make these spaces less desirable by removing items, such as food, that may be attracting the cat. Ensure the cat is not using the elevated surface to escape a fearful stimulus, such as a dog, another cat, or child.

The use of punishment is not recommended and often is ineffective at stopping behavior. Because consistency is important and punishment must be delivered each time the behavior is performed, cats typically learn to avoid climbing on surfaces when the human is present but continue to use these spaces when alone.

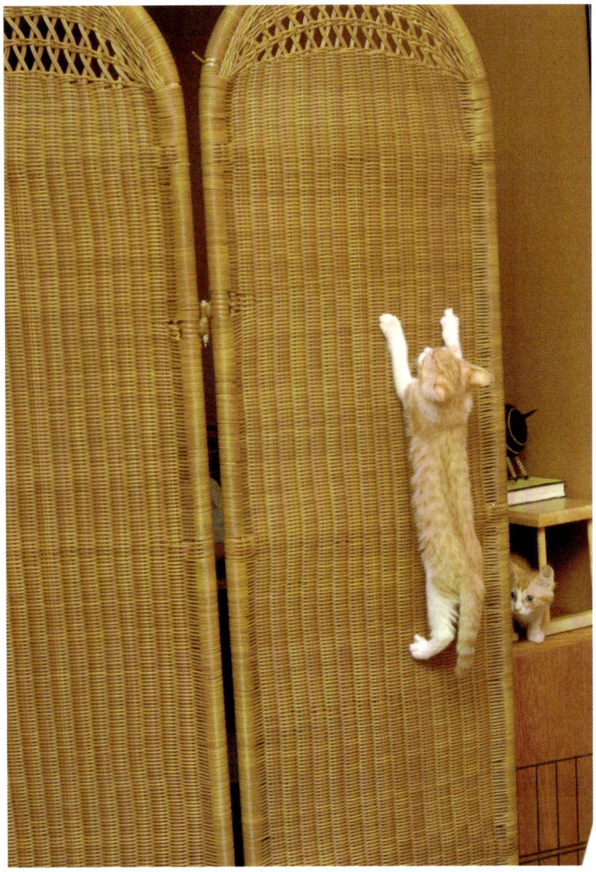

Fig. 6.8 B: Cats are natural climbers and take advantage of any opportunities available to them.

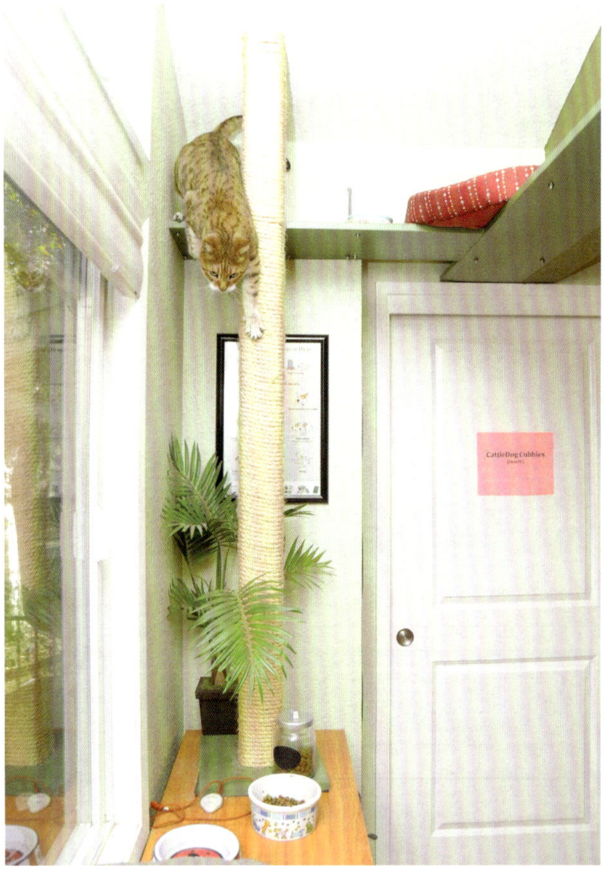

Fig. 6.8 C: Provide cats with desirable locations to climb, look out windows, and perch high up.

Excessive Vocalizing

Meowing is unique to cats and primarily used to communicate with humans, not other cats. This behavior is often reinforced by giving them attention when it occurs. If ignored, different vocalizations may be tried until attention is given. When this happens, the behavior becomes more persistent. Ignoring is not recommended and a more effective method would be to redirect the cat onto a different activity and investigate the primary cause. This behavior can have a medical cause (e.g., pain, hypertension, hyperthyroidism, and sensory decline) or a primary behavioral cause, resulting from environmental stress or anxiety. Ensuring the cat's basic needs are met through enrichment opportunities helps to decrease environmental stress and this behavior.

6.9 Introducing New Pets

Introducing cats to new pets needs to be done gradually and the process pleasant for all involved. It is much easier to build a positive association than it is to reverse a negative one. These introductions can take weeks to months and rushing the process is not recommended.

Introducing Cats to Cats

New cats should be placed in a room separate from resident cats, with all necessary resources. This gives the new cat (or cats) time to adjust to their new surroundings without the added stress of meeting other cats.

The resident cats should have their own core area, in addition to a community space. Each cat, or group of cats, should be given access to this communal space separately.[24] This allows for exploration and habituation to the new environment. When each cat becomes comfortable in the communal space, then intermixing can occur.[24] During these introductions, body language needs to be monitored closely to diffuse conflict early. Food, interactive play, and training of foundation behaviors (e.g., targeting, go to a mat, recall) help to form positive associations among the cats resulting in a smoother introduction.

Introducing Cats to Dogs

When introducing a new dog into the household, use baby gates or a playpen to separate them from resident cats. Cats should always have several escape routes that the dog cannot access (e.g., a baby gate with a cat door, elevated surfaces). A safe area with all resources for the cats needs to be provided. If relocation of resources is required, be sure this is done before the new dog arrives. Teaching both the dog and cat calm behaviors around each other will make these introductions easier.

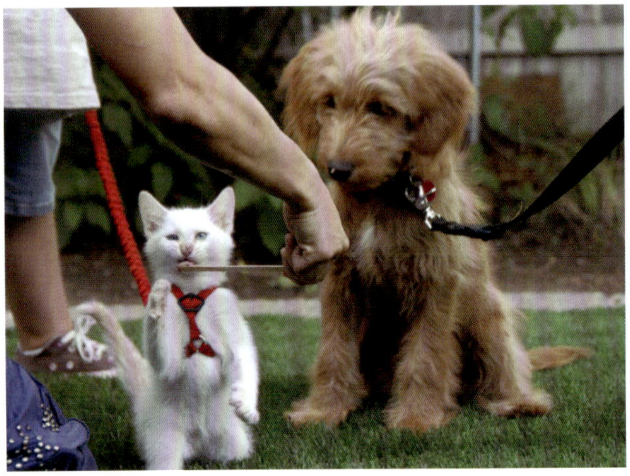

Fig. 6.9 A: During supervised introductions, provide positive experiences between kittens and other pets. Note that both leashes are properly slack here. Taut leashes can create more tension or overstimulation.

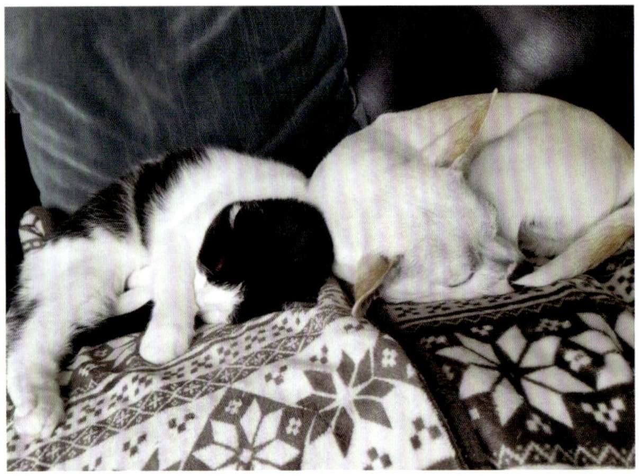

Fig. 6.9 B: Cats can enjoy time spent with other pets. A good way to assess this is to observe the choice of time spent in the same location. (Photo courtesy of Katharine Schwarz).

6.10 Conclusion

Understanding a cat's unique needs is critical to ensure their well-being, both mentally and physically, starting from an early age. Kitty kindergarten serves as a platform to educate caregivers about these needs and prepare their kittens for a thriving adulthood. Proactively addressing these needs not only wards off potential behavioral issues but also paves the way for timely interventions when necessary. This approach does not just benefit the cat, it strengthens the bond between cat and caregiver.

6.11 References

1. Landsberg, G., Radosta, L., & Ackerman, L. (2023). *Behavior Problems of the Dog and Cat* (4th ed.). Elsevier Ltd.

2. Taylor, S., St Denis, K., Collins, S., Dowgray, N., Ellis, S. L. H., Heath, S., Rodan, I., & Ryan, L. (2022). ISFM/AAFP Cat friendly veterinary environment guidelines. *Journal of Feline Medicine and Surgery*, 24(11), 1133–1163.

3. Kolb, B., & Nonneman, A. J. (1975). The development of social responsiveness in kittens. *Animal Behavior*, 23, 368–374.

4. Karsh, E. B., & Turner, D. C. (1988). The human-cat relationship. In *The domestic cat: The biology of its behaviour* (1st ed., pp. 159–177). Cambridge University Press.

5. Casey, R. A., & Bradshaw, J. W. S. (2008). The effects of additional socialisation for kittens in a rescue centre on their behaviour and suitability as a pet. *Applied Animal Behavior Science*, 114(1–2), 196–205.

6. Herron, M. E., Horwitz, D., & Siracusa, C. (2020). *Decoding Your Cat.* Houghton Mifflin Harcourt.

7. Todd, Z. (2022). *Purr: The Science of Making Your Cat Happy.* Greystone Books.

8. Bradshaw, J., & Ellis, S. (2017). *The Trainable Cat: How to Make Life Happier for You and Your Cat.* Basic Books.

9. Sinn, L. (2019, August). Puppy and kitten socialization. *Clinician's Brief.* https://www.cliniciansbrief.com/article/puppy-kitten-socialization Accessed August 31, 2022.

10. Horwitz, D. F., & Mills, D. S. (2018). *BSAVA Manual of Canine and Feline Behavioural Medicine* (2nd ed.). British Small Animal Veterinary Association.

11. Seksel, K. (2008). Preventing behavior problems in puppies and kittens. *Veterinary Clinic of North America Small Animal Practice*, 38(5), 971–982. https://doi.org/10.1016/j.cvsm.2008.04.003

12. Martin, D., & Shaw, J. K. (Eds.). (2023). *Canine and Feline Behavior for Veterinary Technicians and Nurses. (*2nd edition*)* John Wiley & Sons.

13. Wilson, C., Bain, M., DePorter, T., et al. (2016). Owner observations regarding cat scratching behavior: An internet-based survey. *Journal of Feline Medicine and Surgery*, 18(10), 791–797.

14. Strickler, B. L., & Shull, E. A. (2014). An owner survey of toys, activities, and behavior problems in indoor cats. *Journal of Veterinary Behavior*, 9(5), 207–214.

15. Dantas, L. M., Delgado, M. M., Johnson, I., & Buffington, C. T. (2016). Food puzzles for cats: feeding for physical and emotional wellbeing. *Journal of Feline Medicine and Surgery,* 18(9), 723–732.

16. Yuschak, S. (2021, November 15). School is in session: Kittens only! *Today's Veterinary Nurse.* https://todaysveterinarynurse.com/behavior/kitten-socialization-classes/ Accessed August 31, 2022.

17. Little, S., Levy, J., Hartmann, K., et al. (2020). AAFP Feline retrovirus testing and management guidelines. *Journal of Feline Medicine and Surgery*, 22(1), 5–30.

18. Little, S., Bienzle, D., Carioto, L., et al. (2011). Feline leukemia virus and feline immunodeficiency virus in Canada: Recommendations for testing and management. *Canada Veterinary Journal*, 52(8), 849.

19. Turner, D. C., & Bateson, P. (2014). *The Domestic Cat: The Biology of Its Behaviour* (3rd ed.). Cambridge University Press.

20. Kogan, L., Kolus, C., & Schoenfeld-Tacher, R. (2017). Assessment of clicker training for shelter cats. *Animals*, 7(10), 73.

21. Sung, W., & Berger, J. (2022). Training and behavior modification for shelter cats. *Animal Behavior for Shelter Veterinarians and Staff,* 445–475.

22. Rodan, I., Dowgray, N., Carney, H. C., et al. (2022). AAFP/ISFM Cat friendly veterinary interaction guidelines:Approach and handling techniques. *Journal of Feline Medicine and Surgery*, 24(11), 1093–1132. https://doi.org/10.1177/1098612X221128760

23. Bellows, J., Berg, M. L., Dennis, S., et al. (2019). AAHA Dental care guidelines for dogs and cats. *Journal American Animal Hospital Association*, 55(2), 49–69.

24. Ley, J. (2021). Aggression-cats. In: *Small Animal Veterinary Psychiatry*, 180–190. Wallingford UK: CABI.

Author
Katharine Schwarz RVT, KPA-CTP

CHAPTER 7

Recognizing and Managing Protective Emotions

> **Protective Emotions**
>
> The terms ***protective emotions*** and ***repelling behavior*** describe an animal's emotional reaction stemming from fear, anxiety, frustration, or pain indicating the animal's intent to push the threat away. Adopting terms from the Heath Model of Emotional Health, using "protective emotions," "repulsion" or "repulsive" instead of "negative emotional states," "aggressive," and "defensive" can shift the perception and language of veterinary teams and animal professionals, promoting a more empathetic approach to understanding animal behavior.[1,3–5]

7.1 Introduction

While it is impossible for pets to be entirely free from fear during veterinary visits, restraint, and procedures, creating a Low Stress Handling® environment that minimizes stress and encourages humane handling is certainly a realistic goal. To create such an environment, we can start with empathy and adjust the terminology used to describe an animal's behavior. Many animal professionals are familiar with fear, anxiety, stress, phobia, and aggression. These terms are often used interchangeably, as if they all have the same definition; however, each term has a very different meaning and serves a unique purpose.[1,2]

Fear

Fear, considered a normal and adaptive emotion, is a biological response to an actual or perceived threat, with the main goal of self-preservation.[6] Fear and the fear response is influenced by multiple factors including genetics, early learning, and past traumatic experiences. Fears can be environmental (sounds, smells, objects, and places) or in response to humans or other animals. For example, the dog that barks, then runs away when visitors enter the home is exhibiting fear.

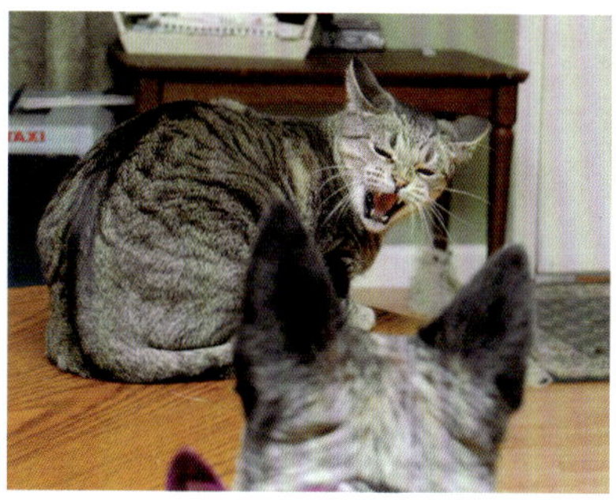

Fig. 7.1 A: This cat is displaying protective emotions and fearful behavior associated with the dog's proximity.

Anxiety

Anxiety, an abnormal or maladaptive response, is the anticipation that something bad is going to happen. It is considered maladaptive because the actual threat is not present, and the behavior does not diminish over time.[6] For example, the dog that avoids getting into the car and pants, drools, and barks while riding could be

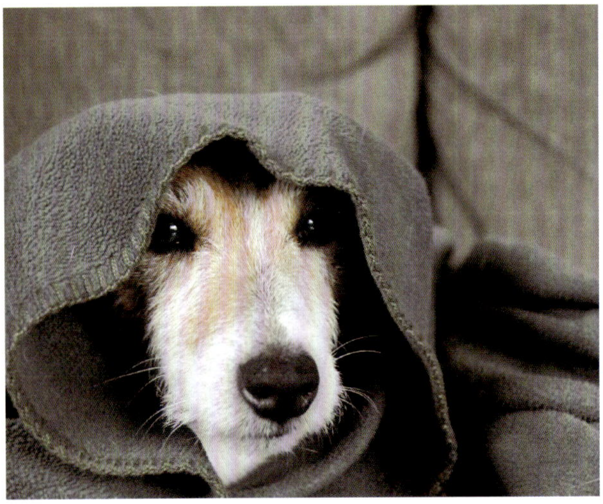

Fig. 8.1 B: This dog tries to hide and cowers when he hears the word "ride," demonstrating anxiety.

exhibiting anxiety. This behavior could also indicate nausea, or a combination of both.

Phobia

Phobia is characterized by an intense, irrational fear of a specific object, situation, or activity that might not pose an immediate threat. This profound fear can lead to avoidance behaviors and significant distress when confronted with the feared stimulus. Repeated avoidance and the relief felt after avoiding the feared object or situation can reinforce the phobic response, even if there is no direct harm to the individual.

Bolt and His Fear of Thunderstorms

One evening, while Bolt, a young Boxer, was playing with his toys, a sudden thunderclap boomed overhead. Startled, Bolt's ears perked up, and his body went rigid. With each subsequent rumble of thunder, he cowered, tucked his tail, and looked around with wide eyes, searching for the source of the noise. His fear reaction was immediate and direct, triggered by the loud noises overhead. Once the thunder stopped, Bolt slowly relaxed and returned to his playful state, although he remained a bit on edge.

Bolt and His Anxiety

Over time, Bolt began to associate certain environmental cues with the onset of a storm. Darkening skies, a drop in temperature, or even his caregiver's actions, such as shutting windows and drawing curtains, would trigger his anxiety as they became predictors of the dreaded thunder. Even before the first clap thunder, Bolt would already show signs of distress. He would pace restlessly, pant, whine, and seek out hiding places. His body would tense up, and he would become hypervigilant to any sounds or changes in his environment. This anticipatory anxiety started well before the actual threat—the thunder—and could linger long after the storm had passed.

Bolt's Phobia

As months passed, Bolt's reactions to thunderstorms intensified beyond normal fear. Even a distant rumble, which most dogs might overlook, would send him into a panic. His reactions became disproportionate to the actual threat, and he would go to extreme lengths to escape the noise, sometimes even injuring himself in the process. For instance, in his frantic state, he often tried to dig through the carpet or squeeze behind furniture, getting stuck. His response was no longer just a fearful reaction to a present threat or an anxious anticipation of a future one. It had escalated to a phobic response—an extreme, irrational fear where the intensity and duration of the reaction are out of proportion to the actual threat.

Note: In the above example, Bolt's ***fear*** was his direct response to thunder, his ***anxiety*** the distress he felt in anticipation of thunder, and his ***phobia*** was the extreme, often irrational, and harmful reaction to thunder and storm related cues that developed with repeated exposure and lack of treatment.

Distress

According to 2022 AAFP/ISFM Cat Friendly Interaction Guidelines, ***distress*** is an umbrella term for the impact of all protective (negative) emotion (e.g., fear, anxiety, pain, frustration) when perceived threats exceed the coping ability of an individual.[4]

Stress

Stress is the physiological response (e.g., the physical changes that take place in the body) that occurs when the body is exposed to a real or perceived threat.[6] This response, which includes physical changes, can be triggered by both engaging (eustress) and protective (distress) emotions.[2,6,7] Common physiological signs of stress include increased body temperature (hyperthermia), elevated heart rate (tachycardia), rapid breathing (tachypnea), and dilated pupils (mydriasis). Additionally, stress can lead to elevated blood glucose levels (hyperglycemia), suppression of the immune system, and delayed healing.[6]

Stress Response

When someone tells you that you have just won the lottery, your heart rate increases, your eyes widen, your pupils dilate, and your cheeks might flush. However, if someone informs you of a large, unexpected debt, you experience the same physiological changes: an increased heart rate, widened eyes, dilated pupils, and flushed cheeks. Despite these identical physical reactions, the experience of these two stress responses is vastly different.

Boo and Cheddar: The Tale of Two Cats

Boo had been the reigning monarch of the Tanner household for four years. A confident and laid-back tabby, she enjoyed lounging on the sunniest windowsill, playing with her favorite toys, and having the undivided attention of her caregivers. Her days were predictable and content.

But all of that changed with the arrival of Cheddar, a young and spirited orange cat. The Tanners had adopted Cheddar from a local shelter, hoping to give Boo a companion to play with. However, they had not anticipated the complexities of feline relationships.

From the outset, territorial disputes arose. Cheddar, curious and eager to explore, would often venture into what Boo considered her space: the top perch of the cat tree, the coziest corner of the couch, and, most sacred of all, the sunny windowsill. Boo would hiss and swat, claiming these spots as hers, while Cheddar, often taken aback, would either retreat or become defensive.

Mealtimes became tense affairs. Despite having separate bowls, Boo would often guard the food area, forcing Cheddar to wait or eat hurriedly under the watchful eye of the older cat.

Cheddar's playful nature also caused conflict. He would often pounce on Boo, mistaking her tail for a plaything or attempting to initiate a play-fight. But Boo, not as playful and more set in her ways, would interpret these actions as threats, leading to skirmishes.

The constant tension created a palpable environmental stress in the household. Both cats became more vigilant, always on the lookout for potential confrontations. Boo started over-grooming, a sign of stress in cats, leading to bald patches on her fur. Cheddar, took to hiding in secluded spots, only coming out when necessary.

Recognizing the signs of stress, the Tanners consulted with a board-certified veterinary behaviorist. They were advised to separate the cats and modify their environment according to the 5 Pillars of a Healthy Feline Environment. This involved creating more vertical space with additional cat trees and shelves, ensuring both cats had ample high perches. Separate feeding stations and litter boxes located in different rooms alleviated mealtime tensions and provided each cat their own space. Gradual, supervised reintroductions, food puzzle toys, and positive reinforcement training (e.g., touch, come when called, station on a mat, and pattern games) helped foster a more harmonious environment for both cats.

Frustration

Frustration in dogs and cats arises when their efforts to achieve a goal (obtain resources, reinforcements, or control) are blocked, leading to accelerated behavioral responses such as excessive vocalization, agitation, or aggression.[2,6–7] This emotion is closely related to fear and anxiety and sometimes hard to differentiate. Over time, consistent frustration can compound and manifest as anxiety.

Jonesy and the Squirrels

Jonesy, a lively Jack Russell terrier, enjoys daily walks with his caregiver through the local park. Known for their boundless energy and strong prey drive, Jack Russells like Jonesy are perpetually alert and ready to chase anything in motion, from swirling leaves to darting small animals. One sunny afternoon, Jonesy caught sight of a squirrel just a few feet away. Sensing Jonesy's focused gaze, the squirrel dashed toward the nearest tree. Instinctively, Jonesy lunged forward, eager to pursue. However, his leash, firmly gripped by his caregiver, restrained him. Frustrated and unable to reach his target, Jonesy started to whine and tug incessantly, his tail wagging with agitation. He jumped and twisted, testing different angles and directions in hopes of escaping the leash's hold. Once the squirrel disappeared from view, Jonesy's frustration turned towards the leash itself, biting and pulling at at the object that had prevented his chase. Recognizing the signs of frustration, his caregiver redirected Jonesy's attention with a "touch" cue, guiding him to touch his nose to his caregiver's hand. This helped him settle and refocus so they could continue their walk.

Rainey and the Laser Pointer

Rainey, an agile tabby cat, enjoys chasing the red dot produced by a laser pointer. One evening, her caregiver played with her using the pointer, making her chase the dot all over the living room. Rainey pounced and swiped, but she could never catch the elusive dot. After several minutes of fruitless chasing, she began to meow loudly and look around in confusion, trying to find where the dot had gone. Eventually, she started swatting at her caregiver's hand holding the laser pointer, displaying her frustration at not being able to catch her intangible prey.

Aggressive Behavior

Aggression has many definitions, with the most common encompassing behaviors such as barking, growling, hissing, lunging, scratching, snarling, snapping, and biting. Less obvious signs of aggression can include staring, a stiff body, piloerection (i.e., hair standing up along the back), and leaning forward or backward. The motivation for aggression often involves increasing distance or stopping an interaction, which is why some animals resort to aggression when cornered or trapped as a means of self-preservation if they cannot escape. Because of this, aggression is often considered a fight or fidget response; however, these behaviors typically share the same underlying motivational state as avoidance and freeze responses.

7.2 Pathophysiology of Fear

The amygdala, the part of thc brain that controls fear and anxiety, receives direct input from sensory pathways in the body. Activation of the sympathetic nervous system, a component of the autonomic system, initiates the flight, fight, fidget, or freeze response, accompanied by the release of stress hormones such as cortisol.

The Hypothalamic-Pituitary-Adrenal (HPA) axis and the Sympathetic-Adreno-Medullary (SAM) axis are central to the body's physiological response to stress. When confronted with a stressor, the HPA axis is activated, leading the hypothalamus to release corticotropin-releasing hormone (CRH). This prompts the pituitary gland to secrete adrenocorticotropic hormone (ACTH), which then signals the adrenal cortex to produce cortisol (GCs), the primary stress hormone. Simultaneously, the SAM axis stimulates the sympathetic nervous system, resulting in the release of the catecholamines: epinephrine and norepinephrine (adrenaline), preparing the body for a fight, flight, freeze, or fidget reaction. Together, these systems prime the body and get it ready to deal with threats, resulting in emotions of fear and anxiety, indicative of heightened alertness and readiness.

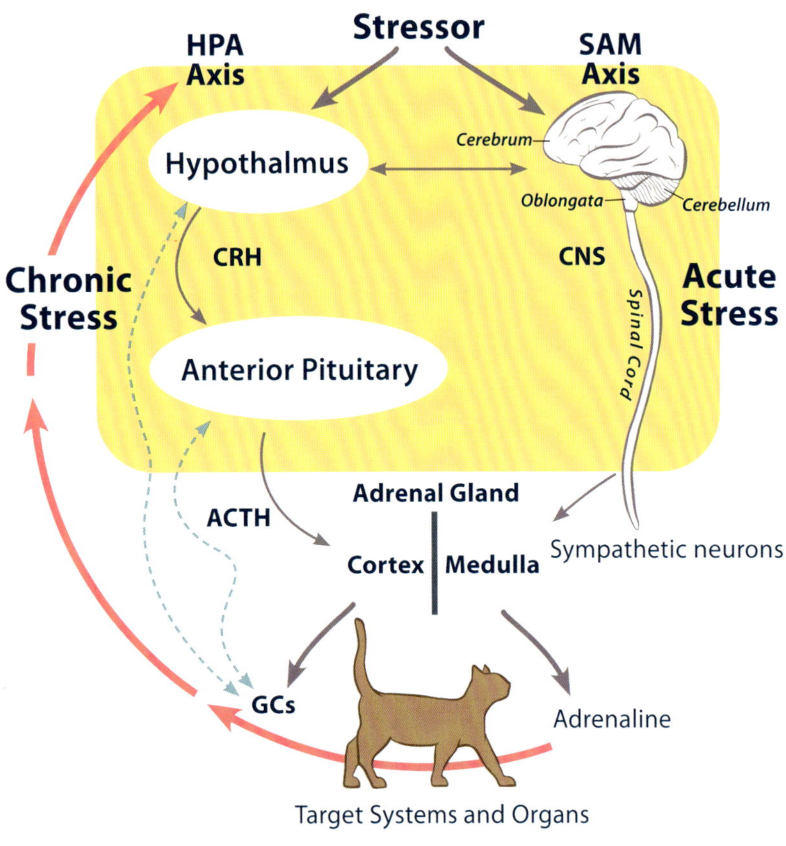

Fig. 7.2 A: The Hypothalamic-Pituitary-Adrenal (HPA) axis and the Sympathetic-Adreno-Medullary (SAM) axis are central to the body's physiological response to stress.

The brain is hardwired for self-preservation. When an animal is anxious or afraid and cannot avoid the stimulus (e.g., human approach, restraint, injection, something painful), they are more likely to anticipate and fear all future interactions with similar circumstances. This process, known as fear conditioning and can make procedures and handling progressively more difficult over time.

Factors That Affect Fear

Other than past experiences or lack thereof, numerous factors affect an individual's response to a fearful stimulus such as genetics, positioning of a fetus in utero, nutritional status of the mother, human influences, and the environment.

Return to Baseline

The time it takes for an animal to return to baseline after a close succession of triggers can vary from minutes in nonanxious animals to days, regardless of the caregiver's expectations.

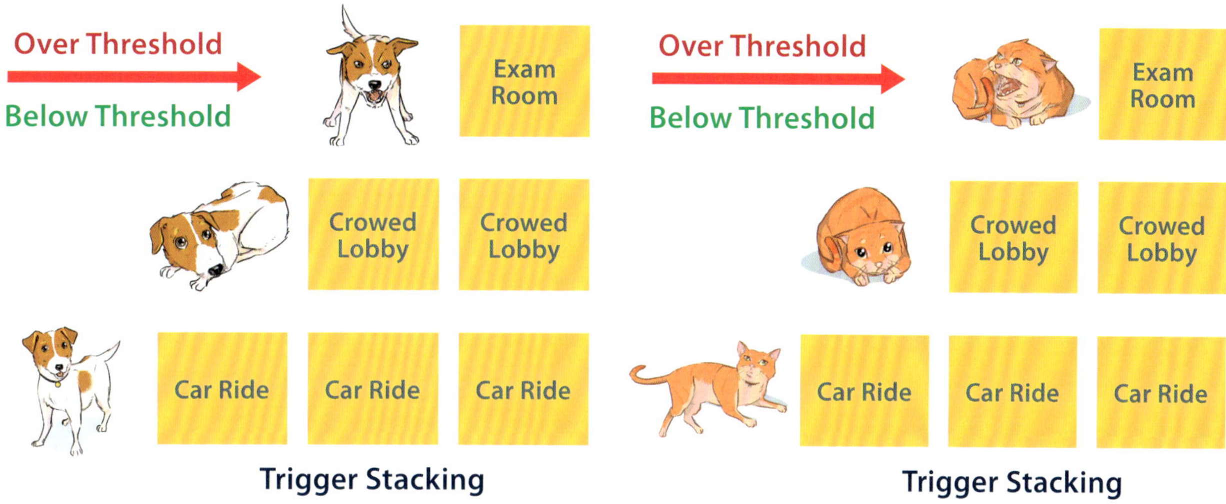

Figs. 7.2 B, C: Examples of trigger stacking in a dog and cat.

Development In Utero

Studies show that the environment within the uterus can play an important role in shaping behavior, including the position of the fetus. For example, the ***Intrauterine Position Effect*** suggests that a female positioned between two males may develop more male behavioral characteristics, such as urine marking.[8] Additionally, the mother nutritional status affects fetal development, cognition, and behavior.[9,10] Adequate energy, protein, fatty acids, and other key nutrients are essential for both fetal and brain development. When these nutrients are lacking, dogs and other animals are more likely to exhibit fearful and anxious behaviors as adults.[11]

In many species, it has been documented that high-stress situations during pregnancy result in an increase in avoidance behaviors and likelihood of aggressive behavior once the fetus reaches adulthood.[12,13] Note that not all stress is considered "bad" for the animal. In humans, moderate amounts of stress during pregnancy have been shown to result in children who are better at solving tasks that require coordination and logical thinking.[14–17] Several studies in mice have demonstrated similar results, suggesting that this may be true for other species of animals as well.[18–21]

Human Influence

Many studies have examined early human interactions with puppies and kittens and their associated long-term behavioral effects. Puppies that have been hand-reared, orphaned, or born by Caesarean section and rejected by their mother tend to develop behavioral issues associated with fear and anxiety.[22] Early weaning appears to have a negative effect on behavior as well.[23–26] In contrast, some studies demonstrate that early and gentle handling of puppies and kittens can have a positive effect on their emotional development, resulting in friendlier dogs and cats that are more comfortable and accepting of human handling later in life.[27–31]

Trigger Stacking

Trigger stacking can occur when an animal is exposed to multiple stressors at once or in close succession without an opportunity for the animal's cortisol levels to return to baseline.[32]

Misty's Visit to the Veterinary Hospital

Misty, a timid domestic shorthair cat, eyed the carrier with suspicion as it was pulled from the storage closet. To her, it signaled the start of an unpleasant experience, something she never enjoyed. Once coaxed into her carrier with food, Misty soon felt a gentle jostling as her caregiver placed her in the car. The motion of the ride, the hum of the engine, and the blur of unfamiliar sights outside only increased her anxiety. By the time they arrived at the veterinary hospital, Misty's eyes were dilated, and she was visibly tense.

Entering the veterinary hospital brought a rush of new scents, sounds, and sights that overwhelmed her sensory system. The lobby was crowded with other animals and their caregivers, adding another layer to her stress. She could hear dogs barking, people talking, and the faint sound of a cat hissing in the distance. Misty tried to shrink back into her carrier, seeking some semblance of comfort.

Once inside the exam room, the space was quieter but still foreign. A veterinary team member approached, opened the carrier door, and reached inside to remove her. She resisted, pressing herself into the far back corner of her carrier, until she was unceremoniously dumped out onto the table. The cold, surface of the table under her paws was frightening and being lifted onto the scale was even more unsettling. The sudden, unfamiliar touch of a thermometer made her tuck her tail around her body in distress.

As she tried to gather herself, the door opened again, and the veterinarian entered. Misty's ears flattened against her head. Although the veterinarian's touch was gentle, it was still a stranger's. Every prod, vaccination, restraint, and slight pinch from drawing blood added to the growing stack of triggers. By the end of the visit, Misty was thoroughly overwhelmed and desperately wanted to retreat to the safety of her carrier.

JoJo's Anxiety at the Veterinary Hospital

JoJo, a spirited golden retriever, wagged her tail excitedly as her caregiver clipped on her leash. She always loved going out, but the car was a different story. The confinement and sensation of movement unnerved her. Upon reaching the car, JoJo froze and flattened herself to the ground, prompting her caregiver to lift her into the back seat. At first, JoJo just watched out the window, but as the journey progressed, she began to whine and restlessly pace in the back seat.

Arriving at the veterinary hospital, the onslaught of smells hit her immediately. There was the scent of other dogs, cats, cleaning products, and a strange smell that she couldn't quite place but found alarming. The waiting room was full, with other dogs on leashes and the occasional cat in a carrier, all accompanied by their caregivers. The variety of sounds, from the high-pitched yips of a Chihuahua to the low growl of a Rottweiler, kept her on edge.

As JoJo's caregiver led her towards the examination room, they passed a scale placed on the floor. A veterinary team member gestured towards it, indicating JoJo should step onto it. Hesitant and unsure, JoJo resisted, but with gentle coaxing and a slight nudge, she was eventually pushed onto the cold, hard, and scary surface. The unfamiliar feeling and the process of getting on the scale added another layer of anxiety to her already growing discomfort.

Inside the examination room, the unfamiliar surroundings made JoJo even more nervous. She sniffed every corner, trying to acquaint herself with the new environment. A veterinary team member approached, preparing her for the upcoming procedures. When the veterinarian entered the room, JoJo's tail tucked slightly between her legs. The physical examination, the sensation of the vaccination, and the unfamiliar restraint and pressure during the blood draw were all uncomfortable and overwhelming experiences for her. Each event was a new stressor, pushing her closer to her threshold. By the end of the appointment, JoJo's usual exuberance and excitement was dampened by the overwhelming series of events she had experienced.

As illustrated by the experiences of both Misty and JoJo, an animal might cope with a single stressful event, but an accumulation of stressors in a brief period called ***trigger stacking***, can overwhelm them. This overwhelming stress can push the animal beyond their threshold, triggering responses such as fight, flight, fidget, or freeze.

Emotional Arousal and Behavioral Thresholds

Every day, the brain is constantly inundated with an enormous amount of information to process and filter. Because sensory input is constant, the brain must determine what is safe and what is threat. When the emotional network is activated, the body prepares to react. The sympathetic nervous system and hypothalamic-pituitary axis (HPA) are put on alert, readying the body and brain to respond if a threat is detected. This state, called emotional arousal, serves to keep an animal alive.

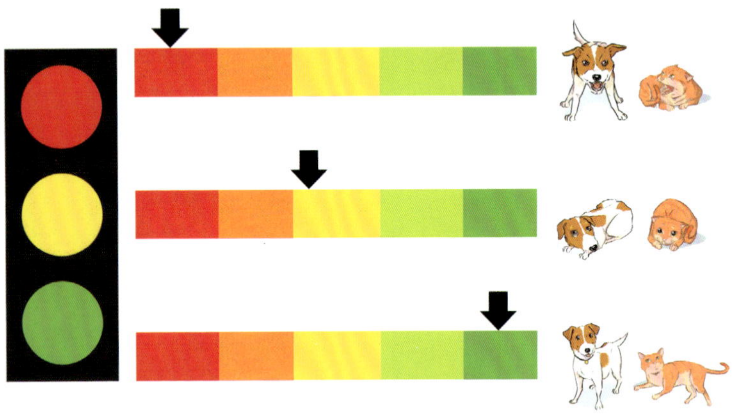

Fig. 7.2 D: Emotional arousal can be likened to a traffic light with three main thresholds: green, yellow, and red.

An animal's arousal can be likened to a traffic light with three main thresholds: green, yellow, and red.[33] Green indicates relaxed behaviors, yellow points to early signs of fear and anxiety such as hypervigilance, avoidance, and attempts to hide or escape, while red denotes intense emotional arousal, including behaviors such as barking, growling, lunging, hissing, swatting, and attempting to bite. The shift between these thresholds varies based on the individual, and is, influenced by genetics, early experiences, environment, and stimulus intensity.[33]

Avoid Labeling

Many different labels are used to describe a fearful or anxious animal, but empathy comes with understanding. Recognizing the true motivation behind an animal's behavior, such as fear, anxiety, or frustration, fosters empathy. While it can be challenging to avoid labels, more descriptive and appropriate terminology should be used when available.[4,33] Erroneously labeling an animal spreads misinformation about their behavior, whereas accurate descriptions provide an opportunity to approach the animal from a different perspective. This approach improves the safety and welfare of both the handler and the animal, while meeting the emotional needs of all involved.

Learn to Listen

When working with animals, constant communication between the human and animal is occurring. Humans need to pay attention to what the animal is trying to say. This means observing and documenting behaviors of the animal throughout an entire interaction. Animals exhibit many ritualized behaviors to request a pause in an action or to express their feelings at any given moment. When these attempts at communication are not recognized, defensive behaviors may escalate. Over time, these can lead to the animal no longer giving warning signs before heightened arousal results in escalated defensive behaviors, such as biting.

Understanding Emotions

Understanding and recognizing emotional states helps to identify ***emotionally withdrawn, shy, or shut-down animals.*** These animals are often just as fearful and anxious as those who display fight or fidget responses, but they express their emotions differently—by freezing, hiding, or avoiding.

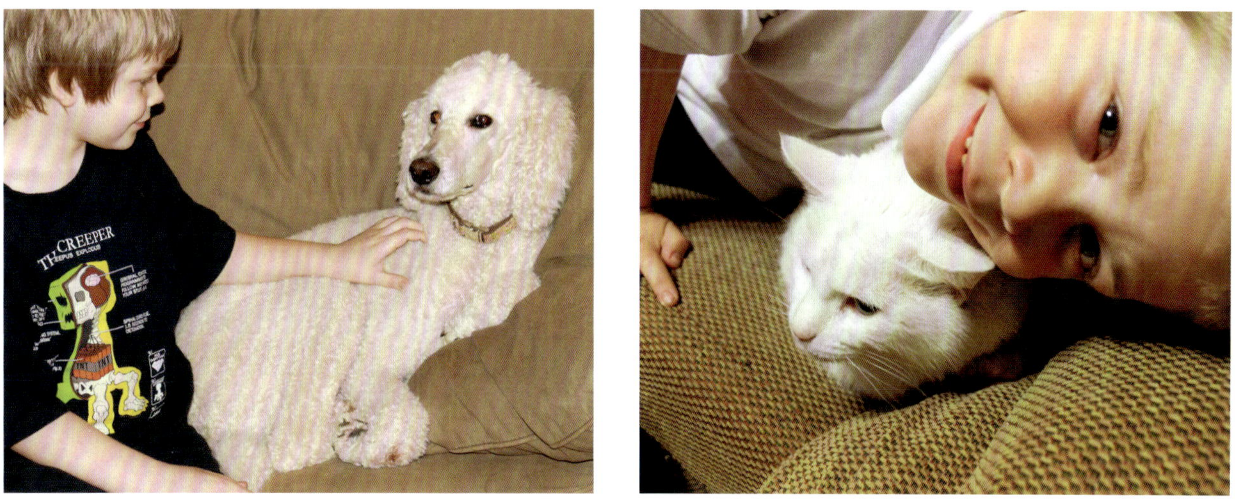

Figs. 7.2 E, F: Dogs and cats may display behaviors like looking away, whale eye, a tight mouth, stiffness, or flattened ears to signal a desire for a pause in the action.

Assessing Welfare

The ***Five Domains Model*** and the ***Five Freedoms*** are two key frameworks in animal welfare. The Five Domains Model, updated in 2020 to include human-animal interactions, evaluates welfare across five areas: *Nutrition, Environment, Health, Behavioral Interactions,* and *Mental State*. The Five Freedoms focus on *freedom from hunger, discomfort, pain,* and *fear*, and *freedom to express normal behavior*.

Both models guide the ethical treatment of animals including dogs and cats, emphasizing their physical, mental, and emotional health. This includes veterinary care, socialization, exercise, mental stimulation, and positive reinforcement training. Importantly, both models advocate for an animal's agency, choice, and control over their environment, representing a modern, comprehensive approach to animal welfare that values overall quality of life.[36]

Choice, Empowerment, and Agency

Agency, the capacity to control one's environment and make choices, is fundamental for emotional health and wellbeing.[6] Without agency, individuals can experience heightened fear, anxiety, frustration, and potentially aggressive (distance increasing) behaviors.[34–36] Flooding, a technique where an individual is exposed to a stressor without an escape option, often stems from excessive handling and restraint. This approach can induce distress and learned helplessness, even if the animal seems outwardly calm, "okay," or "fine."

Cooperative care or consent training enhances communication and teaches animals behaviors that promote elective participation in their own veterinary care or husbandry procedures. When an animal has choice and control, they engage more and the formation of protective emotions diminishes.[2,3–5,34–36] Empowerment can lower emotional arousal, enhance welfare, and increase predictability during procedures.[36]

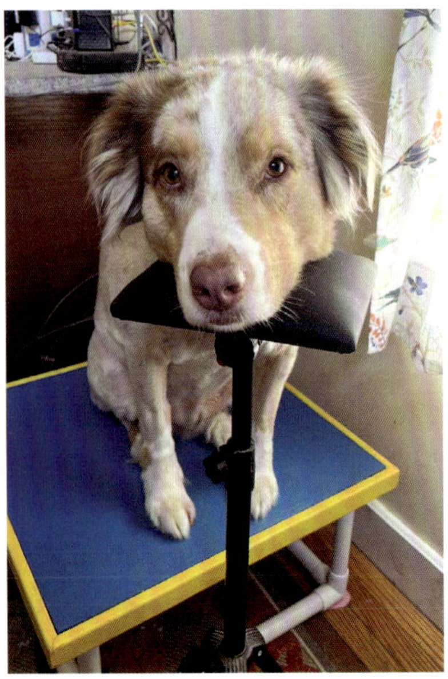

Fig. 7.2 G: This picture illustrates multiple layers of consent behaviors for cooperative care: stationing on a platform, chin rest, and voluntary eye contact.

Start and Stop Behaviors

Cooperative care teaches animals distinct start and stop behaviors to clearly convey their consent for veterinary and common husbandry procedures, signaling either "yes, I'm ready" or "no, I'd like to stop." [35] Both "yes" responses and "no" refusals are reinforced, giving the animal an opportunity to understand they are being heard.[35,37–39] Start behaviors are taught individually before being chained together, creating multiple tiers of consent and genuine voluntary participation.

Once the animal consistently offers these signals, desensitization and counterconditioning can be initiated. These methods can be applied to procedures like nail trims, venipuncture, handling, and examinations.[37–39] Obtaining genuine consent from animals requires both the animal awareness of their choice to participate and the human's to accurately interpret this consent.[35,37–39] An animal's sense of control over these interactions not only enhances communication but makes historically frightening procedures more predictable for the animal.[37–40] This sense of safety reduces anxiety and the need for defensive behaviors.

Empowering Animals

Empowering animals with ***agency***, ***choice***, and ***control*** facilitates the recognition of true consent in cooperative care training. Teaching animals specific behaviors to signal their willingness to participate is fundamental to good welfare. Veterinary team members, trainers, and other animal professionals, along with caregivers, must learn to read and interpret body language. Critical thinking skills are essential to determine when an animal is genuinely consenting to participate, rather than just participating for food, merely enduring the situation, or preferring not to participate at all. For highly food-motivated animals, providing an opt-out option, such as a mat with a food toy, helps reduce coercion and offers a clear indicator that their participation is truly voluntary. Some refer to this as assent.

Table 7.2.1 Examples of Start and Stop Behaviors (Adapted from Sydänheimo et al 2023)

Start	Stop
Chin rest	Chin up
Lying on side, head on the ground	Head up
Nose touch	Turn head away
Offer paw	Move paw away
Step up on a platform	Walk away or avoid the platform
Stand or lie down on a mat	Walk away or avoid the mat

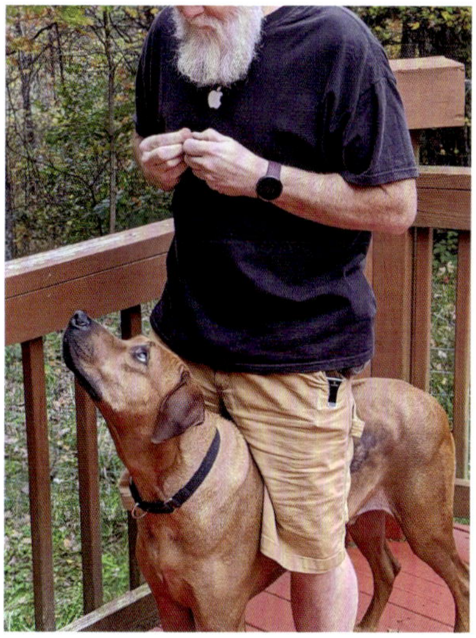

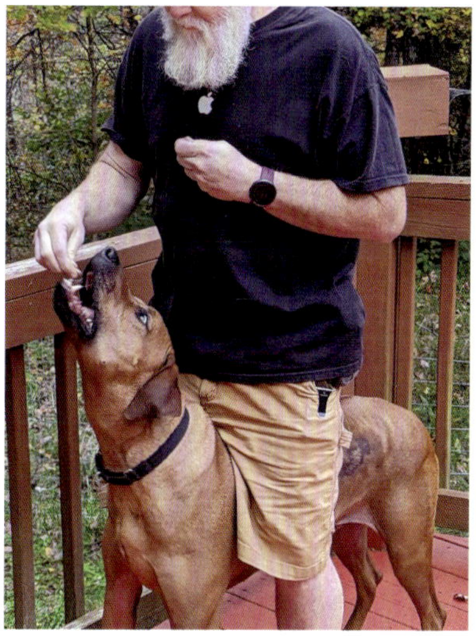

Figs. 7.2 H, I: Cooperative care begins with teaching dogs start and stop behaviors. In the examples shown, the dog has learned to voluntarily offer a specific position, without a specific visual or verbal cue. Eye contact serves as an additional start behavior. Once the dog consistently offers both behaviors, in succession, the training advances to prepare the dog for an actual jugular venipuncture. This preparation involves shaping techniques, desensitization, and counterconditioning. The process starts with just the dog and gradually introduces another person followed by the specific equipment necessary for the actual venipuncture.

7.3 What Do Fear and Anxiety Look Like?

Fear and anxiety stem from the same emotional system and elicit similar behavioral responses. Individual animals express these emotions differently, with behaviors ranging from avoidance to freezing and even antagonistic displays.[6,33] When evaluating emotional states, observe the entire animal. Some animals will clearly signal their emotions, while others may give mixed signals that are harder to interpret.[6,33] Most antagonistic displays come with warning signals when the animal is observed closely.[33,41]

In addition to trigger stacking, numerous factors can affect an animal's tolerance level and response to a real or perceived threat. Underlying medical conditions (e.g., dermatological, gastrointestinal, musculoskeletal, neurological) may cause pain or discomfort and increase irritability. In these cases, the underlying medical conditions must be treated along with addressing the emotional state of the animal.

Body Language of Fear, Anxiety, Frustration, and Pain

Eyes

Close observation of eye position and pupil size is instrumental in discerning an animal's genuine emotional state. Relaxed animals generally have almond-shaped eyes with small, light-responsive pupils.[41–44] Conversely, when an animal feels fearful or stressed, their eyes tend to widen and pupils dilate, becoming less responsive to light.[41–44] These animals may also avoid direct eye contact or briefly engage before quickly looking away.[41–44] In dogs, the term "whale eye" describes a situation where the white part of the eye (sclera) becomes more visible as the animal looks away, while in cats, an increase in blinking behavior can be indicative of stress.[41–43]

Ears

Ear position is often used to gauge emotional states.[41,42–44] Interpreting ear position doesn't always require the observer to be an expert.[7,42–45] However, interpreting ear positioning can be complex due to variations in ear shape and coat color. For instance, cropped or upright ears may pose challenges in interpretation due to loss of behavioral repertoire.[7,41]

Mouth

Fearful dogs typically keep their mouth firmly closed, although some may pant due to fear and anxiety, with their mouth open wide and tongue curled up at the tip.[41,43] Dogs may also grin (retract their lips and show their incisors) when they are in a conflicted state, which can be challenging to interpret accurately. In contrast, cats do not pant, so their mouth usually remains closed and tight when they are fearful and anxious.[7,44] Lip licking and swallowing can be an indicator of fear in both dogs and cats.

Body Position

When assessing an animal's emotional state, consider their body position.[4,41–44] Fearful animals often lower their heads and shift their weight towards their hind end, as if ready for a quick escape.[43] Some may assume a crouched or lowered body position. Cats may tightly wrap their tails around their bodies, which can also indicate abdominal or hind end pain.[44] In extreme cases, both dogs and cats may freeze when overwhelmed by fear. You may also notice piloerection, where their hair stands up, typically along the back and tail in cats, or at the tail base or shoulder blades in dogs.[43,44.] Often mistaken for a request for a belly rub or petting, when dogs or cats roll onto their backs, it is usually not an invitation for further engagement, but rather a cutoff signal or conflict-related behavior asking to end the interaction.[43]

Tail

The way an animal holds and moves their tail is easy to observe, making it a common indicator of their emotional state. However, tail position is just one part of the overall picture when evaluating body language. Fearful dogs tend to lower or tuck their tail, keeping them at or below baseline, and avoiding raising them high over their back.[43] Cats will curl their tail around their body or lower it with piloerection.[44] Quick moving tails are often a sign of high arousal and agitation.[43–44]

Vocalizations

Fearful dogs can exhibit a range of vocalizations, from silence to whining, whimpering, or barking.[41] When they feel threatened and defensive, dogs may also growl and show their teeth.[43] On the other hand, hissing in cats typically occurs when they perceive a threat or are in defensive mode.[44]

Avoidance Behaviors

Arousal thresholds can vary based on numerous factors from the environment to human or animal interactions. When animals show avoidance behaviors like leaning away or avoiding eye contact, they are attempting to distance themselves from perceived threats. Aggressive behaviors such as barking, growling, or biting often arise when avoidance is not effective, or the animal feels cornered. These actions aim to repel the perceived threat, particularly when escape seems impossible.

Table 7.3.1: Body Language and Emotional Arousal in Dogs

Dogs	Green	Yellow	Red
Interaction	Approaches willingly Calmly solicits attention	May be hesitant to approach or approaches then backs away Possible displays include: Hypervigilance Fidgeting Pacing Avoiding interaction Quiet and still, stiff Appears sleepy Shaking & trembling	Will not approach for food, petting, or interactions Actively avoids Hypervigilant, fidgeting, and pacing Urination, defecation, expression of anal glands may occur. May be immobile or frozen
Tail	Horizontal or up slightly Not stiff or tucked May be wagging widely if excited	Tucked or lowered	Tightly tucked between legs or up and wagging stiffly
Body	Relaxed and loose Rests comfortably on the floor Walks into the room fluidly with no hesitation	Somewhat stiff or shaking Head may be down Crouched or lying on the floor or under a bench/chair and does not approach A paw may be raised Roll onto back with abdomen exposed, tail tucked, tight mouth, sideways glance, whale eye, stiff body, ears back	Leaning forward or away Roll onto back as described above Crouched and leaning away May be stiff and still. Trembling may occur Raised hackles
Ears	Forward Relaxed	Slightly back or flat against the head	Ears back or flat against the head
Eyes	Almond shaped Pupils are normal size Soft eye contact	Pupils dilated Avoiding direct eye contact Looks away Whale eye may be present	Open wide Pupils dilated Direct stare

Table 7.3.1: Body Language and Emotional Arousal in Dogs *(continued)*

Dogs	Green	Yellow	Red
Mouth	May be panting but relaxed and not tense	May be open and panting with tip of tongue curled May be closed with corners turned up and tight May growl, snarl, show incisors and canines	Open and panting heavily Tight and closed Wrinkled nose Furrowed brow Growling, snapping, biting
Reinforce-ments	Will take food willingly with a soft mouth May enjoy petting or playing with toy	Will not take food from hand but may eat food from floor Hard mouth (grabby) for treats May refuse food Not interested in playing or touching	Will not eat Will not interact

Table 7.3.2: Body Language and Emotional Arousal in Cats

Cats	Green	Yellow	Red
Interaction	Approaches willingly to interact Seeks attention	Tries to escape or resist handling Hides in carrier, under cabinets, or chairs Some will be hypervigilant attempting to escape the room or get up high	Will not approach Hiding or frantic escape attempts May be immobile or frozen May suddenly bolt
Tail	Candy cane shaped	Flicking or curled around the body Low to the ground	Down, may be curled around the body Piloerection of tail and along spine may occur
Body	Rests comfortably on the floor, in carrier, on table, caregiver's lap, countertop, etc. Explores the room	Crouching down with feet tucked and tail curled around body Attempting to look small Increased respiratory rate Feigned sleep	Crouches or charging and swatting Some freeze when head down; lack of all social interactions Back may be arched Increase in respiratory rate and heart rate
Ears	Up and natural position	Slightly turned back or flattened outward	Pinned back or flat and horizontal

Table 7.3.2: Body Language and Emotional Arousal in Cats *(continued)*

Cats	Green	Yellow	Red
Eyes	Almond shaped Relaxed Soft Pupils are normal sized and not dilated	Pupils dilated Blinking may occur	Direct stare Pupils may be dilated or constricted
Mouth	Whiskers in neutral position slightly to the side or may pull forward and fan out Mouth is closed with loose lips	Whiskers pushed forward or pulled back tightly Lip licking and swallowing	Growling Hissing Spitting Yowling Whiskers flattened against cheeks
Reinforce-ments	Takes food willingly, may enjoy petting or playing with toys	May sniff food but will not eat or engage in play Resists touch or freezes with touch	Will not eat or interact in play

7.4 Sedation as a First Resort

When it comes to physical restraint of animals, it is not uncommon to push animals over their emotional and behavioral thresholds in the name of getting the job done. Arguments such as "it will take too long," "it'll be over quickly," "it's for their own good," or "they are here now" are common phrases uttered by team members to avoid sedation. This leads to reliance on "brutacaine," a method that involves physically overpowering the animal, an approach that is neither ideal nor safe.

Overpowered animals may be mistaken for being "fine," "compliant," or "okay," when in reality, they are frozen in fear.[39,44–45] With each encounter, they learn what keeps them safe, making future visits more challenging and leading to handling resistance, refusal to enter the building, or even biting.

Reservations about sedation arise from concerns about cost (e.g., caregiver's cost or cost to the clinic), time, caregiver opposition, concurrent medical conditions, and lack of knowledge about medications or the sedation process. Because of these reasons,

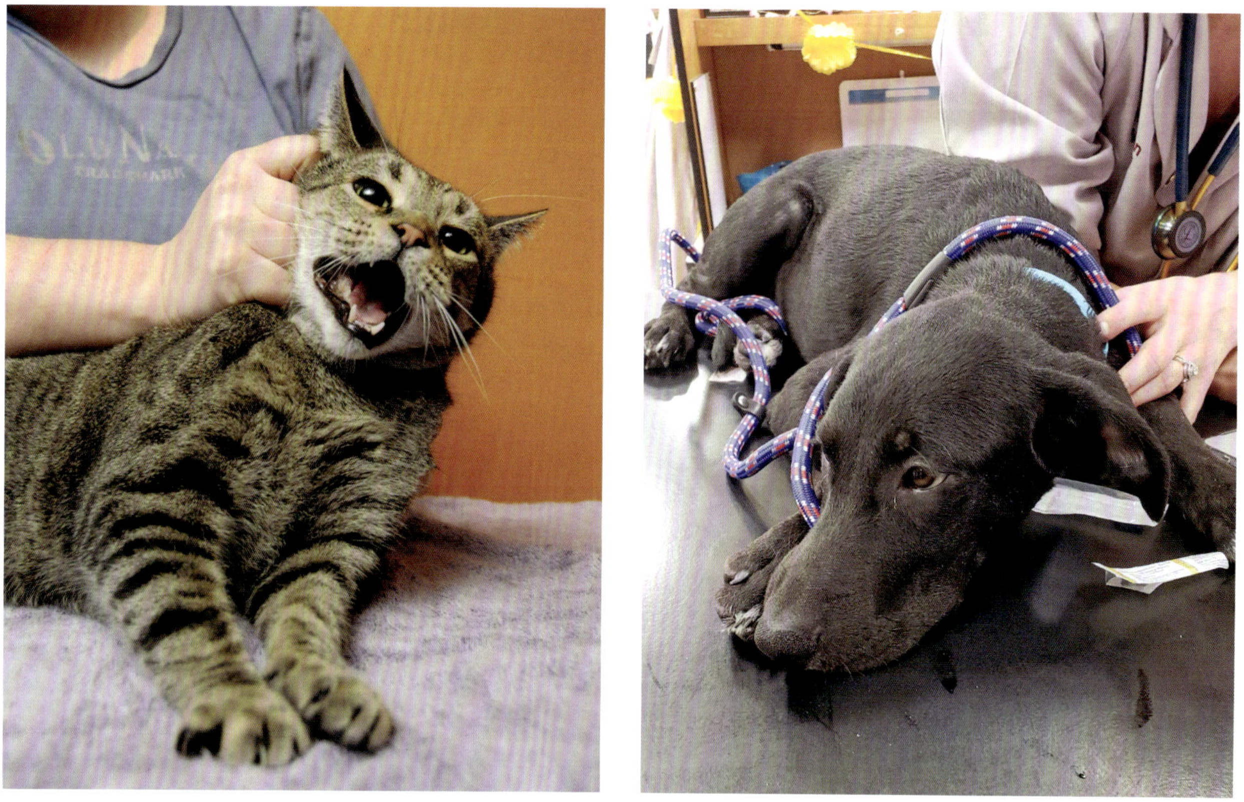

Figs. 7.4 A, B: In the above figures, the cat exhibits signs of resistance, while the dog demonstrates emotional withdrawal, appearing frozen in fear.

many veterinarians and team members tend to offer sedation as a last resort, amplifying the animal's distress and detracting from the best practice of veterinary medicine.

When sedation is needed, the cost should be factored into the treatment plan. Sedation cost can be offset by the ability to schedule the procedure at a convenient time for both the caregiver and the veterinary team. Requiring fewer team members allows them to focus on other revenue producing activities.[46] Communication and education help to make sure everyone shares the same narrative.

Using sedation as a last resort essentially permits wrestling and fighting with the animal until they exceed their arousal threshold. Once over threshold, higher doses of medication may be needed to achieve adequate sedation, increasing the risk of complications and, in some cases, rendering the sedation ineffective. Sedating earlier in the process can ensure these medications are more effective with fewer side effects and decreases the risk of worsening fear over time.

Why Sedation is Important

1. affords convenient scheduling of the procedure.
2. enables efficient utilization of team members.
3. lowers cost, amount of total sedation needed, and potential side effects.
4. reduces fear conditioning, therefore is more likely to improve the animal's behavior over time.

7.5 Creating an Individualized Low Stress Handling® Plan

Individualized Low Stress Handling® plans document each animal's specific needs and preferences.[33] This includes recognizing fearful stimuli, noting favored treats, and handling techniques, and pinpointing preferred locations for different procedures. All these details should be recorded in the medical record.

While clients might deem some procedures, like vaccinations, nail trims, or certain blood tests, as urgent, delaying them allows for desensitization and counterconditioning. Postponing also offers a chance to prescribe and test pre-visit medications. For critical procedures, methods like intramuscular (IM), intravenous (IV), or oral transmucosal (OTM) sedation, or general anesthesia might be necessary.

7.6 Food and the Positive Emotional Response

What Cats Like

Chin scratches, petting behind the ears, and rubbing of acupuncture spots above and between the eyes can have a calming effect.

Fear is not a conscious choice. Thus, to change a fear, it needs to be paired with something that naturally elicits a positive conditioned emotional response (+CER). Palatable food is the easiest and most powerful way to do this. What is palatable to one animal may not be as palatable to another. A variety of choices may need to be offered. Document choices as part of the individualized Low Stress Handling® plan for future reference.

Food Delivery

The timing of food delivery determines whether a positive or negative conditioned emotional response (CER) forms. Counterconditioning works best when food is given while the animal is relaxed, right before handling. Besides food, physical affection and toys can be powerful reinforcers and distract many animals. Involving the caregiver in giving both food and affection can facilitate relaxation, due to the positive emotional conncction already established between the pet and caregiver.

Stressed animals should be fed for the duration of handling to reduce escalation of fear and emotional arousal. For these animals, the food may need to be higher in value (e.g., high-value treat) to keep their interest and maintain a positive conditioned emotional response (+CER). Tools such as lickable mats, cheese boards, food-filled syringes, wooden spoons, or stuffed food toys provide a constant food source. When the handling stops, so does the food. Some animals will not eat at all. For these, postponing the procedure, prescribing oral medications, or sedation would be best.

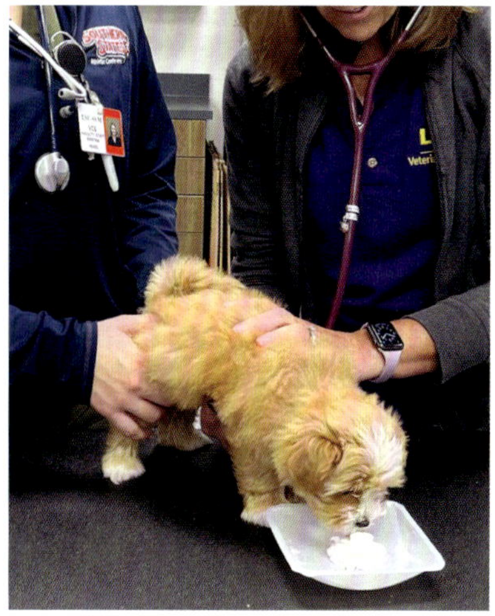

Fig. 7.6 A: The use of food during a physical examination provides an effective distraction and promotes positive and engaging emotions. (Photo courtesy of Louisiana State University School of Veterinary Medicine Community Practice)

Eating While Stressed

Compared to dogs, food intake is a less reliable indicator of stress in cats. While dogs willingly eat when stressed, cats may refuse food even when calm and relaxed. In general, kittens introduced to food distractions during veterinary visits will continue to eat as adults. Sudden refusal of food from a cat that has been previously eating is a clear indicator of escalating stress levels, pain, or disease and should be noted. Some adult cats and kittens show an interest in toys even in mildly stressful situations; therefore, toy acceptance and object play can be another indicator of a cat's emotional state.

Food Presentation

How a food choice is presented is as important as its palatability. Given that unfamiliar team members can be a source of fear and anxiety, leading to mixed emotions, the food should be presented at the end of an object (like a wooden stick), on a blanket, or on a lick mat, rather than directly from the team member's hand. If the animal refuses a treat, it should never be forced onto their nose or in mouth, as this could heighten fear and anxiety. The food should be withdrawn if the animal shows no interest in it.

Good Food Choices for Dogs and Cats

Below are lists of some food choices that dogs and cats may find palatable and can be useful during handling. Be sure to check the pet's dietary restrictions before offering any of the listed foods.

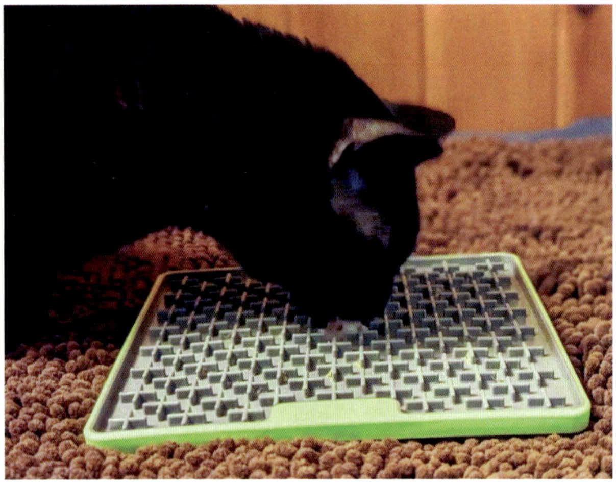

Fig. 7.6 B: Giving special treats on a lickable mat daily can simplify medication administration later in life.

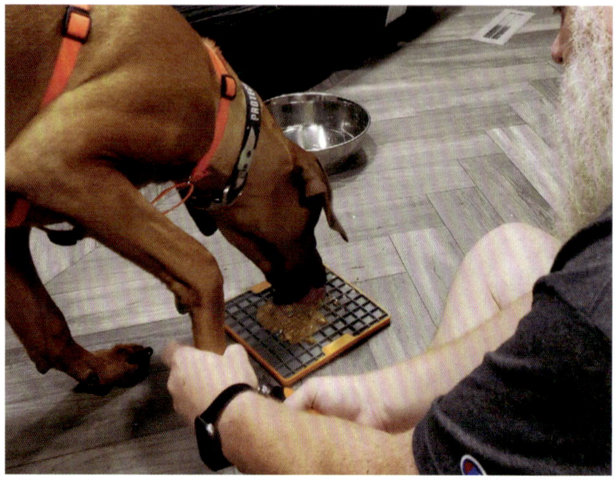

Fig. 7.6 C: Prevention involves using tools like lickable mats during potentially stressful procedures from a young age.

Table 7.6.1: Food Choices for Cats and Dogs

Cats	Dogs
Butter	Chicken treats
Lickable treats (Churu®, Catit®, etc)	Liverwurst
Chicken or turkey baby food	Squeeze cheese
Canned tuna or chicken	Peanut butter
Squeeze cheese	Chicken or turkey baby food
Cream cheese	Greenies™ Pill Pockets™
Whipped cream	Freeze dried liver, chicken, beef, fish, or other flavor
Canned cat food	Cheerios™
Smushed Greenies™ Pill Pockets™	Cream cheese
Royal Canin Pill Assist™	Low sodium turkey hot dogs
Soft cat treats	Dry dog food of various flavors
Dry treats (e.g., Temptations™)	Pupperoni® broken into small pieces
Freeze-dried chicken, fish, beef, shrimp	Braunschweiger/ liverwurst
Broth without onion powder such as Fancy Feast® broth	

7.7 Medications for Fear and Anxiety

When it comes to medications, there is not a ***one size fits all*** approach available for dogs and cats. For most animals, a medication or medication combination does not exist that will completely change their behavior or take away all their fear and anxiety. However, most oral medications can reduce stress and anxiety enough to make a patient less dangerous to themselves and others so oral transmucosal (OTM) or injectable (e.g., IM or IV) sedation can be given. Numerous combinations are available, depending on personal preference and familiarity.

At-Home Medications

Benzodiazepines

Benzodiazepines (e.g., diazepam, alprazolam, lorazepam) are considered true anxiolytics (e.g., help alleviate anxiety), capable of reducing anxiety in dogs and cats.[47–49] These medications may decrease learning or have an amnesic effect, although it can be hard to confirm this in animals. Benzodiazepines can have variable sedative effects, which are sometimes dose-dependent, and can occasionally lead to paradoxical excitement and reduce inhibitions.[47,49] For efficacy, they should be administered before the animal becomes anxious and can be safely combined with other medications.

Gabapentin

Gabapentin, a GABA analogue, reduces both neuropathic pain and anxiety. It has a wide safety margin with sedation as the main side effect. In cats, several studies show reduced stress scores during veterinary examinations and reduced vocalizations during car rides to the veterinary hospital.[50–52]

When used alone, gabapentin has been shown to be less effective in dogs than cats for veterinary visits.[53] However, one study showed gabapentin was effective for the treatment of storm phobia in dogs.[54] The administration of gabapentin two hours before anesthesia maintained with isoflurane demonstrated a MAC_{ISO} sparing effect in dogs.[55] There are no comparable studies in cats.

Currently, no studies have been published on the benefits of combining gabapentin and trazodone.[56] However, they are often co-prescribed and are said to be effective together based on anecdotal evidence. For cats, gabapentin can be mixed with a treat for easier administration. There is no evidence to support dosing the evening before has benefits; however, an additional dose the night before may be beneficial if the cat gets anxious seeing the carrier, especially if they are not previously conditioned to it.

Excreted through the kidneys, the gabapentin dose should be decreased by 50% in cats with renal disease (all IRIS stages) and can sometimes cause prolonged sedation.[57] When combined with injectable sedatives, recovery may be smoother.

Pregabalin

Pregabalin works similarly to gabapentin, but it is more potent. In one study, pregabalin was found to be well tolerated in cats reducing signs of anxiety and fear during transportation in cars.[58] It is speculated to have similar effects during veterinary visits.[59] Follow the same precautions as above when prescribing to cats with renal disease.

Trazodone

Trazodone is often prescribed for veterinary visits, hospital stays, and confinement to alleviate anxiety and provide sedation for both dogs and cats. Research indicates it can reduce stress during veterinary visits.[60,61] Although generally safe with minimal side effects, there is one published case report linking trazodone administration to elevated liver enzymes in a dog, therefore caution is advised for dogs with preexisting liver disease.[62]

Medication Tip

Encouraging dogs to lick something after oral transmucosal medication administration can reduce the likelihood of them licking the gel off their lips.

Dexmedetomidine

Dexmedetomidine oral transmucosal (OTM) gel (Sileo®) has been shown to significantly decrease the likelihood of vocalizations (e.g., whining, yelping, grumbling), avoidance behaviors, and other stress-related activities (e.g., panting, trembling, urinating, defecating) during physical examinations.[63–68] Anecdotally, when applying, it may be more effective if the gel is painted onto the gums as opposed to squirting it in the cheek pouch.

Clonidine

Clonidine has a similar mechanism of action to dexmedetomidine OTM. It is well-tolerated in dogs with fear-based behaviors, and is another in-home medication option to administer to dogs prior to veterinary visits.[69] No studies have currently evaluated its use in cats.

What About Acepromazine?

Acepromazine, a phenothiazine tranquilizer, is *not* an anxiolytic medication. Therefore, it should not be used as a stand-alone medication for veterinary visits or handling purposes. In some animals, acepromazine may be beneficial in combination with other medications like benzodiazepines. While acepromazine can result in mild sedation, the degree of sedation is often not the level needed to safely examine the animal or develop enough compliance to administer additional medications. Acepromazine is thought to have little to no anxiolytic effect and an increase in noise sensitivity has been documented.[70–72] In cats and dogs, acepromazine can cause disinhibition and aggressive behavior.[71] Hyperthermia and hypotension have also been noted.[73] Care should be taken if combining with dexmedetomidine.

The "Chill Protocol"

The GMA protocol, known as "The Chill Protocol," was introduced by clinicians at Tufts University as a case report to aid in the management of aggressive and fearful dogs during an intramuscular (IM) injection and anesthesia.[74] This method involves administering gabapentin the evening prior to the appointment, followed by a combination of gabapentin and melatonin 1–2 hours before the visit. Acepromazine OTM is given 30 minutes before the scheduled examination time.[74]

A recent study revealed that the GMA protocol effectively reduced stress, fear, and aggression in dogs during hospital visits and increased sedation.[74] There was a correlation between older dogs experiencing less stress and more sedation post-GMA.[74] However, individual responses to medications vary, emphasizing the importance of personalized assessments by veterinarians.

Chill Protocol

GMA stands for ***gabapentin***, ***melatonin***, and ***acepromazine***, the medications used as part of the ***Chill Protocol***.

Give a Test Dose

It is important to have caregivers administer a test dose of medication at home before the actual veterinary visit. Start on the low end of the dosage range when administering oral medication, and then titrate up (e.g., increase dose) as appropriate. Once the appropriate dose has been found, a car ride to the veterinary hospital as a trial run is the next step to ensure adequate dosing. These trials give an opportunity to determine which medication and dosages are effective, how long it takes to be effective, how long the medication is effective for, and to document any side effects. These trials also help to determine if other medications are needed in combination to improve effectiveness.

In-Hospital Sedation

As with in-home medications, numerous combinations of injectable medications are available for the sedation of fearful, anxious, or painful animals.[75] If a complete physical exam is not possible before sedation for safety reasons, the pros and cons of each medication or combination should be considered carefully. Common agents used for either intramuscular (IM) or intravenous (IV) administration include dexmedetomidine in combination with various opioids (e.g., morphine, hydromorphone, buprenorphine, butorphanol, methadone), especially when pain is a factor. During procedures when immobilization is needed, the addition of ketamine can be helpful.[76]

Alfaxalone, an induction agent similar to propofol, can be given intramuscular (IM) to small dogs and cats. It tends to cause fewer apneic events compared to propofol.[77–80] For larger dogs, the large volume needed makes intramuscular (IM) injections less than ideal. Alfaxalone should not be used alone because the potential side effects of muscle twitching and myoclonus, may result in poor sedation and a rough recovery. Instead, it is often combined with butorphanol or midazolam, especially in compromised animals.[80]

7.8 Conclusion

This chapter outlines the behavioral indications of protective emotions such as fear, anxiety, and frustration, as well as the physiological stress responses they evoke in the body. Several factors, including genetics, environment, and early life experiences, influence the intensity and impact of these emotions on an animal's actions. When emotionally aroused, dogs and cats can exhibit a range of behaviors from vocal expressions like barking or hissing to physical reactions such as biting or avoiding. While most are familiar with the fight or flight responses, the lesser recognized freeze response, marked by emotional withdrawal, holds equal importance. In this context, it is easy to mistakenly label animals as fine or obedient when they are actually immobilized by fear.

Recognizing and understanding these everchanging emotional states during interactions with animals is vital. Instead of simplifying their states with labels, empathy should be applied and animals given choice and control over those choices. Such empowerment promotes predictable interactions and assures them that if they choose to say no, they will be heard. Every animal possesses distinct preferences and necessities. Recognizing and addressing these with a specialized Low Stress Handling® plan ensures their well-being, guarantees safety, and fosters client comprehension and compliance.

Moreover, medications are indispensable in managing deep-seated emotions like fear, anxiety, and frustration. Determining when to use sedation to boost an animal's well-being is essential. Instead of being an afterthought, pre-visit medication interventions and sedation should often be the primary strategy, particularly to guarantee that animals receive all the care they require.

7.9 References

1. Tooley, C., & Heath, S. E. (2023). Emotional arousal impacts physical health in dogs: A review of factors influencing arousal, with exemplary case and framework. *Animals*, 13(3), 465.

2. McMillan, F. D. (2005). Stress, distress and emotion: Distinctions and implications for mental well-being. In F. D. McMillan (Ed.), *Mental Health and Well-Being in Animals* (pp. 93–111). Blackwell Publishing.

3. Heath, S. (2018). Understanding feline emotions . . . and their role in problem behaviours. *Journal of Feline Medicine and Surgery*, 20(5), 437–444.

4. Rodan, I., et al. (2022). AAFP/ISFM Cat friendly veterinary interaction guidelines: Approach and handling techniques. *Journal of Feline Medicine and Surgery,* 24(11):1093–1132.

5. Taylor, S., et al. (2022). SFM/AAFP Cat friendly veterinary environment guidelines. *Journal of Feline Medicine and Surgery*, 24(11), 1133–1163.

6. Mills, D., Karagiannis, C., & Zulch, H. (2014). Stress—its effects on health and behavior: A guide for practitioners. *Veterinary Clinics: Small Animal Practice*, 44(3), 525–541.

7. Grigg, E. K., Hetts, S., & Shanan, A. (2023). Recognizing distress. In *Hospice and Palliative Care for Companion Animals: Principles and Practice* (pp. 44–61).

8. Ryan, B. C., & Vandenbergh, J. G. (2002). Intrauterine position effects. *Neuroscience & Biobehavioral Reviews*, 26(6), 665–678.

9. Morgane, P. J., Mokler, D. J., & Galler, J. R. (2002). Effects of prenatal protein malnutrition on the hippocampal formation. *Neuroscience & Biobehavioral Reviews*, 26(4), 471–483.

10. Weaver, I. C., Cervoni, N., Champagne, F. A., D'Alessio, A. C., Sharma, S., Seckl, J. R., Dymov, S., Szyf, M., & Meaney, M. J. (2004). Epigenetic programming by maternal behavior. *Nature Neuroscience*, 7(8), 847–854.

11. Bosch, G., Beerda, B., Hendriks, W. H., Van der Poel, A. F., & Verstegen, M. W. (2007). Impact of nutrition on canine behaviour: Current status and possible mechanisms. *Nutrition Research Reviews*, 20(2), 180–194.

12. Appleby, D. L., Bradshaw, J. W., & Casey, R. A. (2002). Relationship between aggressive and avoidance behaviour by dogs and their experience in the first six months of life. *Veterinary Record*, 150(14), 434–438.

13. Glover, V. (2015). Prenatal stress and its effects on the fetus and the child: Possible underlying biological mechanisms. In *Perinatal programming of neurodevelopment* (pp. 269–283).

14. Van den Bergh, B. R., Mulder, E. J., Mennes, M., & Glover, V. (2005). Antenatal maternal anxiety and stress and the neurobehavioural development of the fetus and child: Links and possible mechanisms. A review. *Neuroscience & Biobehavioral Reviews*, 29(2), 237–258.

15. Talge, N. M., Neal, C., Glover, V., (2007). Antenatal maternal stress and long-term effects on child neurodevelopment: How and why? *Journal of Child Psychology and Psychiatry*, 48(3–4), 245–261.

16. Bale, T. L. (2005). Is mom too sensitive? Impact of maternal stress during gestation. *Frontiers in Neuroendocrinology*, 26(1), 41–49.

17. Son, G.H., Geum, D., Chung, S., Kim, E. J., Jo, J. H., Kim, C. M., Lee, K. H., Kim, H., Choi, S., Kim, H. T. & Lee, C. J., (2006). Maternal stress produces learning deficits associated with impairment of NMDA receptor-mediated synaptic plasticity. *Journal of Neuroscience*, 26(12), 3309–3318.

18. Akatsu, S., Ishikawa, C., Takemura, K., Ohtani, A., & Shiga, T. (2015). Effects of prenatal stress and neonatal handling on anxiety, spatial learning and serotonergic system of male offspring mice. *Neuroscience Research*, 101, 15–23.

19. Chan, J. C., Nugent, B. M., & Bale, T. L. (2018). Parental advisory: maternal and paternal stress can impact offspring neurodevelopment. *Biological psychiatry*, *83*(10), 886–894.

20. Meek, L. R., Dittel, P. L., Sheehan, M. C., Chan, J. Y., & Kjolhaug, S. R. (2001). Effects of stress during pregnancy on maternal behavior in mice. *Physiology & behavior*, 72(4), 473–479

21. Parker, V. J., & Douglas, A. J. (2010). Stress in early pregnancy: maternal neuro-endocrine-immune responses and effects. *Journal of reproductive immunology*, 85(1), 86–92.

22. Jagoe, A., & Serpell, J. (1996). Owner characteristics and interactions and the prevalence of canine behaviour problems. *Applied Animal Behaviour Science*, 47(1–2), 31–42.

23. Guardini, G., Mariti, C., Bowen, J., et al. (2016). Influence of morning maternal care on the behavioural responses of 8–week-old Beagle puppies to new environmental and social stimuli. *Applied Animal Behaviour Science*, 181, 137–144.

24. Foyer, P., et al. (2013). Early experiences modulate stress coping in a population of German shepherd dogs. *Applied Animal Behaviour Science*, 146(1–4), 79–87.

25. Foyer, P., Wilsson, E., & Jensen, P. (2016). Levels of maternal care in dogs affect adult offspring temperament. *Scientific Reports*, 6(1), 19253.

26. Santos, N. R., Beck, A., & Fontbonne, A. (2020). A review of maternal behaviour in dogs and potential areas for further research. *Journal of Small Animal Practice*, 61(2), 85–92.

27. Casey, R. A., & Bradshaw, J. W. S. (2008). The effects of additional socialisation for kittens in a rescue centre on their behaviour and suitability as a pet. *Applied Animal Behaviour Science*, 114(1–2), 196–205.

28. Boone, G., et al. (2022). The effect of early neurological stimulation on puppy welfare in commercial breeding kennels. *Animals*, 13(1), 71.

29. Battaglia, C. L. (2009). Periods of early development and the effects of stimulation and social experiences in the canine. *Journal of Veterinary Behavior*, 4(5), 203–210

30. Schoon, A., & Berntsen, T. G. (2011). Evaluating the effect of early neurological stimulation on the development and training of mine detection dogs. *Journal of Veterinary Behavior*, 6(2), 150–157.

31. Gazzano, A., Mariti, C., Notari, L., Sighieri, C., & McBride, E. A. (2008). Effects of early gentling and early environment on emotional development of puppies. *Applied Animal Behaviour Science*, 110(3–4), 294–304.

32. Hargrave, C. (2015). Anxiety, fear, frustration and stress in cats and dogs—implications for the welfare of companion animals and practice finances. *Companion Animal*, 20(3), 136–141.

33. Herron, M. E., & Shreyer, T. (2014). The pet-friendly veterinary practice: a guide for practitioners. *Veterinary Clinics: Small Animal Practice*, 44(3), 451–481.

34. Englund, M. D., & Cronin, K. A. (2023). Choice, control, and animal welfare: definitions and essential inquiries to advance animal welfare science. *Frontiers in Veterinary Science*, 10.

35. Horowitz, A. (2021). Considering the “dog” in dog–human interaction. *Frontiers in Veterinary Science, 8*, 642821.

36. Littlewood, K. E., Heslop, M. V., & Cobb, M. L. (2023). The agency domain and behavioral interactions: assessing positive animal welfare using the Five Domains Model. *Frontiers in Veterinary Science*, 10. https://doi.org/10.3389/fvets.2023.1284869

37. Sydänheimo, A., Freeman, M., & Hunt, K. (2023). Cooperative Care Does Not Scare–Use of Cooperative Care Training in Routine Husbandry in Dogs. *Animal Behaviour and Welfare Cases*, abwcases20230010.

38. Jones, E. (2023). Cooperative care for companion dogs: emotional health and wellness. *Companion Animal, 28*(7), 1–6.

39. Jones, E. (2023). Preparing fearful dogs for vaccinations with cooperative care. *Animal Behaviour and Welfare Cases*, abwcases20230011.

40. Wess, L., Böhm, A., Schützinger, M., Riemer, S., Yee, J. R., Affenzeller, N., & Arhant, C. (2022). Effect of cooperative care training on physiological parameters and compliance in dogs undergoing a veterinary examination–A pilot study. *Applied Animal Behaviour Science*, 250, 105615.

41. Siniscalchi, M., d'Ingeo, S., Minunno, M., & Quaranta, A. (2018). Communication in dogs. *Animals*, 8(8), 131.

42. Flint, Hannah E., et al. Effect of training for dog fear identification on dog owner ratings of fear in familiar and unfamiliar dogs. *Applied Animal Behaviour Science* 208 (2018): 66–74.

43. Hargrave, C. (2017). Canine stress in a nutshell—why does it occur, how can it be recognised, and what can be done to alleviate it?. *The Veterinary Nurse*, 8(3), 140–147.

44. Hargrave, C. (2017). Feline stress in a nutshell—why does it occur, how can it be recognised, and what can be done to alleviate it? *The Veterinary Nurse*, 8(4), 192–199.

45. Wan, M., Bolger, N., & Champagne, F. A. (2012). Human perception of fear in dogs varies according to experience with dogs. *PLoS ONE*, 7(12), e51775.

46. Barletta, M., & Raffe, M. (2016). Behavioral response and cost comparison of manual versus pharmacologic restraint protocols in healthy dogs. *The Canadian Veterinary Journal*, 57(3), 258.

47. Sherman, B., & Papich, M. (2009). Drugs affecting animal behavior. In J. Reviere & M. Papich (Eds.), *Veterinary Pharmacology and Therapeutics* (9th ed., pp. 509–540). Wiley-Blackwell.

48. Posner, L., & Burns, P. (2009). Sedative agents: tranquilizers, alpha-2 agonists and related agents. In J. Riviere & M. Papich (Eds.), *Veterinary Pharmacology and Therapeutics* (9th ed., pp. 337–380). Wiley-Blackwell.

49. Crowell-Davis, S. L., Murray, T. F., & de Souza Dantas, L. M. (2019). *Veterinary psychopharmacology*. John Wiley & Sons.

50. Van Haaften, K. A., Forsythe, L. R. E., Stelow, E. A., et al. (2017). Effects of a single pre appointment dose of gabapentin on signs of stress in cats during transportation and veterinary examination. *Journal of the American Veterinary Medical Association*, 251(10), 1175–1181.

51. Pankratz, K. E., Ferris, K. K., Griffith, E. H., et al. (2018). Use of single-dose oral gabapentin to attenuate fear responses in cage-trap confined community cats: A double-blind, placebo-controlled field trial. *Journal of Feline Medicine and Surgery*, 20(6), 535–543.

52. Kruszka, M., Graff, E., Medam, T., et al. (2021). Clinical evaluation of the effects of a single oral dose of gabapentin on fear-based aggressive behaviors in cats during veterinary examinations. *Journal of the American Veterinary Medical Association*, 259(11), 1285–1291.

53. Stollar, O. O., Moore, G. E., Mukhopadhyay, A., Gwin, W., & Ogata, N. (2022). Effects of a single dose of orally administered gabapentin in dogs during a veterinary visit: a double-blinded, placebo-controlled study. *Journal of the American Veterinary Medical Association*, 260(9), 1031–1040.

54. Elsner, S., Medam, T., & Masson, S. (2021). Effects of a single oral dose of gabapentin on storm phobia in dogs: A double-blind, placebo-controlled crossover trial. *Veterinary Record*, 189(7)

55. Johnson, B. A., Aarnes, T. K., Wanstrath, A. W., Pereira, C. H. R., Bednarski, R. M., Lerche, P., & McLoughlin, M. A. (2019). Effect of oral administration of gabapentin on the minimum alveolar concentration of isoflurane in dogs. *American Journal of Veterinary Research*, 80(11), 1007–1009.

56. Tucker, L. E., Sanchez, A., Valverde, A., Blois, S., Uccello, O., Rutherford, A., Monteith, G., et al. (2023). Pharmacokinetic, sedative, and physiological effects of oral compounded formulations of trazodone alone or in combination with gabapentin in male cats. *Journal of Veterinary Pharmacology and Therapeutics*, 46(5), 300–310.

57. Quimby, J. M., Lorbach, S. K., Saffire, A., Kennedy, A., Wittenburg, L. A., Aarnes, T. K., Creighton, K. J., Jones, S. E., Paschall, R. E., King, E. M., & Bruner, C. E. (2022). Serum concentrations of gabapentin in cats with chronic kidney disease. *Journal of Feline Medicine and Surgery*, 24(12), 1260–1266.

58. Lamminen, T., Korpivaara, M., Aspegrén, J., Palestrini, C., & Overall, K. L. (2023). Pregabalin alleviates anxiety and fear in cats during transportation and veterinary visits—A clinical field study. *Animals*, 13(3), 371.

59. Lamminen, T., Doedée, A., Hyttilä-Hopponen, M., et al. (2022). Pharmacokinetics of single and repeated oral doses of pregabalin oral solution formulation in cats. *Journal of Veterinary Pharmacology and Therapeutics*, 45(4), 385–391.

60. Kim, S. A., Borchardt, M. R., Lee, K., Stelow, E. A., & Bain, M. J. (2022). Effects of trazodone on behavioral and physiological signs of stress in dogs during veterinary visits: a randomized double-blind

placebo-controlled crossover clinical trial. *Journal of the American Veterinary Medical Association*, 260(8), 876–883.

61. Stevens, B. J., Frantz, E. M., Orlando, J. M., et al. (2016). Efficacy of a single dose of trazodone hydrochloride given to cats prior to veterinary visits to reduce signs of transport-and examination-related anxiety. *Journal of the American Veterinary Medical Association*, 249(2), 202–207.

62. Arnold, A., Davis, A., Wismer, T., & Lee, J. A. (2021). Suspected hepatotoxicity secondary to trazodone therapy in a dog. *Journal of Veterinary Emergency and Critical Care*, 31(1), 112–116.

63. Cohen, A. E., & Bennett, S. L. (2015). Oral transmucosal administration of dexmedetomidine for sedation in 4 dogs. *The Canadian Veterinary Journal*, 56(11), 1144.

64. Dent, B. T., et al. (2019). Pharmacokinetics and pharmacodynamic effects of oral transmucosal and intravenous administration of dexmedetomidine in dogs. *American Journal of Veterinary Research*, 80(10), 969–975.

65. Gioeni, D., et al. (2020). Oral transmucosal or intramuscular administration of dexmedetomidine–methadone combination in dogs: Sedative and physiological effects. *Animals*, 10(11), 2057.

66. Hauser, H., Campbell, S., Korpivaara, M., et al. (2020). In-hospital administration of dexmedetomidine oromucosal gel for stress reduction in dogs during veterinary visits: A randomized, double-blinded, placebo-controlled study. *Journal of Veterinary Behavior*, 39, 77–85.

67. Hopfensperger, M. J., et al. (2013). The use of oral transmucosal detomidine hydrochloride gel to facilitate handling in dogs. *Journal of Veterinary Behavior*, 8(3), 114–123.

68. Messenger, K. M., Hopfensperger, M., Knych, H. K., & Papich, M. G. (2016). Pharmacokinetics of detomidine following intravenous or oral-transmucosal administration and sedative effects of the oral-transmucosal treatment in dogs. *American Journal of Veterinary Research*, 77(4), 413–420.

69. Ogata, N., & Dodman, N. H. (2011). The use of clonidine in the treatment of fear-based behavior problems in dogs: An open trial. *Journal of Veterinary Behavior*, 6(2), 130–137.

70. Väisänen, M., Raekallio, M., Kuusela, E., et al. (2002). Evaluation of the perioperative stress response in dogs administered medetomidine or acepromazine as part of the preanesthetic medication. *American Journal of Veterinary Research*, 63, 969–975.

71. Piotti, P., Uccheddu, S., Alliani, M., et al. (2019). Management of specific fears and anxiety in the behavioral medicine of companion

animals: Punctual use of psychoactive medications. *Dog Behavior*, 2, 23–30.

72. Bergeron, R., et al. (2002). Physiology and behavior of dogs during air transport. *Canadian Journal of Veterinary Research*, 66(3), 211.

73. Rankin, D. C. (2015). Sedatives and tranquilizers. In K. A. Grimm, L. A. Lamont, W. J. Tranquilli, et al. (Eds.), *Veterinary Anesthesia and Analgesia* (5th ed., pp. 196–206). Ames, Iowa: Wiley Blackwell.

74. Costa, R. S., Jones, T., Robbins, S., Stein, A., & Borns-Weil, S. (2023). Gabapentin, melatonin, and acepromazine combination prior to hospital visits decreased stress scores in aggressive and anxious dogs in a prospective clinical trial. *Journal of the American Veterinary Medical Association*, 1(10), 1–6.

75. Simon, B. T., & Steagall, P. V. (2020). Feline procedural sedation and analgesia: When, why, and how. *Journal of Feline Medicine and Surgery*, 22(11), 1029–1045.

76. Grubb, T., Sager, J., Gaynor, J. S., Montgomery, E., Parker, J. A., Shafford, H., & Tearney, C. (2020). 2020 AAHA anesthesia and monitoring guidelines for dogs and cats. *Journal of the American Animal Hospital Association*, 56(2), 59–82.

77. Wiese, W. Muir P. Lerche A., and L. Nelson K. Pasloske T. Whittem (2008). Cardiorespiratory and anesthetic effects of clinical and supraclinical doses of alfaxalone in dogs. *Veterinary Anaesthesia and Analgesia*, 35(6), 451–462.

78. Maney, J. K., Shepard, M. K., Braun, C., Cremer, J., & Hofmeister, E. H. (2013). A comparison of cardiopulmonary and anesthetic effects of an induction dose of alfaxalone or propofol in dogs. *Veterinary anaesthesia and analgesia*, 40(3), 237–244.

79. Warne, L. N., Beths, T., Whittem, T., Carter, J. E., & Bauquier, S. H. (2015). A review of the pharmacology and clinical application of alfaxalone in cats. *The Veterinary Journal*, 203(2), 141–148.

80. TTamura, J., Ishizuka, T., Fukui, S., Oyama, N., Kawase, K., Miyoshi, K., Sano, T., Pasloske, K., & Yamashita, K. (2015). The pharmacological effects of the anesthetic alfaxalone after intramuscular administration to dogs. *Journal of Veterinary Medical Science*, 77(3), 289–296.

Author
Christine D. Calder DVM, DACVB

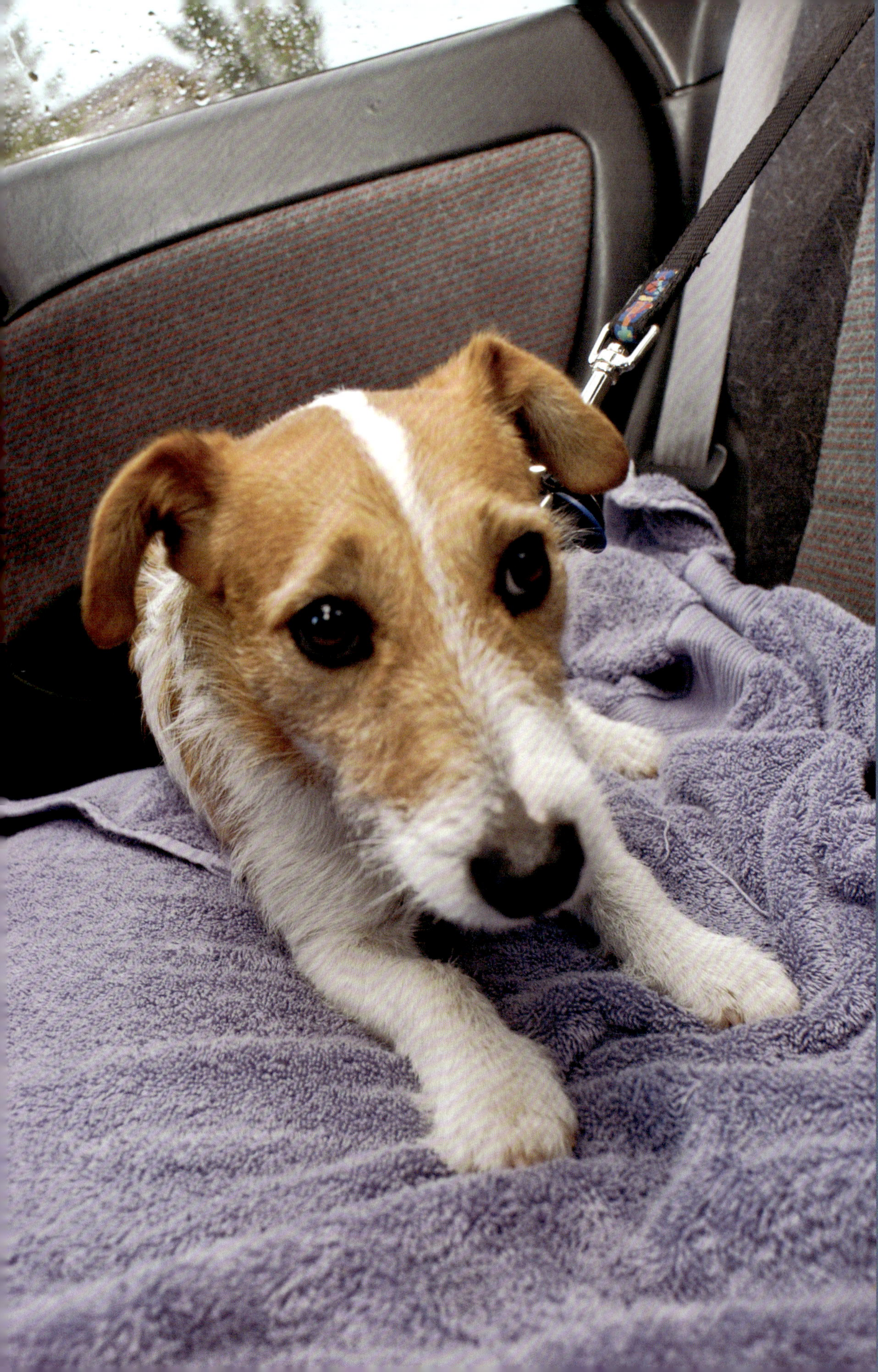

CHAPTER 8

Low Stress Handling®: Home to the Hospital

8.1 Introduction

Veterinary visits can be stressful for both animals and caregivers, often leading to postponed care. Veterinary teams can minimize that distress by creating a low stress environment and applying Low Stress Handling® techniques during visits. Preparation begins at home and continues through the car journey to the veterinary hospital.

8.2 Creating a Low Stress Handling® Environment

When caring for animals, addressing all sensory needs throughout the hospital visit is vital to reduce stress and anxiety.[1–4]

The Waiting Room

Since waiting rooms can be a stressful environment, making modifications to this space can help ensure a low stress experience.[5] Patients that can see other animals and people may become frightened or overstimulated quickly. If possible, a separate, dedicated waiting room or corner for cats is ideal. Cats in carriers should be covered, elevated, and arranged to minimize and avoid contact with other cats and dogs.

Table 8.2.1: Sensory Considerations in the Hospital

Auditory	• Exam rooms should be in low traffic areas and separate from other animals. • White or brown noise machines mask noise. • Species-specific music • Keep human voices low. Turn down or off cellphone ringers. • Use draft protectors to minimize outside sound.
Olfactory	• Clean rooms thoroughly between patients with an unscented cleaner. • Use dedicated cat examination and waiting room • Pheromone products (diffusers, sprays) on towels and bandanas • Catnip or silver vine products for cats if not overly arousing
Visual	• Window film • Walls, shelves, screens, and furniture to divide waiting room • Remove artwork with animal likenesses.
Taste	• Treats with different delivery methods (syringes, squeeze pouches, pretzels, lickable mats or tubes) • Food filled puzzle toys
Tactile	• Non-slip mats and rugs on slippery surfaces, exam room tables, and scales • Monitor response to touch and petting. • Keep constant contact when touching and examining (don't lift hands on and off).

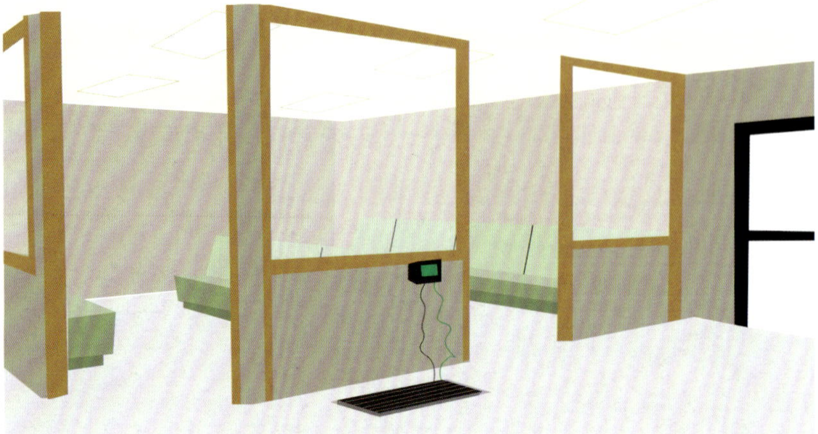

Fig. 8.2 A: For feline patients, a separate room, entrance, and waiting area is ideal.

Clinic Cats

Clinic cats should not be permitted in the waiting room, examinations rooms, or left free in cat wards since this may cause conflict with pets in carriers or on leashes.

Strategically adding partial walls or rearranging furniture minimizes visibility and provides safe areas to elevate cat carriers. Maintain seating areas far apart to prevent accidental encounters. Small collapsible screens are economical and make great visual barriers when needed.

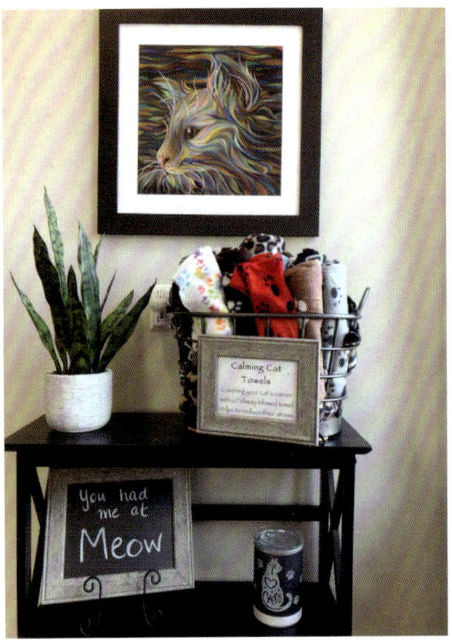

Fig. 8.2 B:. Provide towels or blankets to cover cat carriers. These can be sprayed with synthetic pheromones to help improve comfort levels. (Photo courtesy of Colleen Koch)

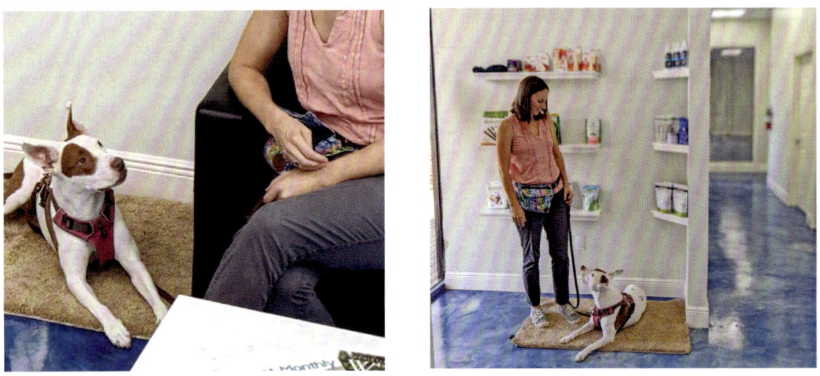

Figs. 8.2 C, D: A portable mat can help a dog relax while waiting for their appointment. (Photos courtesy of Laura Ansel)

Flooring Considerations

In hospitals, floors that are easy to clean and disinfect are essential. However, slippery, shiny, or uneven surfaces can pose risks for dogs. Smooth floors, for instance, can be challenging for those with orthopedic or neurological issues, leading to slips, falls, and hesitations. Placing non-slip mats or rugs, particularly in thresholds, hallways, and examination areas, provides safer footing.

Weight Scale

Scales are often shiny, stainless steel, and raised off the floor, creating an unappealing and potential physical obstacle. A recessed or low-profile scale is preferred. Placing a rubber mat on the scale improves traction. Teaching patients how to station on a raised surface is a cooperative care skill that can be useful. A stocked treat jar near the scale or snuffle mat on the scale provides a quick and immediate opportunity to reward patients in position.

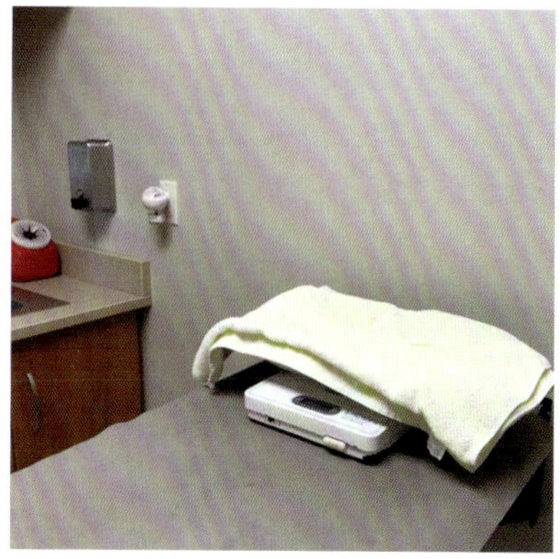

Fig. 8.2 E: For cats, a pheromone-infused towel should be placed on the scale before weighing. To entice a cat onto the scale, use treats or wand toys. (Photo courtesy of Dr. Colleen Koch)

Weighing Smokey Inside His Carrier

Smokey, a cautious tabby cat, had always been a bit wary of the veterinary hospital. His caregiver, Lou, understood Smokey's fears and anxieties and did his best to make each visit as low stress as possible. Today, however, Smokey was due for a procedure that required sedation, and that meant getting weighed.

Lou gently set Smokey's carrier, wrapped in a pheromone-infused towel he had selected from the basket at the entrance, on a low table in the cat waiting area. From inside the carrier, Smokey's wide eyes indicated his fear. Lou leaned in closer and spoke softly to his anxious feline companion, "Don't worry, Smokey. We'll face this together, and it'll be alright."

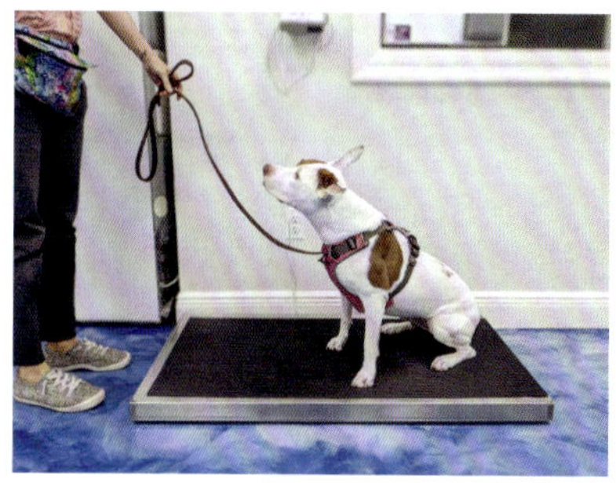

Fig. 8.2 F: A non-slip mat on the weight scale improves traction. (Photo courtesy of Laura Ansel)

The veterinary technician, Sarah, approached to offer her assistance. Recognizing Smokey's unease, she gently proposed, "If it would make Smokey more comfortable, we can weigh him inside his carrier. We have the weight of his carrier from his previous visit documented in his chart. Is this the same carrier you used at that visit?"

Lou nodded gratefully, realizing this might be the best approach for their anxious feline friend. Sarah carefully lifted the carrier with Smokey inside and placed it on the scale. She noted the weight displayed on the digital screen.

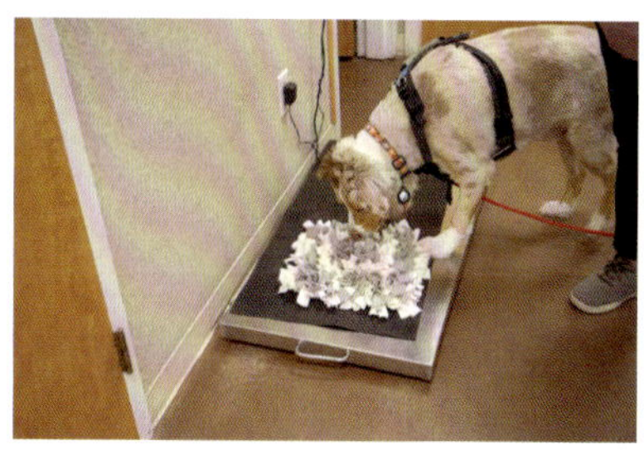

Fig. 8.2 G: A snuffle mat on the weight scale encourages engagement with the scale, making the dog more likely to step up on their own.

"Alright, Smokey's carrier with him inside weighs 15.2 pounds," Sarah announced as they walked into the examination room. In the room, she verified that the carrier itself weighs 3.1 pounds. Sarah did some quick math. "So, Smokey weighs 15.2 pounds inside the carrier, and the empty carrier weighs 3.1 pounds. To determine Smokey's weight, we need to subtract the weight of the carrier from today's weight with Smokey inside."

Lou watched as Sarah performed the calculation. "15.2 minus 3.1 equals . . . 12.1 pounds. Smokey weighs 12.1 pounds," Sarah confirmed.

Lou breathed a sigh of relief. "Thank you, Sarah. That's a clever way to weigh him without causing too much stress. Smokey will be back to his normal self in no time."

With the weight measurement complete, Smokey was ready for his sedation. Lou left smiling knowing Smokey was in good hands. He would return later after Smokey had awaken from his procedure.

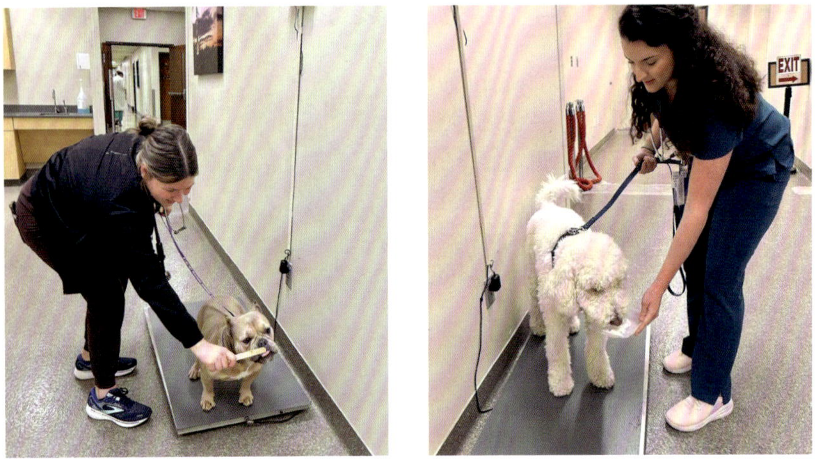

Figs. 8.2 H, I: A lure can be used to position dogs onto the scale and encourage them to briefly stand still for the most accurate weight. (Photos courtesy of Louisiana State University School of Veterinary Medicine Community Practice)

Max's Scale Challenge

In a busy veterinary hospital, Sophia faced a unique challenge with her dog, Max. Since his last visit as a puppy, Max had grown considerably, and obtaining his current weight was necessary. But there was a problem: Max was terrified of the scale.

Sophia knew she needed a creative solution to get Max on the scale; therefore, she prepared an array of distractions, including a snuffle mat, a lickable mat for the wall, and Max's favorite treat—chicken. She knew that she had the option of using a "touch" or "feet up" cue to encourage Max to voluntarily step onto the scale, if needed.

Sophia decided to start with Max's favorite walking game, the Control Unleashed® 1-2-3 Game. Starting simply, the game began in the parking lot as she counted "1, 2" then "3" in a slightly higher pitch, immediately handing Max a chicken reward after every "3." This game not only distracted Max but also helped establish a predictable rhythm for his walk into the hospital and onto the scale.

After entering the veterinary hospital, Sophia gently directed Max toward the scale while keeping up the rhythm of the game. As they moved around the room and onto the scale, she continued counting, "1," "2," and then "3," promptly rewarding Max with a piece of chicken as he stood still on the scale. This approach helped to maintain engagement they waited for the scale to record his weight. Engrossed in the game and the tantalizing scent of chicken, Max barely realized he was standing on the scale.

Once the weight was recorded, Sophia didn't break stride. She continued the counting game as they moved off the scale and walking down the hallway to the examination room. Max, motivated by the treats and the familiar pattern, stayed engaged throughout the process.

Treatment Area

The treatment area of a veterinary hospital can be stressful and overstimulating for many patients.[6] If possible, patients should remain in the examination room with clients for all procedures including vaccinations and venipuncture.[7–13] If a visit to the treatment area cannot be avoided, cats should be transported in carriers and dogs on leashes for safety reasons.

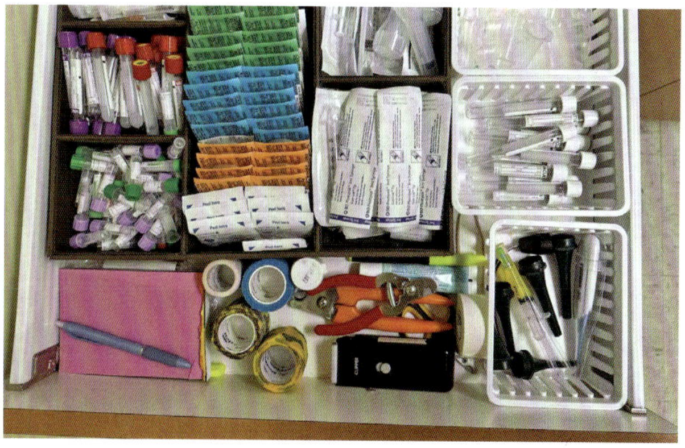

Fig. 8.2 J: Drawers should be fully stocked and ready to use. (Photo courtesy of Eliot Veterinary Hospital)

Each examination room and station in the treatment area should be well stocked with high-value treats and all necessary medical supplies. This helps to avoid a wait or the need to carry the patient around the area while collecting equipment and supplies. For cats, a dedicated area should be created that is secure and quiet; however, if a quiet area cannot be found, wait until one is available.

Kennels and Cages

Many veterinary hospitals and animal care facilities will house and hospitalize animals in the treatment area. Often centrally located, this area tends to be full of activity with the movement of dogs, cats, and people passing through the hospital. Animals housed in this area should be arranged in such a way to reduce overstimulation and emotional arousal. Placement of lightweight towels or sheets on kennel and cage doors provides privacy and opportunities to hide.[14,15] Plastic partitions, glass walls, frosted window film, or opaque barriers allow for direct observations while still considering the comfort level of animals.

If immediate care or monitoring during recovery from anesthesia is not needed, animals should be moved to different wards. House cats in kennels or cages arranged to prevents them from seeing other animals on treatment tables or in adjacent cages. Cover half of the kennel door with towels or sheets, offers both cats and dogs the option to either hide or observe their surroundings. A transparent or sheer drape can provide visual access to the animal while maintaining a sense of privacy.

Exam Room Sedation

Whenever possible, cats should remain in the examination room for all procedures (e.g., blood draw, cystocentesis, ultrasound). If the treatment room cannot be avoided, sedation should occur in the examination room and the cat moved into the treatment area once fully sedated. An alternative is to ask the caregiver to wait outside until the procedure is complete instead of removing the cat from the room. If sedation is needed, and a room is not readily available, the cat should be transported to a quiet area of the hospital in their carrier for the sedation process.

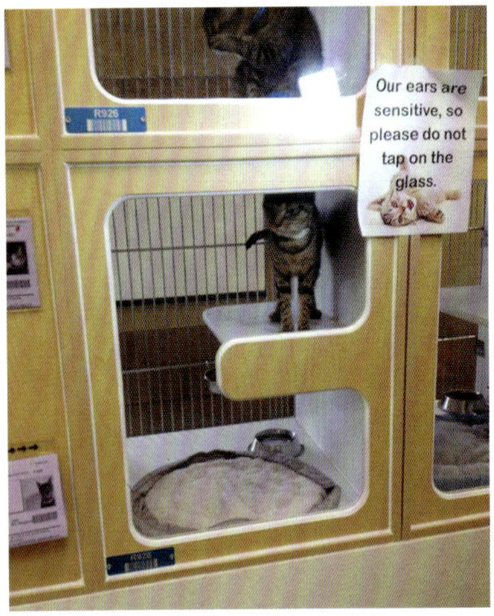
Our ears are
sensitive, so
please do not
tap on the
glass.

Fig. 8.2 K: Steel walls can be highly reflective, potentially causing stress. Brushed steel helps to reduce these reflections. For cats, non-metal options are preferable due to their non-reflective nature (photo courtesy of Riverside County Department of Animal Services)

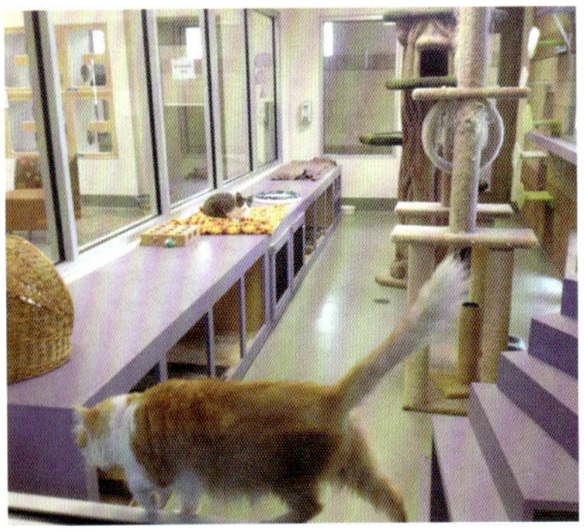

Fig. 8.2 L: In the shelter, providing an enriched environment is of the utmost importance. Cats should have the opportunity to select their resting and hiding spots (photo courtesy of Riverside County Department of Animal Services).

Kennels and Cages

Kennel and cage doors with metal components tend to be loud, resulting in a startle effect and elevated stress levels. Clipboards and caddies attached to the doors can contribute to this sound aversion. For some brands of kennels and cages, sound dampening devices are commercially available. Training team members to open and close these doors with care to minimize noise.

Boarding and Kennel Areas

If boarding or grooming services are offered, a low stress environment should be standard. The same is true in a shelter setting. To minimize stress, dogs should not have visual or direct contact through walls, fences, or gates. Additionally, extraneous noises (e.g., drying fans on kennel doors) should be limited, especially around cats. Whenever possible, cats should be accommodated in a designated cat-only boarding room, with specialized enrichment opportunities tailored to the needs of shelter cats and those with extended stays.

Resting Areas

Elevated beds with soft bedding provide dedicated resting places for cats especially those with arthritis. Towels or pet beds are easy to replace and clean. However, raised hammock-style beds may pose a lower risk for dogs that tend to consume bedding.

Hospitalized and Boarding Cats

Hospitalized and boarding cats, need access to hiding and resting areas separate from their food and water. These areas should be distinct from the litterbox.[16–19] For kennels with limited space, low-sided cardboard boxes, high-sided cat beds, or carrier bottoms can be used to create these spaces, ensuring adequate separation between the litterbox and feeding area.[20]

Audio Enrichment

In shelters, boarding facilities, and veterinary clinics, some types of music and audiobooks have been shown to have a calming effect on animals and people. Music broadcasted from a computer, tablet, or phone, via hardwired or portable Bluetooth® speakers, helps to reduce ambient noises and promote quiet time.[6,21]

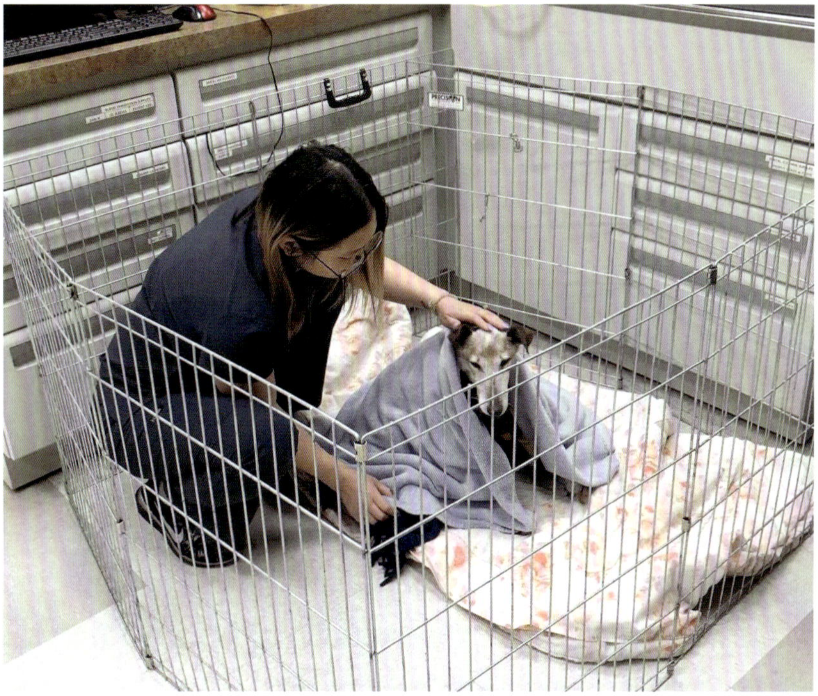

Fig. 8.2 M: For larger dogs, dogs with confinement anxiety, or those with mobility concerns, an exercise pen may be more suitable during their stay. (Photo courtesy of Jessica Benoit)

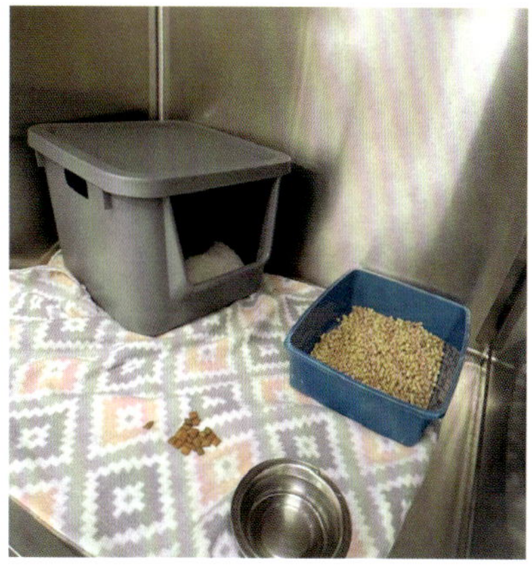

Fig. 8.2 N: Hospitalized and boarding cats need hiding and resting areas. Their food and water should be located away from their litterbox. (Photo courtesy of Sara Berger, LVT, FFCP, CFVP).

Cleaning Between Patients

In between patients, rooms should be cleaned and disinfected to remove debris and minimize other animal scents.[22] In hospitals with a high percentage of feline patients, a dedicated cat room can shorten the amount of time it takes to air out the room between appointments. Rooms can be stocked with species-specific treats, toys, and for cats, hiding boxes, that are easy to disinfect and clean.

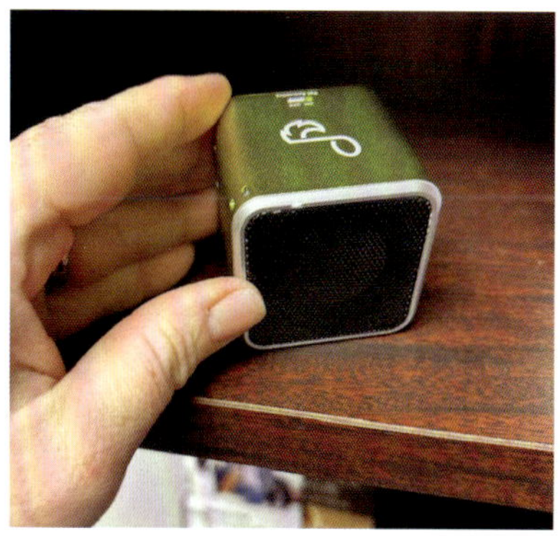

Fig. 8.2 O: Bluetooth speakers can be used in exam rooms, hospital wards, and boarding areas. Music and audiobooks have been shown to have a calming effect on some animals and people. (Photo courtesy of Sara Berger, LVT, FFCP, CFVP)

8.3 Preparing for Low Stress Handling® Veterinary Visits

The Low Stress Handling® preparation process begins when scheduling with the customer service representative (CSR). The CSR should check the medical record for prior notes, including the pet's handling plan. Discussing the pet's behavior before departure, during the car ride, and at the hospital with the client aids in planning the visit.

During scheduling, the script should have questions such as:

- Is your pet cautious or fearful of the carrier or their harness/collar/leash when getting ready?
- In the car, does your pet vocalize, pant, drool, or vomit?
- Does your pet hesitate at the entrance?
- Does your pet bark, hiss, or growl at other animals?
- Is a muzzle necessary for your dog?
- Does your pet require pre-visit medications or sedation for the appointment?

Scheduling Appointments

Effective communication during the scheduling of the appointment starts the preparation to keep stress to a minimum during veterinary visits.

If the client answers "yes" to any questions, consider scheduling the pet during quieter times or having the client wait in the car until an exam room is ready. This helps the pet enter the hospital without confronting other animals or people, preserving their emotional well-being. A follow-up call might be necessary to discuss further options, including medications and supplements. Prescribing medication requires an established veterinary-client-patient relationship as per their state's Veterinary Practice Act. Inform new clients that an examination might not be possible during the initial visit, and a subsequent appointment may be required once medications are prescribed.

Checklist for the Veterinary Visit

When confirming appointments, provide clients with a checklist for the visit. This may include:

- appropriate travel equipment such as a pet-safe carrier, collar or harness, and non-retractable leash
- a basket muzzle (if the dog has been conditioned to wear a muzzle)
- multiple types of treats, including high-value treats (e.g., chicken, fish, or fish paste, Churu®, tripe, peanut butter).
- favorite toys
- pheromone-infused cloth items (e.g., towel or bandana)

- a favorite mat, blanket, or bed
- puzzle toys or enrichment items (e.g., stuffed frozen Kong®, Toppl®, lickable mat, or snuffle mat)
- catnip, silvervine, Tatarian honeysuckle, or valerian root; catnip has no effect for some cats, and others can become agitated[4,23]

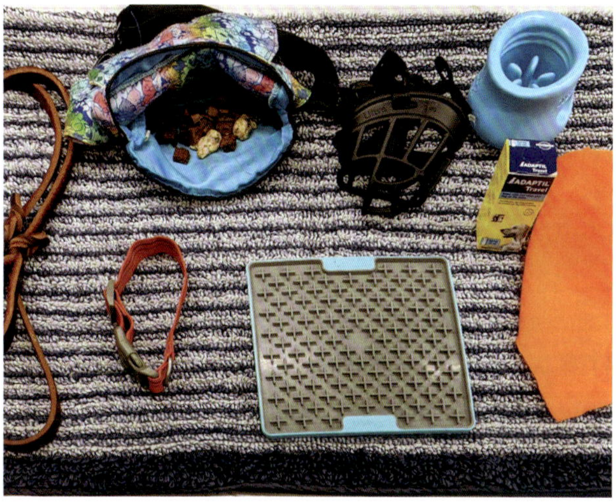

Fig. 8.3 A: Items to pack for a dog may include a mat for stationing, well-fitted collar and leash, pheromone-sprayed bandana, high-value treats, a previously conditioned muzzle, and puzzle toys. (Photo courtesy of Laura Ansel)

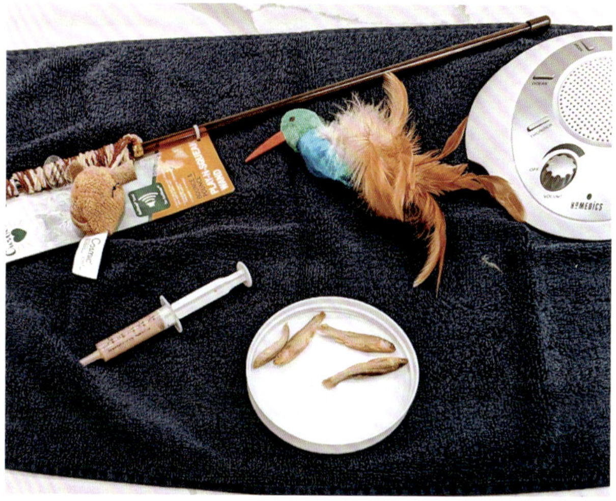

Fig. 8.3 B: Items to pack for a cat may include feather toys, catnip toys, pheromone-sprayed towel, and high-value treats. A sound machine may be useful in the room. (Photo courtesy of Laura Ansel)

Benefits of Carrier Training

For cats, carrier training reduces signs of stress during car rides and leads to shorter veterinary examinations.[24–27] Caregivers should be encouraged and instructed how to train their cats using positive reinforcement.[25,26] Discussions on how to carrier train should be introduced during kitten visits.

The ideal carrier should have multiple openings and a removable top. These types of carriers are commercially available and allow for disassembling for Low Stress Handling® examinations and sedation. The addition of a pheromone-infused towel, catnip (only if calming), and favorite toy increases a cat's willingness to enter. If the cat is harness and leash trained, remove the leash once in the carrier for safety reasons.

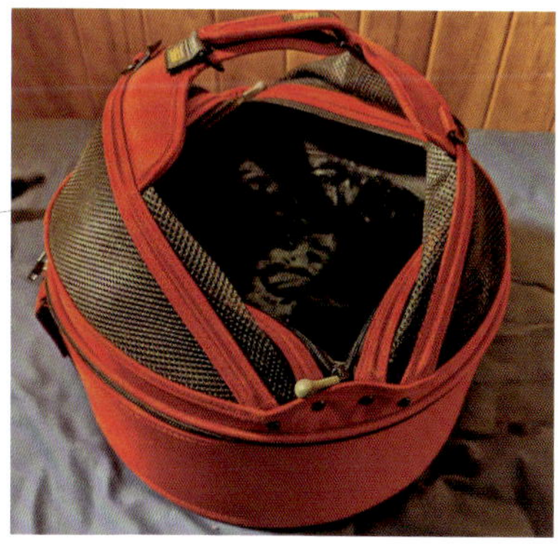

Fig. 8.3 C: For cats and small dogs, a round carrier may be preferred.

Carrier Training

Carriers are also beneficial for some dogs. Just as with cats, carrier training should be done when they are young. Information on carrier training can be found here:

https://veterinarypartner.vin.com/doc/?id=10282561&pid=19239

Walking Equipment

At home, dogs and cats should be fitted with appropriate equipment. These items improve ease of handling during transport and in the hospital, minimizing the risk of escape or injury.

Basic equipment includes a:

- well-fitted flat buckle or quick snap collar allowing for two fingers to fit easily between the collar and neck (dogs).
- four-to-six-foot standard leash with working snap or clasp (dogs and cats).
- well-fitted harness (dogs and cats).
- appropriately fitted head harness (dogs only).
- basket muzzle that allows the dog to pant, eat treats, and drink water but does not rub their eyes or fall off their nose when the head is tilted downward (dogs only).

For escape artists, additional equipment includes:

- a coupler connecting the collar and harness. a separate leash for each separate piece of equipment (e.g., collar, harness, head halter) (dogs only).

This equipment should be conditioned well in advance of the veterinary visit and should be on the dog or cat before leaving the house. For those clients that arrive without a carrier, one can be

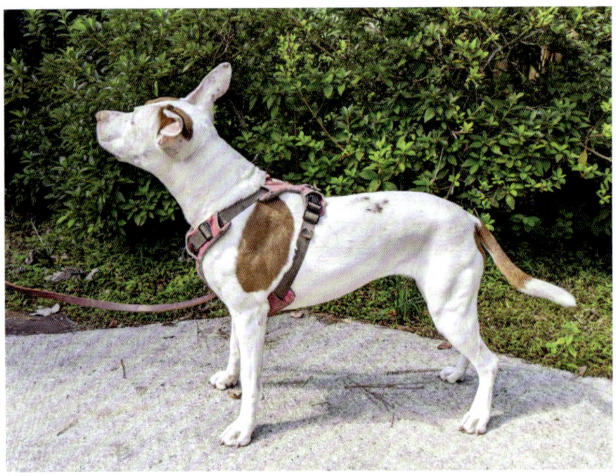
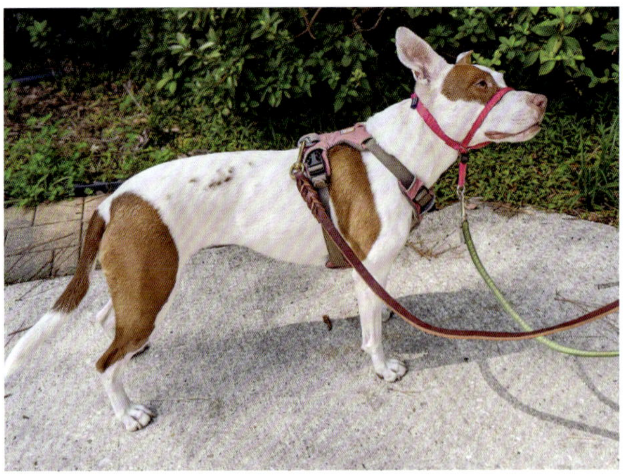

Figs. 8.3 D, E: Use a well-fitted harness with a six-foot leash attached. This dog is wearing two devices (head halter and harness), each with a separate leash. (Photos courtesy of Laura Ansel)

gifted, sold, or loaned. The return of loaned carriers should not be expected until after the cat is safely back home.

Avoid equipment that relies on pain, fear, or discomfort to inhibit behavior. Such tools are not aligned with the Low Stress Handling® methodology and should not be used in stressful settings like the veterinary hospital. In fact, if a patient enters the hospital wearing these tools, they should be removed at every visit. This proactive measure serves a dual purpose: it provides an opportunity for caregiver education and ensures that patients do not endure additional stressors and pain during the visit, thereby reducing the risk of fear conditioning and promoting a more positive experience for the pet.

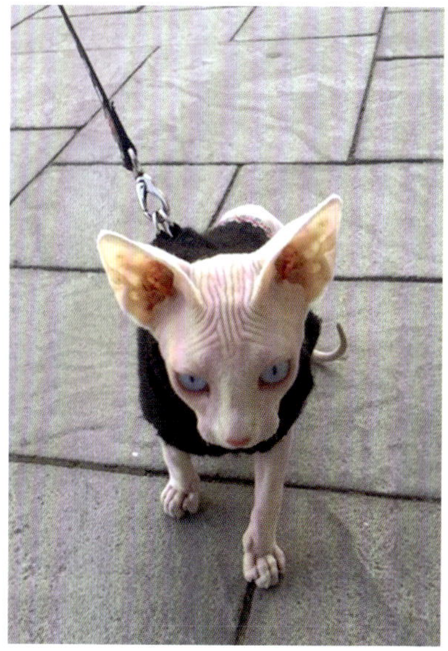

Fig. 8.3 F: Leashes and harnesses are not just for dogs. Teaching cats to be comfortable walking and wearing a harness and leash has many benefits.

Equipment to avoid includes:

- prong or pinch collars
- chain or choke collars that tighten around the neck
- retractable leashes
- nylon sleeve and Comfort® (Coastal Pet Products) muzzles
- shock (static) collars that provide electric, vibration, or beeping corrections
- citronella, ultrasonic, or anti-bark collars

Using Food

Food is a primary reinforcer and essential for survival. It serves as an effective distraction, alters emotional responses, and rewards specific behaviors.[28] While many dogs are open to a variety of foods, some, along with many cats, can be more selective, particularly when stressed.[29] Each animal has its own reinforcement hierarchy, which may include food, toys, praise, or petting.

Caregivers often understand their pets' food preferences. In stressful environments, some animals may willingly eat their regular kibble as treats, whereas others might need higher-value items. Encourage caregivers to bring a variety of treats and toys to each appointment. In addition, the facility should stock their own selection.

Cut treats into pea-sized pieces for quick consumption and minimal chewing. Items like hot dogs, cheese, and chicken can be prepared at the beginning of the week and stored in the fridge.

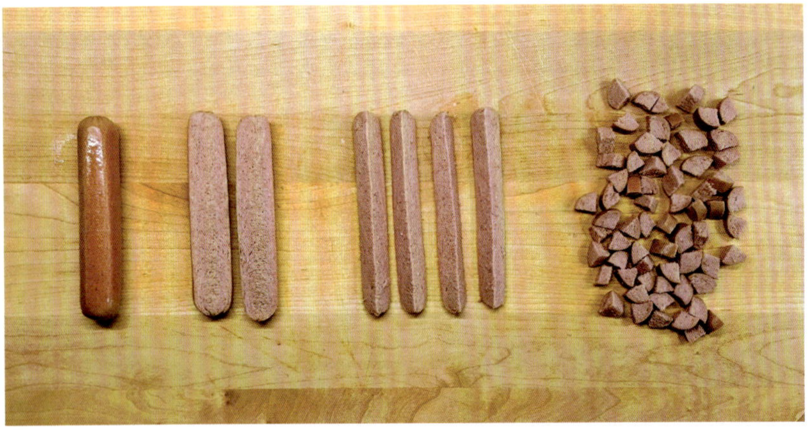

Fig. 8.3 G: A single, standard-size hot dog can be sliced and chopped into 64 pieces, yielding small, easily consumed treats for dogs. (Photo courtesy of Laura Ansel)

Some animals prefer crunchy treats. Withholding meals to encourage eating during a visit is not advised.

Cats and some dogs often show reluctance towards unfamiliar foods. Introducing them to new foods early on can pique their interest and broaden their dietary preferences, making them more adaptable to various foods. Offering pill pockets as treats from a young age, helps to make mediation administration easier as they age.

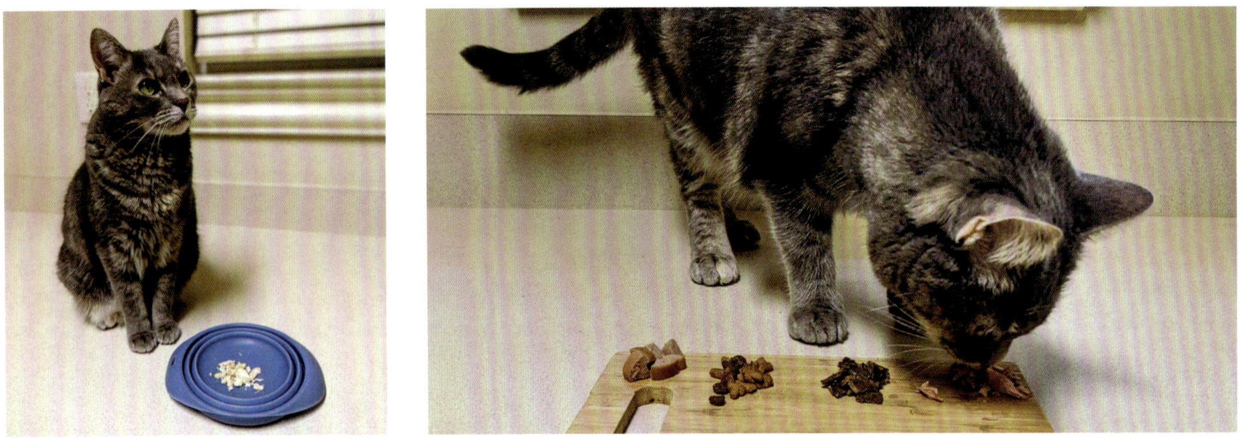

Figs. 8.3 H, I: Regularly offer cats at least one new food item to encourage broadening their food preferences. Treat buffets give an opportunity to observe treat preferences. (Photos courtesy of Laura Ansel)

Food Choices

Introducing small amounts of new foods with regular meals can encourage cats and picky dogs to try different options. Offering a variety of kibble or canned foods that feature diverse flavors and textures can effectively broaden their dietary choices.

Dietary Considerations

Some animals have dietary restrictions due to medical conditions (e.g., diabetes mellitus, food intolerance, weight concerns) or client concerns (food allergies, cultural restrictions, their own preferences). These restrictions and preferences should be noted in the medical record so that veterinary team members can accommodate them.

8.4 The Car Ride

Car ride anxiety is common in pets and can sometimes be difficult to differentiate from motion sickness. For animals experiencing this type of anxiety or those experiencing motion sickness (e.g., drooling, vomiting, panting, vocalizing), pre-visit medications can help reduce both nausea and anxiety.[30,31]

Additional ways to reduce anxiety on car rides includes:

- playing species-specific calming music[32–34]
- spraying pheromone products on the floor mats, a towel, or bandana[1]
- using lavender spray on a towel or car diffuser (dogs only)
- applying a compression vest (e.g., ThunderShirt® or calming wrap)
- offering enrichment toys (e.g., snuffle mat, lickable mat, frozen food puzzles)
- remote-activated treat dispenser

Carriers should be properly secured in the vehicle. For cats, the safest location for the carrier, is on the floor behind the passenger seat to minimize movement. Secure larger carriers in the back seat or interior cargo area of a vehicle. Impact-resistant crates are available in various sizes, and some can be permanently secured inside vehicles.

Animals should never be allowed to roam freely or ride in the front seat for safety reasons. Do not transport carriers or crates in a truck bed or in a non-climate-controlled cargo space (e.g., car trunks). Puppies and kittens should be trained from an early age to accept the seatbelt or carrier.

Offering a long-lasting food toy helps to occupy the pet. A remote treat dispensing device can be used to safely deliver treats without distracting the driver. Products that offer both automatic and remote button dispensing options are available.

If overly stimulated by activity outside the vehicle, reducing visual access may be needed.[35] Use a lightweight, breathable sheet or towel to cover the crate or carrier. When seat belted, window shades and wearable products (e.g., tinted goggles, eye shades) may be beneficial.

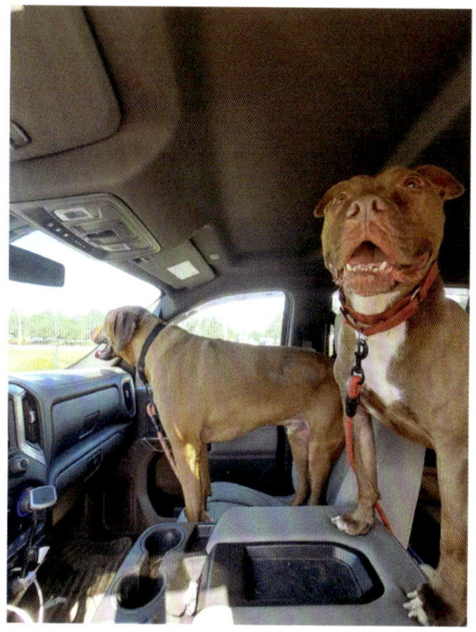

Fig. 8.4 A: Car ride anxiety is common and should be addressed to decrease veterinary visit stress.

Safety First

See ***centerforpetsafety.org*** for more information regarding which carriers and seat belt harness have passed crash testing.

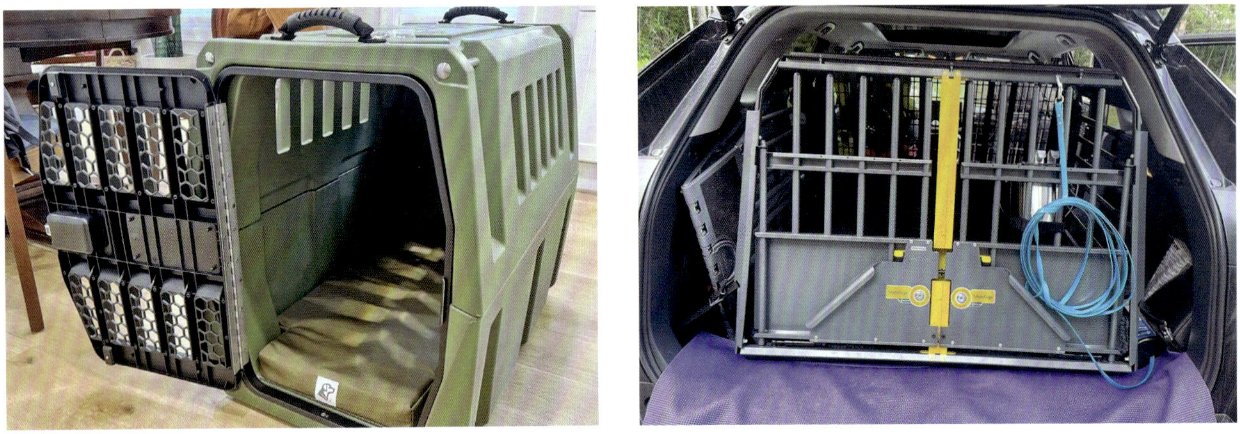

Fig. 8.4 B, C: Two different styles of impact resistant crates for car safety.

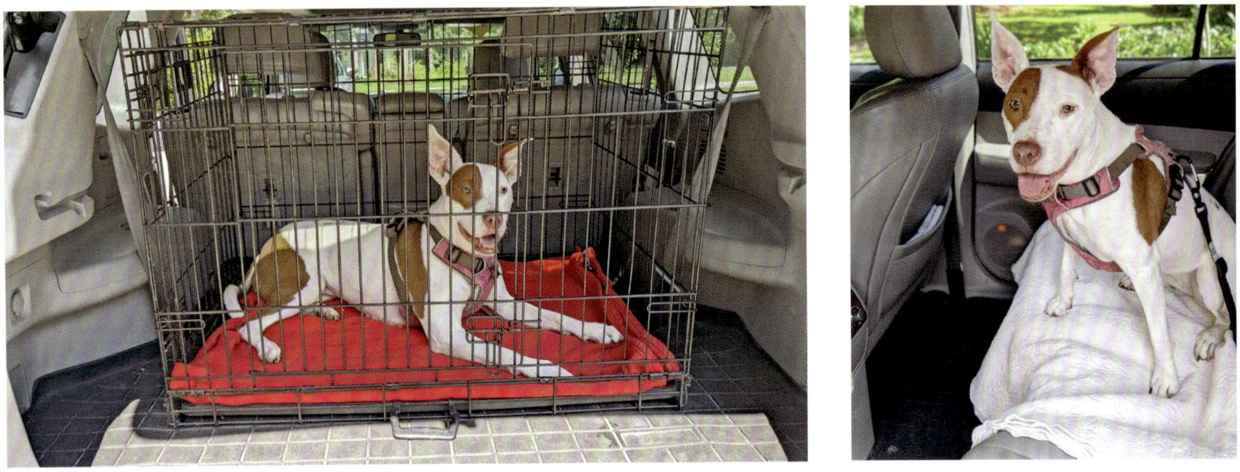

Figs. 8.4 D, E: Crates can be placed in cargo areas for safe travel. Alternatively, seat belt restraints can keep dogs confined to the backseat. (Photos courtesy of Laura Ansel)

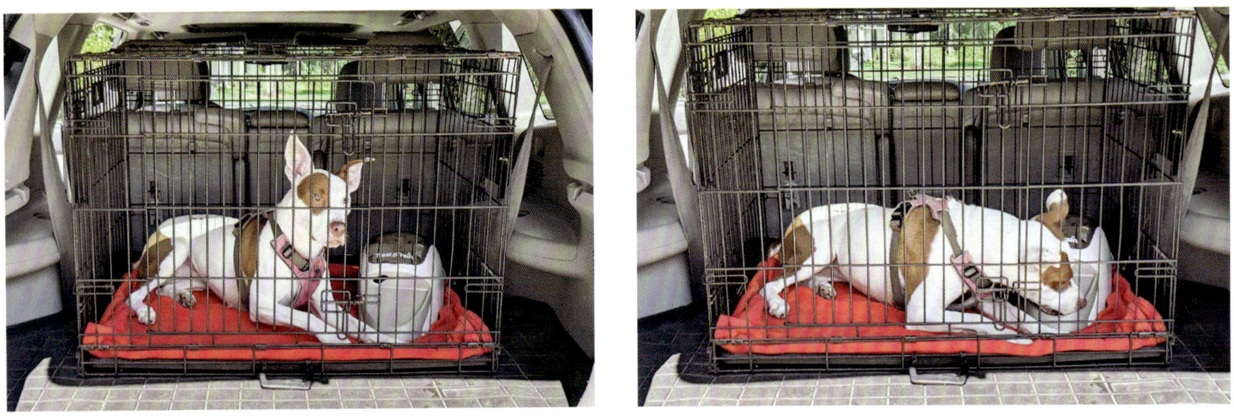

Figs. 8.4 F, G: A remote treat dispenser is used to dispense treats to a dog in a crate while riding in the car. (Photos courtesy of Laura Ansel)

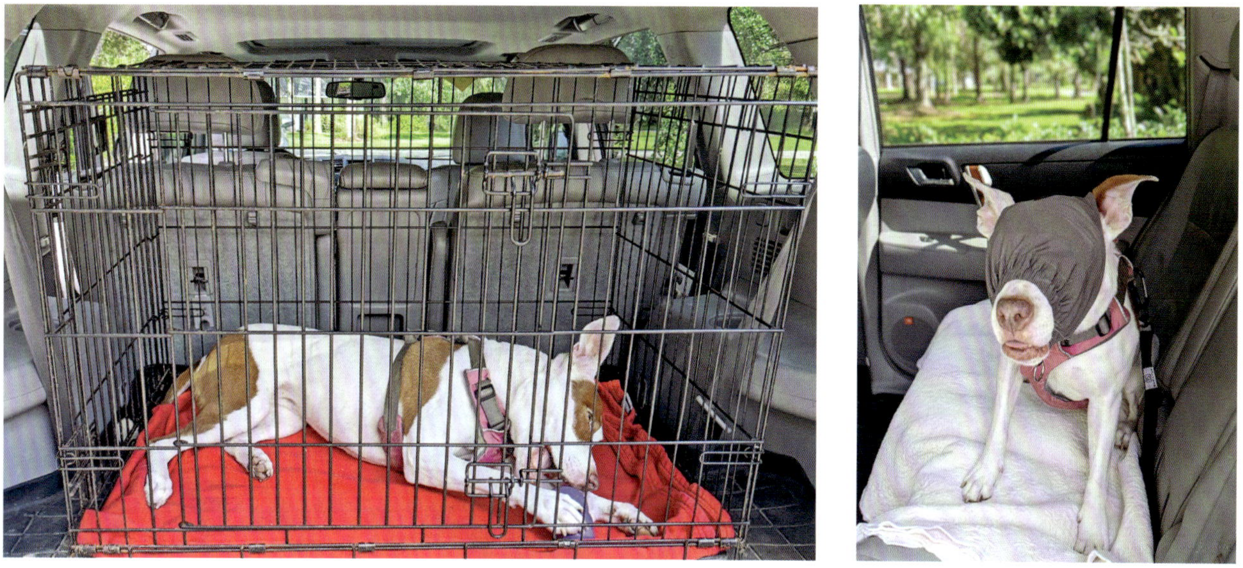

Figs. 8.4 H, I: Food toys provide distraction from outside activity. Masks (Thundercap®) help to keep dogs calm by reducing visual input. (Photos courtesy of Laura Ansel)

8.5 Arrival

The waiting room is a stressful place for many patients, especially during busy times.[36] Remaining in the car or walking around a quiet area outside can minimize stress and trigger stacking. When scheduling, identify those patients who benefit from remaining in a temperature-controlled vehicle until an examination room opens. The caregiver can then call to check in upon arrival and wait for a team member to escort them to a room.

Before opening the vehicle door to exit, a leash should already be in place to reduce the risk of escape. For dogs that require and have been conditioned to wear a basket muzzle, caregivers should also apply it before leaving home or upon arrival in the car.[37]

If a client chooses to stay outside, transferring the pet to a veterinary team member will be necessary. This transfer should occur outside the vehicle so the team member does not reach inside to take the pet. This may need to occur several feet from the vehicle, on the sidewalk, or a nearby grassy area. If removing an animal from the car, make sure the pet is in a covered carrier before lifting.

When approaching dogs, team members should face away and toss treats beyond the dog to prevent motivational conflict. When passing the leash, the client should hand it to the team member

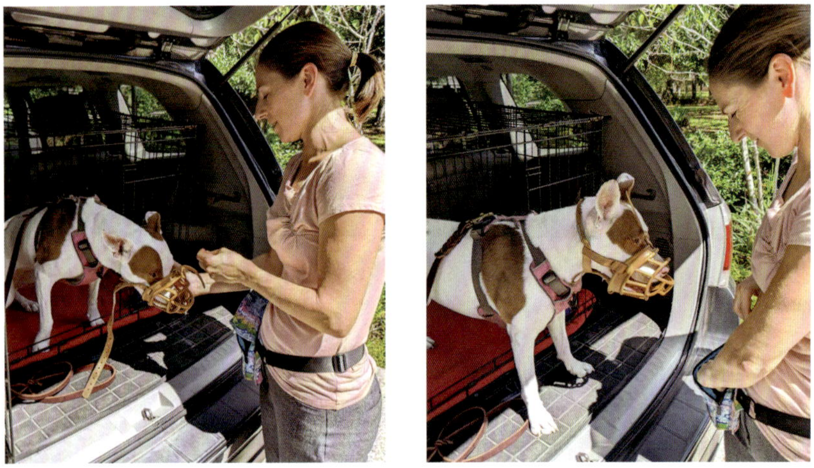

Figs. 8.5 A, B: Muzzles can be applied before exiting the care and entering the clinic. Appropriately sized muzzles allow for panting, drinking, and consuming treats. (Photos courtesy of Laura Ansel)

in a way that avoids reaching over the dog. For small dogs that need to be carried, transfer their hind end first to the other person. If this is too stressful, place the dog on the ground and do a leash transfer instead.

Scenario 1: Mrs. Smith and Sugar

On a bright, sunny morning, Mrs. Smith arrived at the veterinary hospital, unable to carry her cat, Sugar, after a recent surgery. The veterinary team was ready to assist, and Sugar's carrier, covered with a pheromone-infused towel was safely tucked on the floor behind the passenger seat. Waiting anxiously in her car, Mrs. Smith hoped for the best for Sugar. Ashley, a veterinary team member, approached with a gentle smile, knowing that her calm and relaxed behavior would be reassuring for both Mrs. Smith and Sugar. She carefully reached for the carrier taking extra care to avoid startling Sugar and securely carried it inside. In the examination room, Ashley opened the carrier to let Sugar explore as they waited for Mrs. Smith to join them.

Scenario 2: Anita and the Stray German Shepherd

Anita had just spotted a stray German Shepherd wandering her neighborhood. The dog seemed a bit shy, and not much was known about him but she was able to get a leash on him. Concerned, she was able to coax him into the car and drive to the local animal shelter for assistance.

Upon arrival, Katie, a shelter team member, arrived and cautiously approached the dog, tossing treats beyond the dog to avoid startling him. The German Shepherd, enticed by the treats, began to cautiously approach Katie. She waited patiently, giving him time to build trust at his own pace.

Soon the dog was taking treats from Katie and it was time to transfer the leash from Anita to Katie. To start this process, Anita, the German Shepherd, and Katie started walking parallel in the same direction away from the car and the shelter doors. Once comfortable, Anita handed the leash to Katie, and the handover went smoothly. Katie continued to engage the dog with treats as they walked back to the shelter to scan for a microchip and possibly reunite him with his caregiver.

Scenario 3: Pete and Chewy's Dental Visit

Pete arrived at the veterinary hospital with his small dog, Chewy, for a dental procedure. Chewy was nervous, so Pete carried him inside. After checking in, Clay, a veterinary team member, came to take Chewy to the prep area.

Since Chewy was a small dog, Pete initially planned to transition Chewy by transferring him hind end first but Chewy seemed stressed by this approach. Adapting quickly, Pete set Chewy down and handed the leash to Clay for a smoother transition. Chewy, more comfortable on the ground, walked with Clay to the treatment room. Pete stayed until they entered the room and then left, planning to return when Chewy was ready for pickup.

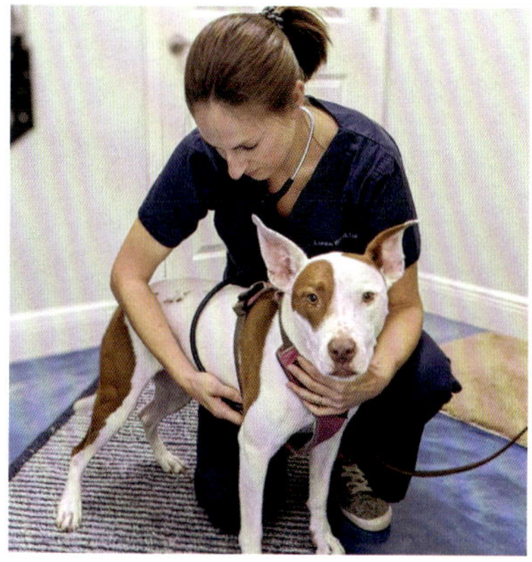

Fig. 8.6 A: A non-slip mat on the floor helps patients feel more secure. (Photo courtesy of Laura Ansel)

8.6 A Low Stress Handling® Appointment

Animals should have the choice of where their examinations and procedures take place. If they prefer the floor, they should be free to move away as desired. Ramps, steps, platforms, and lift tables enable animals to independently access the examination table, increasing their comfort and sense of control. Towels and non-slip mats on these surfaces prevent slipping and enhance stability. Many dogs and cats may choose to jump onto a bench or chair, likely because it reminds them of the couches they use at home.

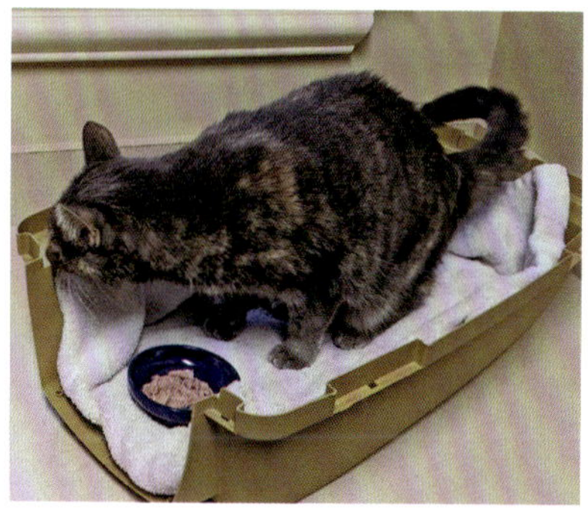

Fig. 8.6 B: Many cats prefer to be examined in their carrier. Removing the top eliminates the need to physically remove the cat. Loosely draped towels and food can further reduce stress in this situation. (Photo courtesy of Laura Ansel)

Exam and Procedure Location

For cats, examinations and procedures should be conducted in their preferred location, whether it be in the bottom half of a carrier, on someone's lap, or on a counter or table equipped with a non-slip mat. During physical examinations, lightly draped towels may be used to improve a cat's comfort. Loosely draped towels allow for selective exposure of areas of the cat for examination as needed. All equipment, including a scale and extra towels, should be kept in the room for easy access.

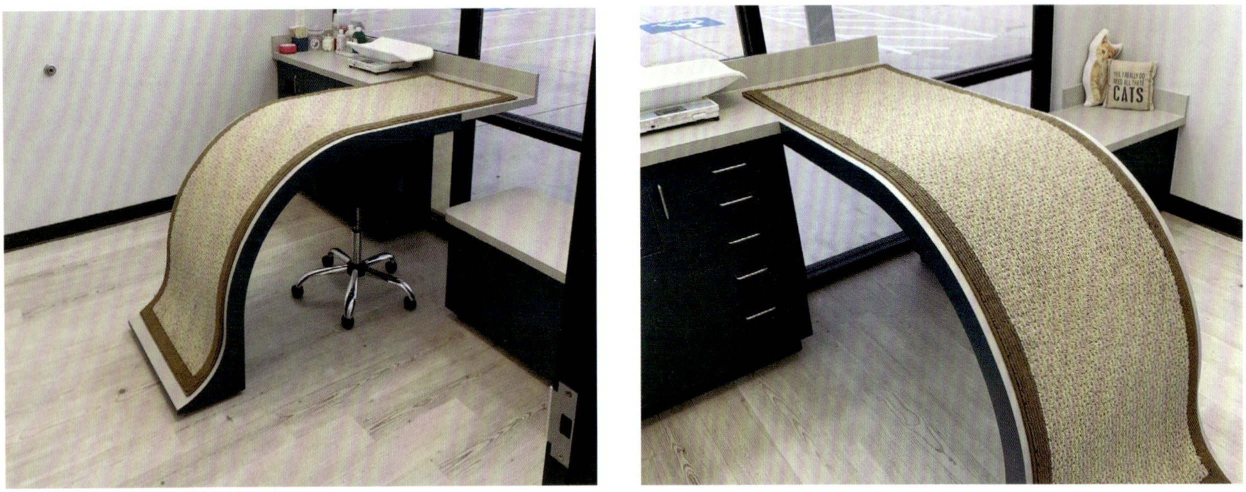

Figs. 8.6 C, D: Examination rooms dedicated to feline patients provide an opportunity to make customizations that improve comfort levels throughout the visit. (Photos Courtsey of Jennifer Le and A Couple of Vets)

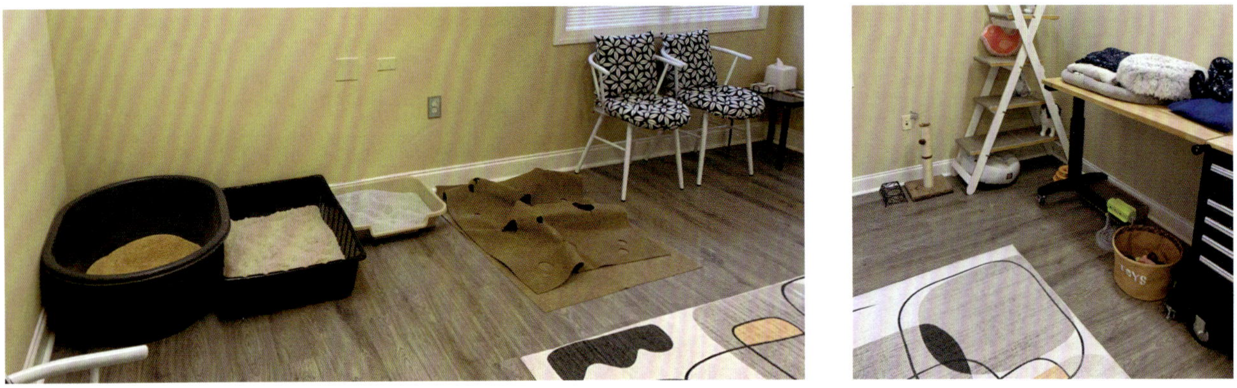

Figs. 8.6 E, F: Example of a feline only consultation room. (Photos courtesy of Lynne Seibert, DVM, DACVB)

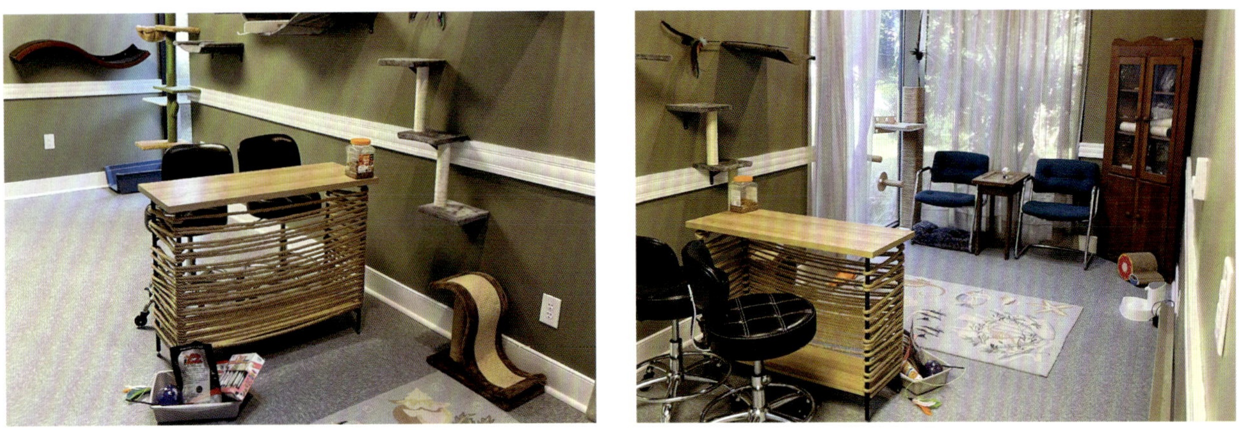

Figs. 8.6 G, H: Feline consultation/waiting area. (Courtesy of Amy Learn, VMD, DACVB, Animal Behavior Wellness Center-Richmond, VA)

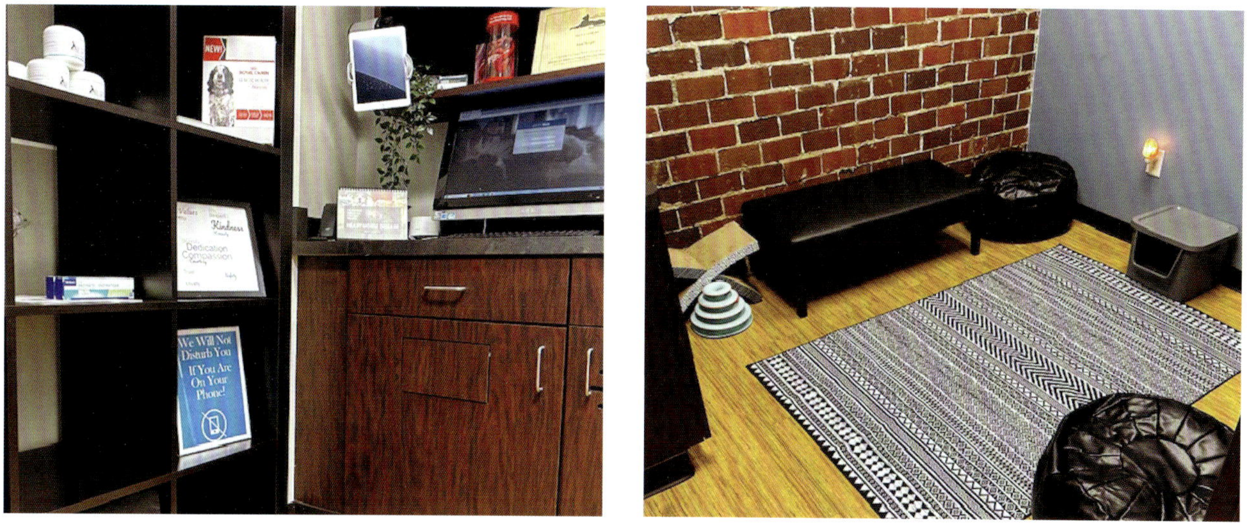

Figs. 8.6 I, J: A hiding space in the examination room helps cats feel safer. (Photos courtesy of Sara Berger, LVT, FFCP, CFVP)

Table 8.6.1: General Greeting Guidelines

DO	DO NOT
• **Assess body language**: Before approaching, observe the patient's body language to gauge their comfort level and readiness for interaction. • **Positioning**: Team members should position their bodies parallel to or slightly away from the patient, which is less intimidating than directly facing them. • **Controlled movements**: Keep arms close to the body and avoid making large or rapid movements that could startle the animal. • **Approach method:** Squat or kneel when interacting with patients to avoid looming over them, which can be perceived as threatening. • **Respect personal space**: To build trust, always encourage the animal to enter your personal space voluntarily, rather than invading their space. • **Use of treats:** Encourage clients to offer treats to their pets during visits, as this can create a positive association. • **Behavioral cues**: Cue for known behaviors, like "sit" or "touch," for positioning. • **Carrier interactions**: Invite patients to come out of their carriers on their own. If needed, remove the tops or open the lids of carriers.	• **Approach method**: Avoid approaching directly from the front of the patient, as this can be perceived as confrontational or intimidating. • **Respecting personal space**: Refrain from reaching for or leaning towards the patient, which could be seen as an invasion of their personal space and cause stress. • **Handling with care**: Do not physically push, pull, or try to manipulate the patient into a position. Such actions can cause fear or discomfort. • **Use of treats**: Avoid forcing patients to take treats directly from hands. This can be threatening for some animals, especially if they are anxious or unfamiliar with the person. • **Carrier interaction**: Do not reach into carriers to touch or remove animals. This space is often seen as a safe haven for pets and invading it can result in distress.

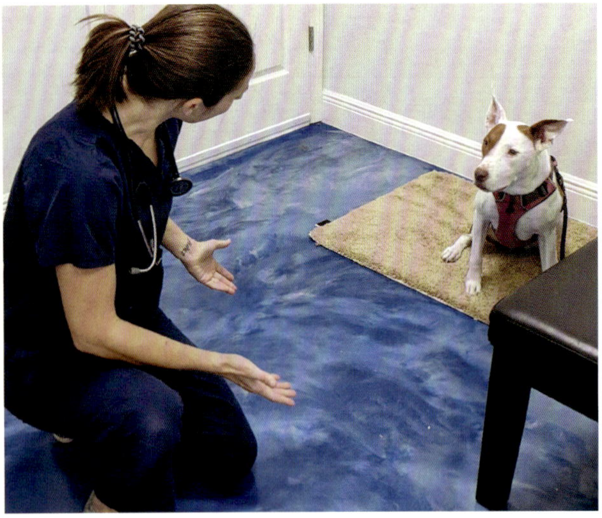

Fig. 8.6 K. A team member squatting down with their body angled away from the patient is less threatening. (Photo courtesy of Laura Ansel)

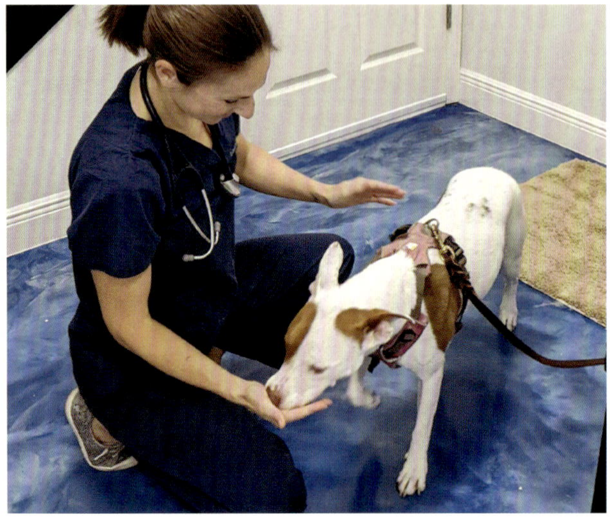

Fig. 8.6 L. Team members should give an opportunity for the animal to approach them rather than reaching for or looming over them. (Photo courtesy of Laura Ansel)

How to Greet Patients in the Hospital

Since the first interaction many animals have in a hospital is with a team member, all staff should be knowledgeable about canine and feline body language. Approaching fearful patients directly can escalate their fear, resulting in negative outcomes.[35] Team members should refrain from reaching into carriers or extracting animals from behind their caregiver's legs or from under furniture. Instead, allow them time to acclimate and explore their environment during the initial check-in and history-taking process.

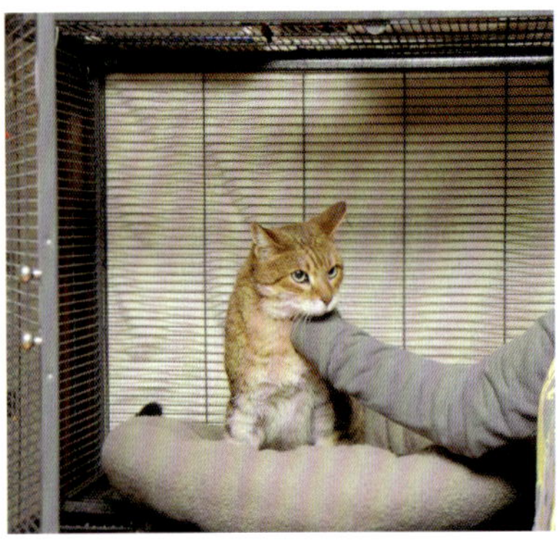

Fig. 8.6 M: When greeting cats, it is important for the cat to initiate the greeting. A hand can be offered but the cat should decide whether to interact or not.

Greeting Cats

Cats generally prefer to be pet in the temporal region, between their eyes and ears, rather than the caudal region near their tail.[38,39] To assist caregivers and veterinary team members in accommodating this preference, the Human-Cat Interaction (HCI) guidelines, also known as the "CAT" guidelines, were developed. These guidelines emphasize three key aspects: providing the cat with choice and control "C", paying attention "A" to the cat's behavior and body language, and limiting touch "T", primarily to their temporal regions. Following guidelines has been shown to reduce protective emotions in cats.[38]

Table 8.6.2: The key principles of the "CAT" interaction guidelines

Choice and Control "C"	**Provide the cat with choice and control during the interaction.**
	1 **Initiating contact**: In a seated position, gently offer a hand to the cat, allowing them to approach and decide whether to interact or not. 2 **Recognizing the cat's choice**: If a cat wants to be touched, they will typically indicate this by rubbing against a person. If there is no such contact, it is advisable to avoid petting. 3 **Respecting the cat's space**: Allow the cat to move away if they choose to do so. Do not follow the cat. 4 **Monitoring the interaction**: When petting a cat, pause briefly every 3–5 seconds to assess the cat's reaction. If the cat does not seek more contact after pausing, a break is needed.
Attention "A"	**Pay attention to the cat's behavior and body language.**
	Recognizing when a cat needs a break during interaction is key for their comfort. Here are signs to look out for: 1 **Avoidance behaviors**: The cat may turn their head or move away. 2 **Ear position**: Ears that flatten or rotate backwards can indicate discomfort. 3 **Head shaking**: A cat that shakes their head may be indicating they need space. 4 **Fur movement**: A rippling effect on the fur along their back can be a stress indicator. 5 **Nose licking**: A cat licking their nose is often a subtle sign of needing a break. 6 **Change in activity**: The cat may become still, stop purring, or cease rubbing against objects or people. 7 **Head turning:** A sharp turn of the head to face a person or their hand can signal discomfort. 8 **Brief grooming:** Sudden, short grooming sessions are sometimes a stress response. 9 **Tail movement**: Vigorous tail twitching or swishing, especially when the tail is held horizontally or close to the ground, is a clear sign of agitation.
Touch "T"	**Consider where the cat is being touched.**
	1 **Preferred touch areas**: Most relaxed cats enjoy being touched at the base of their ears, around their cheeks, and under their chin. 2 **Areas to avoid**: Avoid touching the base of the tail and the ventral abdomen as many cats find contact in these areas uncomfortable. 3 **Exercise caution**: When touching a cat's back, flank, legs, and tail, proceed cautiously. These areas can be sensitive for some cats. 4 **Observing body language**: Always pay close attention to the cat's body language to make sure they appear comfortable and relaxed during the interaction. Signs of discomfort or agitation suggest stopping or changing the approach.

Adapted from Haywood et al (2021). Providing humans with practical, best practice handling guidelines during human-cat interactions increases cats' affiliative behaviour and reduces aggression and signs of conflict. *Frontiers in Veterinary Science*, 8, 835.

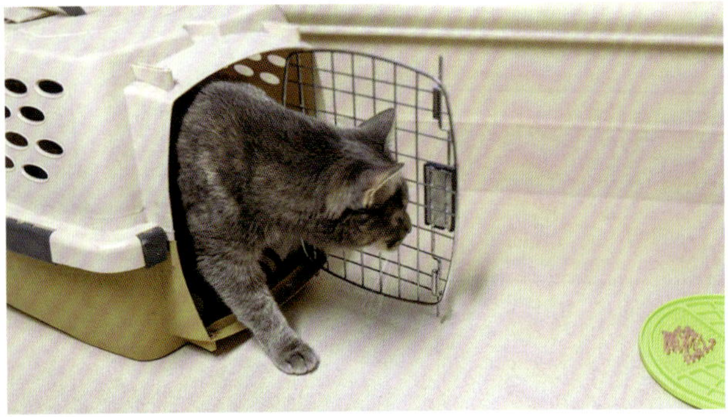

Fig. 8.6 N: Ideally carriers should be placed on the floor. Once in an enclosed room, open the carrier door for safe exit and exploration of the environment. This is especially important in elderly, sick, weak, or hurt cats to minimize the risk of falling off or jumping from the table. (Photo courtesy of Laura Ansel)

Using Cues

Handling and restraint techniques used during physical examinations and other procedures to stabilize and manipulate animals into certain positions can be a painful and confusing process. Force is never appropriate and is not considered a part of Low Stress Handling®. Luring and cueing animals into the desired positions is the preferred approach, as it allows them to make choices and maintain a sense of control.

Team members should inquire with caregivers about the behavior cues their pets are familiar with and these cues should be documented in the medical record. Behaviors such as "sit," "touch," "down," "step-up," or "chin" enable patients to be positioned using positive reinforcement and this hands-off method, minimizing stress and discomfort.

Examination

How an animal is approached for examination matters. They should always have the choice to move closer, and when they choose to do so, they should be rewarded. When providing treats, avoid feeding them directly from your hand; instead, gently toss the treats away to reduce any motivational conflict. For patients that are more at ease on the floor, consider kneeling and conducting the examination

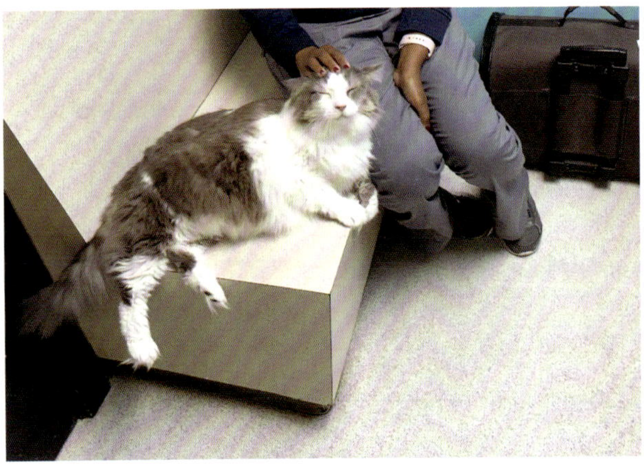

Fig. 8.6 O: Benches are great for healthy cats with good mobility and allow an opportunity to be near their caregiver for comfort.

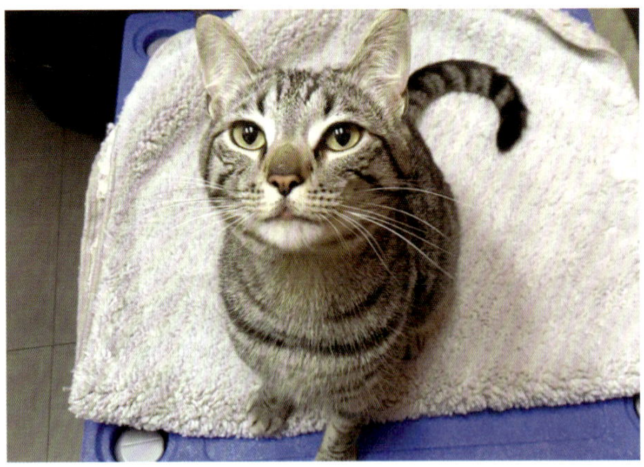

Fig. 8.6 P: Training cats to station on a platform, as part of cooperative care, offers numerous benefits. (Photo courtesy of Jessica Benoit)

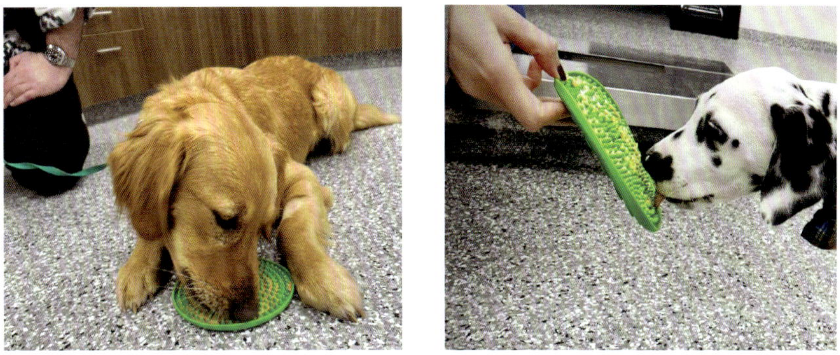

Figs. 8.6 Q, R: Using minimal handling and restraint during examinations reduces stress for many patients. Providing food distractions enhances the experience. (Photo courtesy of Louisiana State University School of Veterinary Medicine Community Practice)

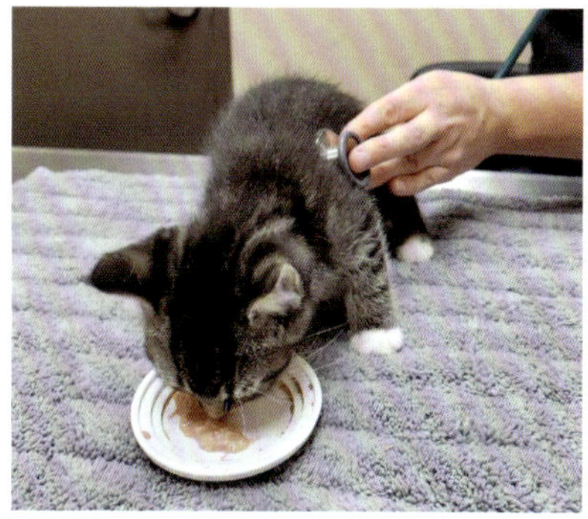

Fig. 8.6 S: Food distractions help make auscultation easier especially for wiggly kittens. (Photo courtesy of Jessica Benoit)

at their level. Use food as a distraction and offer treats throughout the examination. A food toy or a remote treat dispenser can keep patients engaged and relaxed during the process, which is the goal.

Alternative Examination Locations for Cats

Cats are often examined on tables, but alternatives like benches, high-sided cat beds, or perches can be better options. Some cats may prefer being on the floor or inside the bottom half of their carrier. If a table is necessary, using a non-slip mat on the surface provides stability and comfort. Offering treats or food toys during handling helps make the experience more pleasant for the cat.

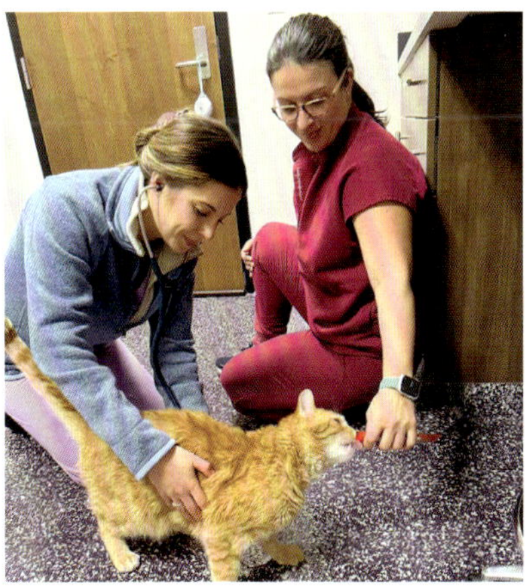

Fig. 8.6 T: Some cats are comfortable being examined on the floor with minimal handling. (Photo courtesy of Louisiana State University School of Veterinary Medicine Community Practice)

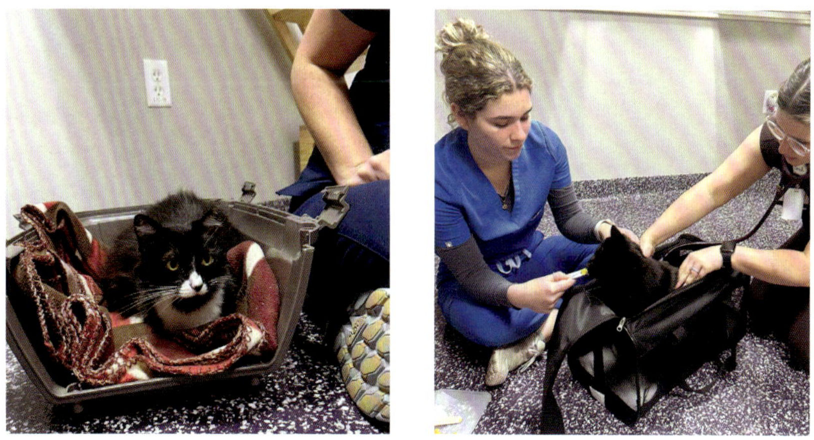

Figs. 8.6 U, V: Cats may prefer to sit on a bed, shallow-sided box, or bottom of their carrier. Some cats and dogs might like hiding under towels during exams. Uncovering one body section at a time can reduce stress and establish a predictable pattern. (Photos courtesy of Louisiana State University School of Veterinary Medicine Community Practice)

8.7 Low Stress Handling® Individualized Plan

After each visit, create an individualized handling plan documenting all preferences identified during the visit.[35] Recording the plan in the medical record allows for easy reference at future visits and includes detailed information such as:

1. **Pre-visit Medications and Sedation Plan:** Include any specific medications and dosages required for the animal, along with instructions for their administration. Detail any necessary sedation, specifying the type, dosage, and administration methods, to facilitate appropriate scheduling of the appointment.

2. **Veterinarian and Team Member Preference**: Note any preferences the animal has for certain veterinarians or staff members. This can help reduce stress and improve the overall experience for the animal, caregiver, and team members.

3. **Arrival Protocols:** Detail the most suitable way to bring the animal into the veterinary hospital. This may include using a specific entrance for anxious pets, bringing them in carriers or on specific types of leashes, or scheduling visits at quieter times.

4. **Preferred Reinforcements**: Documenting what types of positive reinforcements work best for each animal, such as treats (from high value to low value), gentle petting, grooming, or toys, to help prepare the room before the animal and caregiver arrive.

5. **Familiar Behavioral Cues:** Document known cues, such as touch, step-up, stationing, and positioning, to facilitate a smooth visit by minimizing the need for heavy restraint or manual manipulation.

6. **Examination and Procedural Location**: Some animals may feel more at ease in a particular room or setting. For example, cats might prefer a quiet, enclosed space, while dogs might be more relaxed in a larger, open area.

7. **Exit Plan:** Plan how the animal will leave the clinic, especially if they are particularly anxious or stressed post-visit. This might include a quiet exit route or assistance to the car.

Oreo's Veterinary Visit

Oreo, a 6-year-old neutered male black and white domestic short-haired cat, was terrified of the veterinary hospital. He was due for his annual wellness exam, vaccinations, and bloodwork. Three weeks before the scheduled exam, his caregiver called the veterinary hospital. Aware of Oreo's previous unease around other dogs and cats, she knew the hospital environment was particularly stressful for him.

Fortunately, the hospital had documented a handling plan for Oreo the previous year. During the call, the customer service representative reviewed this plan with his caregiver, ensuring she was well-prepared. Kristen confirmed her readiness and arranged to pick up the prescribed gabapentin later that week to help alleviate Oreo's anxiety during the car ride, examination, and during the visit itself.

Oreo's appointment was scheduled with his preferred veterinarian, Dr. Koch, on a Saturday, allowing plenty of time for preparations. Two weeks before Oreo's appointment, it was time for his caregiver to give a trial dose of the gabapentin. This trial would help determine the appropriate dose for Oreo, the optimal timing for administration, the duration of its effectiveness, and whether there were any side effects.

Table 8.7.1 Individualized Handling Plan for Oreo

Medications and Sedation Plan	Oreo requires gabapentin 100 mg, given 2 hours, by mouth, before his visit.
Veterinarian and Team Member Preference	Oreo prefers Dr. Koch due to the special lickable treats she gives him and her predictable greetings using the "touch" cue.
Arrival Protocol	Oreo's caregiver, arrives at the hospital with Oreo but waits in the car until the special examination room is ready. The customer service representative will text when it is time for Oreo's appointment.
Preferred Reinforcements	Oreo enjoys lickable treats.
Familiar Behavioral Cues	Oreo is familiar with the "touch" cue which can be used for greetings and to move him around the room, on and off the examination table if needed.
Examination and Procedural Location	Oreo prefers the end examination room with a window and bench. He likes to perch on the windowsill during his examination and look out at the flower garden. A non-slip mat should be placed there in preparation.
Exit Plan	His caregiver will check out and pay for the appointment in the examination room before exiting through a side door and returning to her car.

Appointment Day

Two hours before the appointment, Oreo received his prescribed gabapentin on a lickable mat with some wet canned food. This medication would reduce his vocalizations in the car and help him feel less anxious during the examination. Oreo's caregiver, carefully drove him to the hospital, placing his covered carrier on the floor behind the passenger seat. Upon arrival, she sent a text message to the hospital, notifying them of their arrival. They waited patiently in the car until the customer service representative responded, indicating that Oreo's special examination room was ready.

Once receiving the text message, Oreo and his caregiver made their way to the examination room, which had a window and a cozy bench, just as Oreo liked. To make Oreo's experience even more comfortable, the hospital staff had placed a soft, non-slip mat on the windowsill for him. Upon entering the room, Oreo immediately leaped onto the mat, initially showing signs of stress as he began grooming himself. However, he soon started to relax on his preferred perch. From his vantage point by the window, Oreo could observe the garden outside and watch the butterflies, providing him with a welcome distraction.

Dr. Koch entered the room with a warm and welcoming smile. Her familiarity with Oreo was an immediate source of comfort for both Oreo and his caregiver. Dr. Koch initiated their interaction by asking for a "touch," a familiar cue where Oreo's nose gently touched her outstretched finger. She then presented Oreo's favorite lickable treats, helping him to relax even more. Throughout the examination, Oreo remained remarkably calm and engaged, demonstrating the effectiveness of the carefully planned approach. This included administering gabapentin, using the familiar "touch" cue, and offering high-value treats.

Dr. Koch conducted a thorough wellness check as Oreo comfortably perched by the window. Remarkably, Oreo hardly seemed to notice the examination taking place. Thanks to the documented handling plan, the entire experience was as low stress as possible. After the examination was complete, Oreo's caregiver efficiently checked out and settled the bill right in the examination room. This arrangement ensured that Oreo did not have to encounter any other cats or dogs before exiting through the side door.

8.8 Leaving the Hospital

Just as with arrival, departure from the hospital should follow a similar protocol, especially for patients with heightened fear, anxiety, and stress. When discharging patients after hospitalization or sedated procedures, follow a structured process beginning with a review of at-home instructions and the collection of payment in an examination room, prior to reuniting the patient with their caregiver.

Comprehensive Behavioral Plan

A comprehensive behavioral plan should include documentation of the day's procedures, the patient's hospital stay, and the home environment. This plan should address the need for anti-anxiety medications, postoperative limitations, and pain relief, even for minor procedures.

Enhancing the Return Car Trip Experience

To make the return car trip more comfortable and enjoyable for the patient, provide a food-dispensing or puzzle toy in the car. This not only serves as a distraction but can also make the experience more enjoyable for the pet.

Creating a Designated Safe Space at Home

Upon arriving home, a designated safe space so the pet has a place to relax before reintegrating with other household pets. This strategy helps minimize the risk of redirected aggression resulting from heightened emotional arousal upon returning home. These post-hospitalization practices are designed to ensure the patient's well-being and comfort during their transition back to their familiar environment.

8.9 Conclusion

Using the Low Stress Handling® techniques detailed in this chapter allows for an understanding of the experience from the animal's viewpoint. By altering the environment, emotional arousal can be reduced, creating a safer and more enjoyable experience for everyone.

8.10 References

1. Anseeuw, E., Apker, C., Ayscue, C., & et al. (2006). Handling cats humanely in the veterinary hospital. *Journal of Veterinary Behavior: Clinical Applications and Research*, 1(2), 84–88.

2. King, T., Flint, H. E., Hunt, A. B., Werzowa, W. T., & Logan, D. W. (2022). Effect of music on stress parameters in dogs during a mock veterinary visit. *Animals*, 12(2), 187.

3. Zhang, L., & McGlone, J. J. (2020). Scratcher preferences of adult in-home cats and effects of olfactory supplements on cat scratching. *Applied Animal Behaviour Science*, 227, 104997.

4. Bol, S., Caspers, J., Buckingham, L., Anderson-Shelton, G. D., Ridgway, C., Buffington, C. A. T., Schulz, S., & Bunnik, E. M. (2017). Responsiveness of cats (Felidae) to silver vine (Actinidia polygama), Tatarian honeysuckle (Lonicera tatarica), valerian (Valeriana officinalis) and catnip (Nepeta cataria). *BMC Veterinary Research*, 13(1), 70.

5. Caney, S. M., Robinson, N. J., Gunn-Moore, D. A., & Dean, R. S. (2022). Happy cats: stress in cats and their carers associated with outpatient visits to the clinic. *Journal of Feline Medicine and Surgery*, 24(12), e551–e557.

6. Furgala, N. M., Moody, C. M., Flint, H. E., Gowland, S., & Niel, L. (2022). Veterinary background noise elicits fear responses in cats while freely moving in a confined space and during an examination. *Behavioral Processes*, 201(104712). https://doi.org/10.1016/j.beproc.2022.104712

7. Csoltova, E., Martineau, M., Boissy, A., & Gilbert, C. (2017). Behavioral and physiological reactions in dogs to a veterinary examination: Owner-dog interactions improve canine well-being. *Physiology & behavior*, 177, 270–281.

8. Dawson, L. C., Dewey, C. E., Stone, E. A., Guerin, M. T., & Niel, L. (2016). A survey of animal welfare experts and practicing veterinarians to identify and explore key factors thought to influence canine and feline welfare in relation to veterinary care. *Animal Welfare*, 25(1), 125–134.

9. Griffin, F. C., Mandese, W. W., Reynolds, P. S., Deriberprey, A. S., & Blew, A. C. (2021). Evaluation of clinical examination location on stress in cats: A randomized crossover trial. *Journal of Feline Medicine and Surgery*, 23(4), 364–369.

10. Mandese, W. W., Griffin, F. C., Reynolds, P. S., Blew, A. C., Deriberprey, A. S., & Estrada, A. H. (2021). Stress in client-owned dogs related to clinical exam location: a randomised crossover trial. *Journal of Small Animal Practice*, 62(2), 82–88.

11. Mariti, C., Ricci, E., Zilocchi, M., & Gazzano, A. (2013). Owners as a secure base for their dogs. *Behaviour*, 150(11), 1275–1294.

12. Stellato, A. C., Dewey, C. E., Widowski, T. M., & Niel, L. (2020). Evaluation of associations between owner presence and indicators of fear in dogs during routine veterinary examinations. *Journal of the American Veterinary Medical Association*, 257(10), 1031–1040.

13. Stellato, A. C., Flint, H. E., Dewey, C. E., Widowski, T. M., & Niel, L. (2021). Risk-factors associated with veterinary-related fear and aggression in owned domestic dogs. *Applied Animal Behaviour Science*, 241, 105374.

14. Arrandale, L., & Buckley, L. (2017). Towels versus hides: which are best at reducing acute stress in the newly hospitalised domestic cat (Felis sylvestris catus)? *Veterinary Nursing Journal*, 32(10), 285–288.

15. Buckley, L. A., & Arrandale, L. (2017). The use of hides to reduce acute stress in the newly hospitalised domestic cat (Felis sylvestris catus). *Veterinary Nursing Journal*, 32(5), 129–132.

16. Ellis, J. J., Stryhn, H., & Cockram, M. S. (2021). Effects of the provision of a hiding box or shelf on the behaviour and faecal glucocorticoid metabolites of bold and shy cats housed in single cages. *Applied Animal Behaviour Science*, 236, 105221.

17. Stella, J., Croney, C., & Buffington, T. (2014). Environmental factors that affect the behavior and welfare of domestic cats (Felis silvestris catus) housed in cages. *Applied Animal Behaviour Science,* 160, 94–105.

18. Stoneburner, R. M., Naughton, B., Sherman, B., & Mathews, K. G. (2021). Evaluation of a stimulus attenuation strategy to reduce stress in hospitalized cats. *Journal of Veterinary Behavior,* 41, 33–38.

19. Wright, C., & Baugh, S. (2018). Effectiveness of providing a box, or partially covering the cage front, on reducing cat stress. *The Veterinary Nurse*, 9(6), 328–332.

20. Pereira, G. D. G., Fragoso, S., Morais, D., de Brito, M. T. V., & de Sousa, L. (2014). Comparison of interpretation of cat's behavioral needs between veterinarians, veterinary nurses, and cat owners. *Journal of Veterinary Behavior*, 9(6), 324–328.

21. Wells, D., Graham, L., & Hepper, P. (2002). The influence of auditory stimulation on the behavior of dogs housed in a rescue shelter. *Animal Welfare,* 11(4), 385–393. doi:10.1017/S0962728600025112

22. Weese, J. S. (2015). Cleaning and disinfection of patient care items, in relation to small animals. *Veterinary Clinics: Small Animal Practice*, 45(2), 331–342.

23. Flematti, G. R. (2022). Behavioral differences among domestic cats in the response to cat-attracting plants and their volatile compounds reveal a potential distinct mechanism of action for actinidine. *BMC biology*, 20(1), 1–38.

24. Argüelles, J., Echaniz, M., Bowen, J., & Fatjó, J. (2021). The impact of a stress-reducing protocol on the quality of pre-anaesthesia in cats. *Veterinary Record*, 188(12).

25. Gruen, M. E., Thomson, A. E., Clary, G. P., Hamilton, A. K., Hudson, L. C., Meeker, R. B., & Sherman, B. L. (2013). Conditioning laboratory cats to handling and transport. *Lab Animal*, 42(10), 385–389.

26. Pratsch, L., Mohr, N., Palme, R., Rost, J., Troxler, J., & Arhant, C. (2018). Carrier training cats reduces stress on transport to a veterinary practice. *Applied Animal Behaviour Science*, 206, 64–74.

27. Tateo, A., Nanni Costa, L., & Padalino, B. (2022). The welfare of dogs and cats during transport in Europe: a literature review. *Italian Journal of Animal Science*, 21(1), 539–550.

28. Westlund, K. (2015). To feed or not to feed: Counterconditioning in the veterinary clinic. *Journal of Veterinary Behavior*, 10(5), 433–437.

29. Mariti, C., Bowen, J. E., Campa, S., Grebe, G., Sighieri, C., & Gazzano, A. (2016). Guardians' perceptions of cats' welfare and behavior regarding visiting veterinary clinics. *Journal of Applied Animal Welfare Science*, 19(4), 375–384.

30. Spano, V., Springer, C. M., Christensen, E., & Albright, J. D. (2023). Effects of transdermal mirtazapine and oral gabapentin as pre-veterinary visit pharmaceuticals for shelter cats. *Journal of Veterinary Behavior*, 64–65, 47–53. https://doi.org/10.1016/j.jveb.2023.06.001

31. van Haaften, K., Forsythe, L., Stelow, E., & others. (2017). Effects of a single preappointment dose of gabapentin on signs of stress in cats during transportation and veterinary examination. *Journal of the American Veterinary Medical Association*, 251, 1175–1181.

32. Hampton, A., Ford, A., Cox III, R. E., Liu, C. C., & Koh, R. (2020). Effects of music on behavior and physiological stress response of domestic cats in a veterinary clinic. *Journal of Feline Medicine and Surgery*, 22(2), 122–128.

33. Paz, J. E., da Costa, F. V., Nunes, L. N., Monteiro, E. R., & Jung, J. (2022). Evaluation of music therapy to reduce stress in hospitalized cats. *Journal of Feline Medicine and Surgery*, 24(10), 1046–1052.

34. Snowdon, C. T., Teie, D., & Savage, M. (2015). Cats prefer species-appropriate music. *Applied Animal Behaviour Science*, 166, 106–111.

35. Herron, M. E., & Shreyer, T. (2014). The pet-friendly veterinary practice: a guide for practitioners. *Veterinary Clinics: Small Animal Practice*, 44(3), 451–481.

36. Mariti, C., Raspanti, E., Zilocchi, M., Carlone, B., & Gazzano, A. (2015). The assessment of dog welfare in the waiting room of a veterinary clinic. *Animal Welfare*, 24(3), 299–305.

37. Arhant, C., Schmied-Wagner, C., Aigner, U., & Affenzeller, N. (2021). Owner reports on the use of muzzles and their effects on dogs: An online survey. *Journal of Veterinary Behavior*, 41, 73–81.

38. Haywood, C., Ripari, L., Puzzo, J., Foreman-Worsley, R., & Finka, L. R. (2021). Providing humans with practical, best practice handling guidelines during human-cat interactions increases cats' affiliative behaviour and reduces aggression and signs of conflict. *Frontiers in Veterinary Science*, 8, 835.

39. Soennichsen, S., & Chamove, A. S. (2002). Responses of cats to petting by humans. *Anthrozoös,* 15(3), 258–265. https://doi.org/10.2752/089279302786992577

Contributing Authors
Laura Ward-Ansel DVM
Christine D. Calder DVM, DACVB

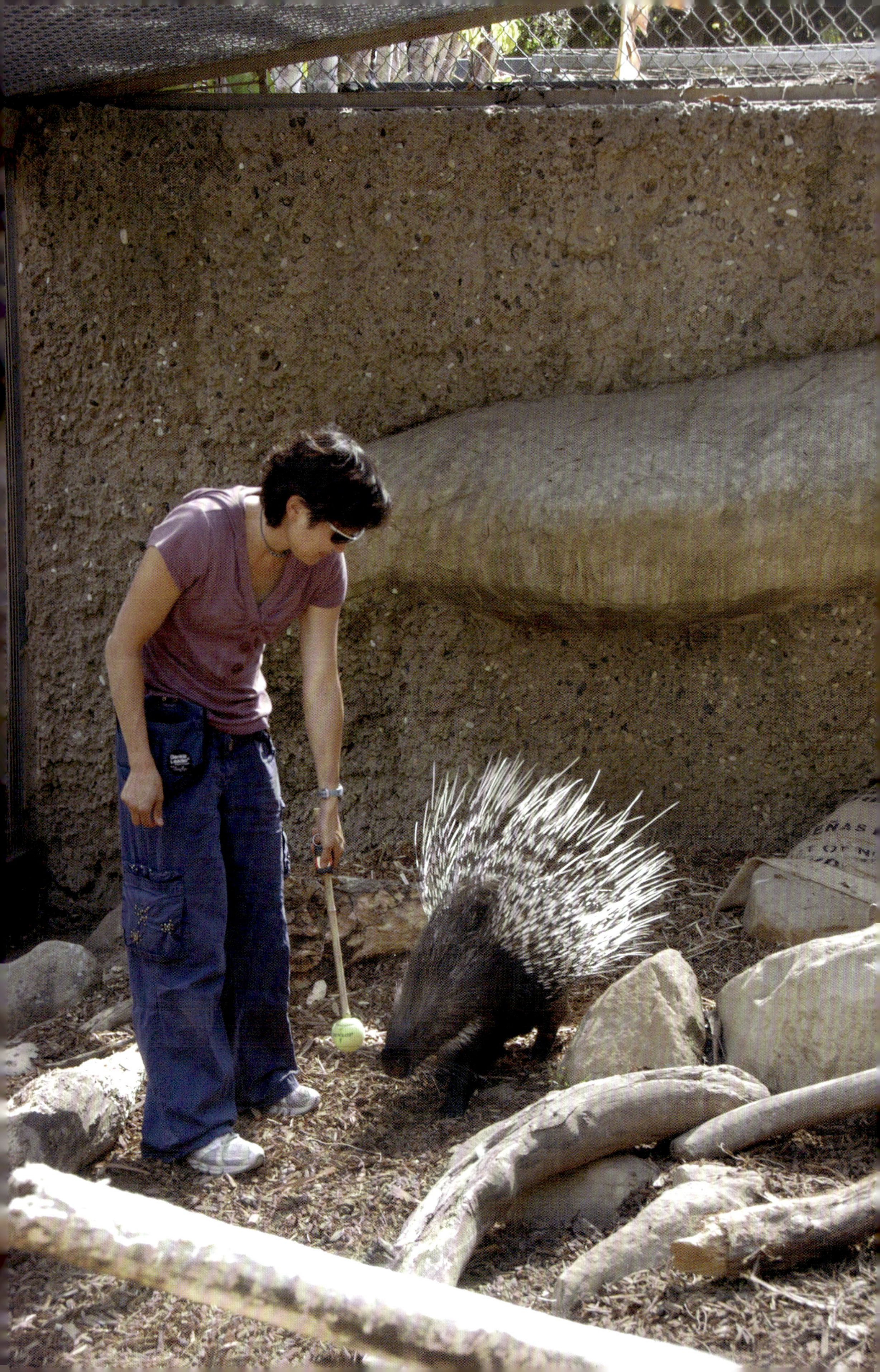

CHAPTER 9

Low Stress Handling® Movement of Cats and Dogs

9.1 Introduction

Veterinary hospitals, shelters, and other animal facilities are full of slippery floors, cold surfaces, novel sounds, smells, and unfamiliar people and animals, which can increase fear and anxiety. Every action by a handler conveys a message to the animal. Even subtle variations in greetings, handling techniques, and how animals are placed into or removed from cages, kennels, and runs influence their behavioral responses. To establish trust, handlers must understand body language and observe the animal carefully. This chapter offers guidelines for safely and efficiently moving and handling dogs and cats.

9.2 Equipment for Low Stress Handling®

Various tools assist in restraining and containing animals for transport within veterinary hospitals or facilities.[1] Safety for both the animal and handler is essential when selecting equipment.[1] Equipment requiring specialized skills should be used exclusively by those trained to do so.[1]

Safe Collar Choices for Dogs and Cats

Only flat buckle or martingale collars (no-slip or slip-limited) are appropriate. Other collars should be removed and either set aside or given to the caregiver to take home. Pinch, prong, choke, or electronic collars are unsafe and should always be removed. For cats, only breakaway collars should be used.

Table 9.2.1 Equipment options

Dogs	Cats
harness	harness
collar	collar
carrier	carrier
towels or blankets	towels or blankets
Elizabethan collars*	soft variety of Elizabethan collars*
muzzles	
head halters	
leashes	

*Denotes emergency only or post-surgical care. These require cooperative care training before use. Muzzles are not recommended in cats even for emergency use.[2–5]

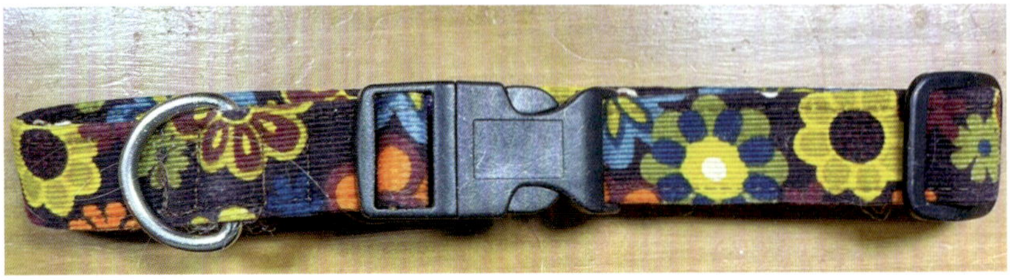

Fig. 9.2 A: Flat buckle collar

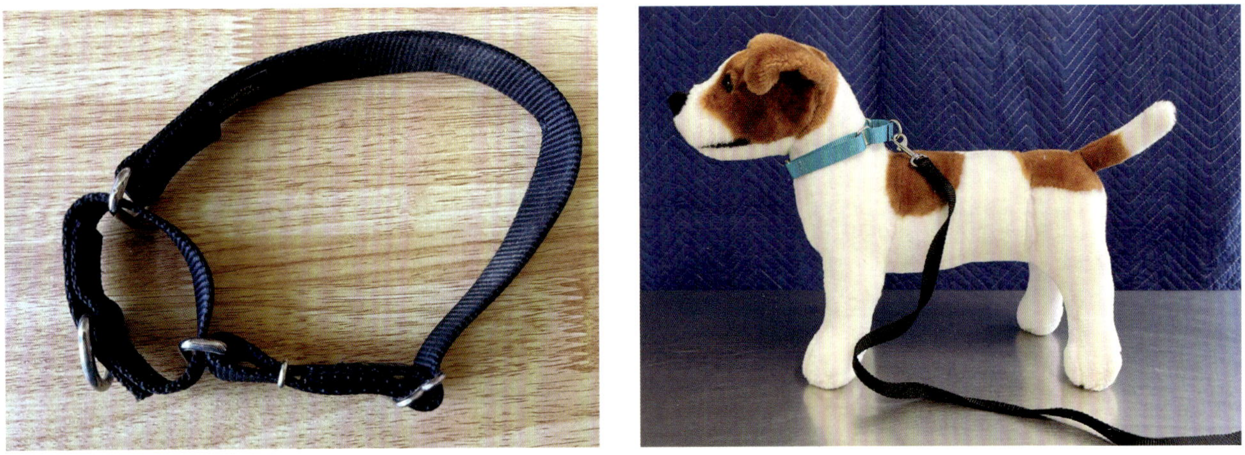

Fig. 9.2 B, C: Martingale Collars

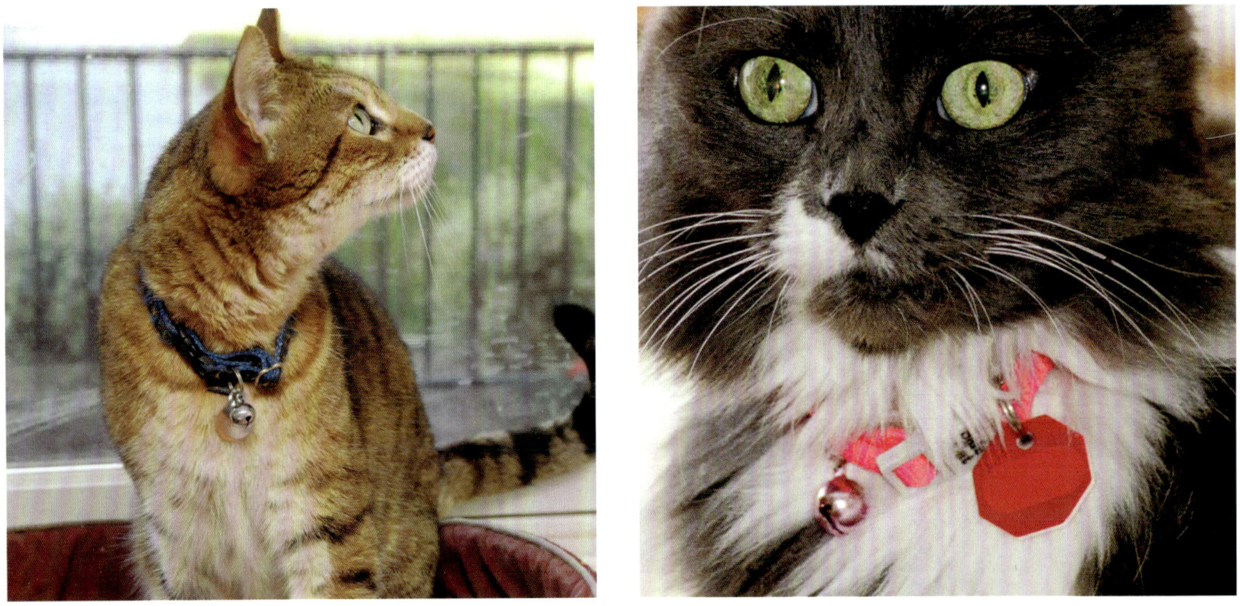

Figs. 9.2 D, E: Cats wearing breakaway collars. Do not hold these collars for restraint since they come apart easily.

Harness Selection and Benefits for Dogs and Cats

A supply of harnesses in multiple sizes should be available. Front clip harnesses tend to reduce pulling and encourage engagement with their handlers, in contrast to back clip versions.[6] Dogs that may benefit from a harness include those that pull excessively on the leash, have neck or back pain or injury, increased intracranial or intraocular pressure, permanent tracheostomies, or are brachycephalic.[6,7] Using a properly sized harness reduces the risk of tracheal damage and excessive cervical trauma.[6,7] For cats, keep preferred brands and styles on hand to recommend to clients and adopters.

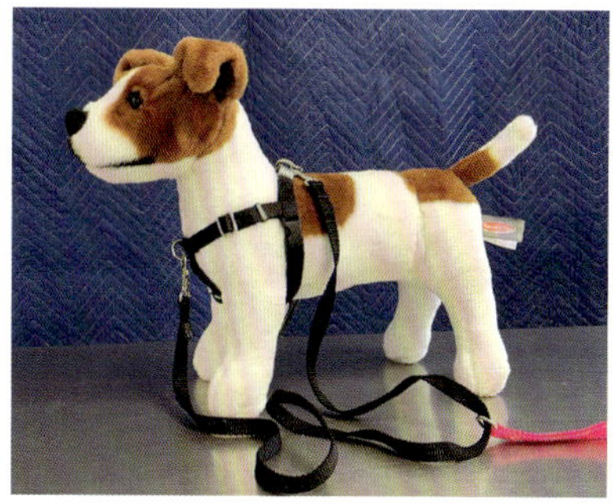

Fig. 9.2 F: Appropriately sized harness with a double clip leash.

Head Halters

Various head halters are available on the market, designed to help manage a dog's behavior without causing distress.[8] Dogs that tend to pull on leashes attached to flat collars or slip leads, and those that have not shown improvement with a harness might be suitable candidates for head halters. Both head halters and harnesses require proper conditioning before use.

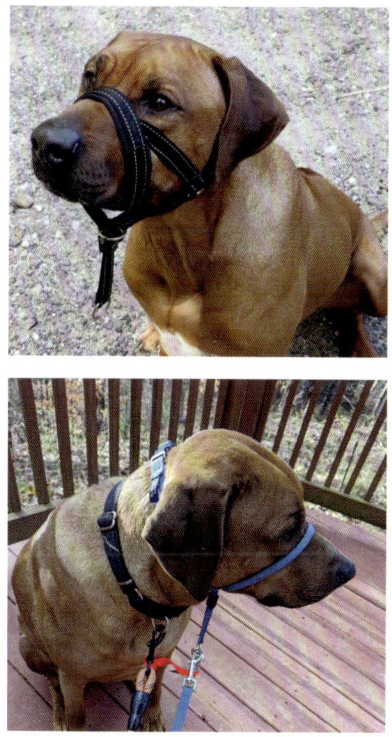

Figs. 9.2 G, H: Head halter variety.

Slip Leads

In animal care facilities and veterinary hospitals, slip leads are often preferred due to their convenience in both application and removal. They are best suited for brief transfers, such as moving between runs, and not for extended outdoor walks or training sessions. Dogs should voluntarily put their head through the slip lead or be lured with treats. The same method can be applied when removing the lead. While slip leads can function without collars, they can also be paired with a harness or looped behind one leg when a neck lead is not appropriate. A slip lead is never appropriate for a cat.

A wide variety of slip leads are available. The ideal slip lead is thick, made from soft material, and at least 4–6 feet long. The increased surface area of a thicker leash tends to be more comfortable than a thinner lead and is preferred. Softer material offers greater comfort for both the dog and handler. Retractable leashes are never appropriate in a veterinary hospital or animal care facility.

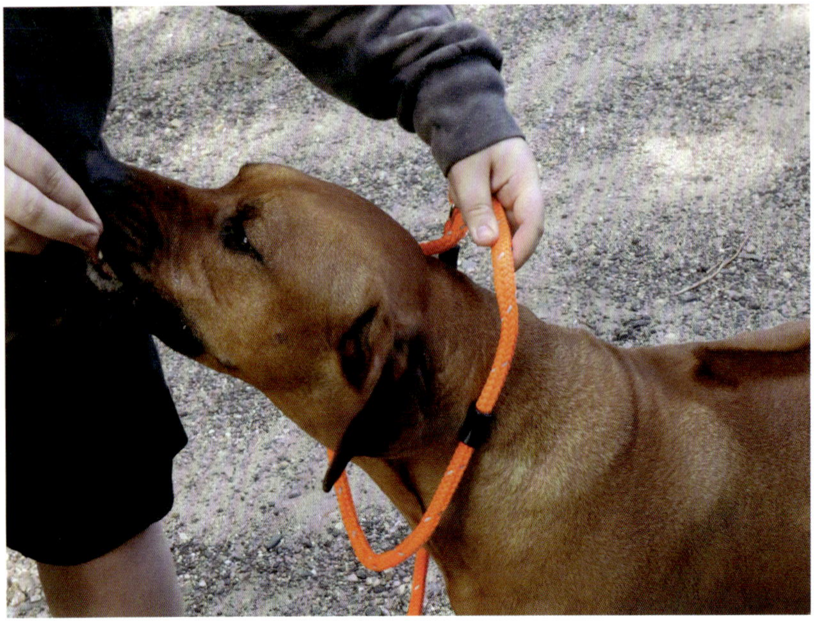

Fig. 9.2 I: Slip leads should be thick, made from soft material, and at least 4–6 feet long.

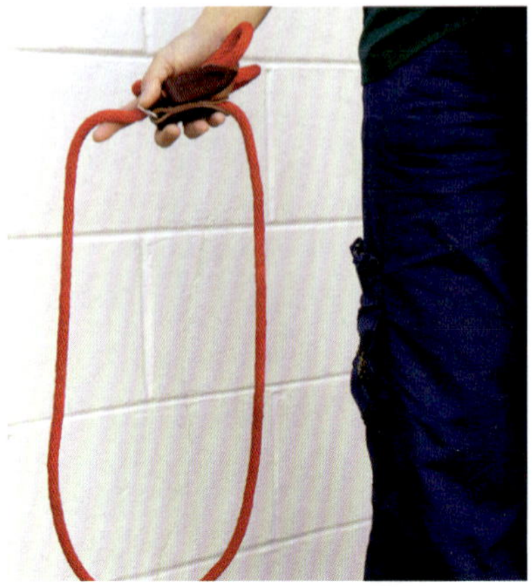

Fig. 9.2 J: When transferring dogs in and out of kennels, create a large loop with the leash, holding it in one hand. This leaves the other hand available to provide treats and handle the kennel door.

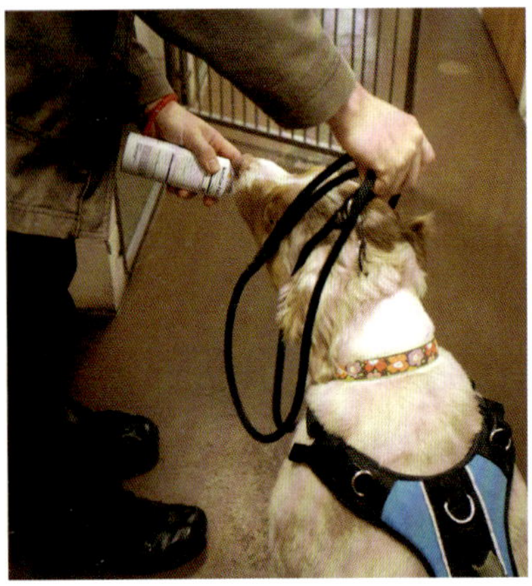

Fig. 9.2 K: The dog should be encouraged to voluntarily place their head through the lead using a food lure.

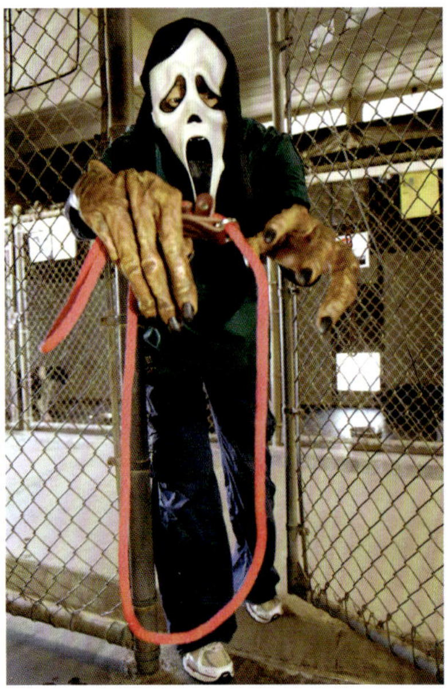

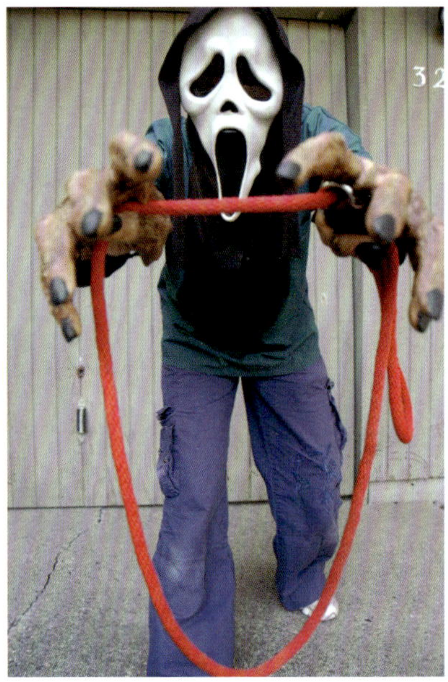

Figs. 9.2 L, M: Incorrect Even the friendliest person can seem intimidating to a dog. Approaching with a leash and making direct eye contact can be perceived as threatening, increasing the dog's fear and potentially triggering a defensive response.

Safe Leash Removal Techniques

Do not reach over the dog's head to take off the leash. Instead, use food during leash removal. While the dog consumes the treat, slide the leash over their head. If the dog refuses food, consider using an alternate technique involving a second leash attached to the O-ring.

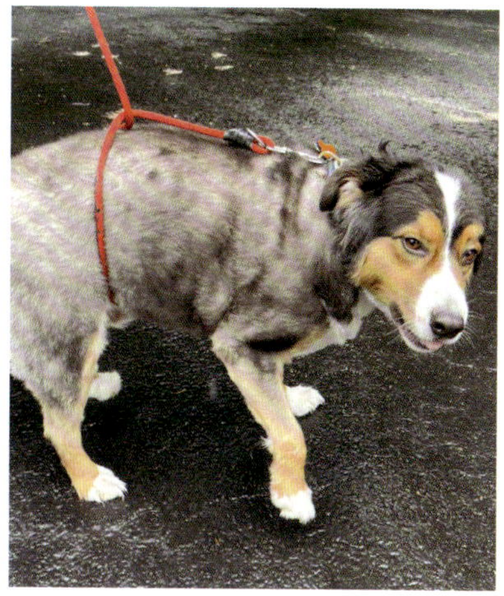

Fig. 9.2 N: Incorrect Slip leads should never be wrapped around the waist. This practice is unsafe and can lead to discomfort, as evident from this dog's body language.

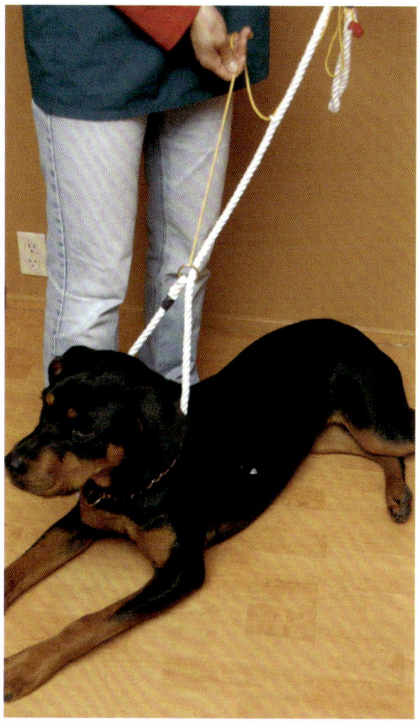

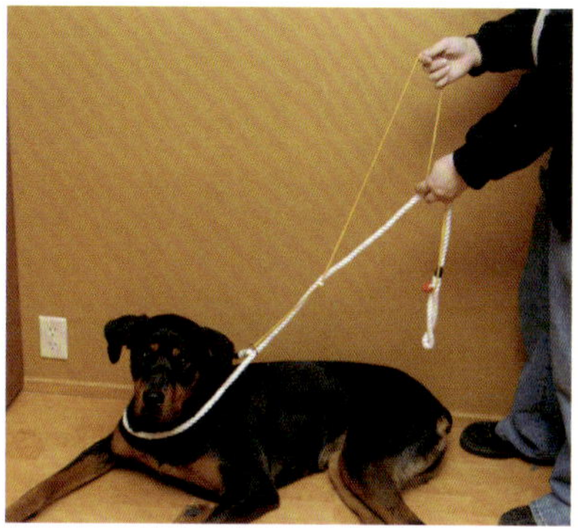

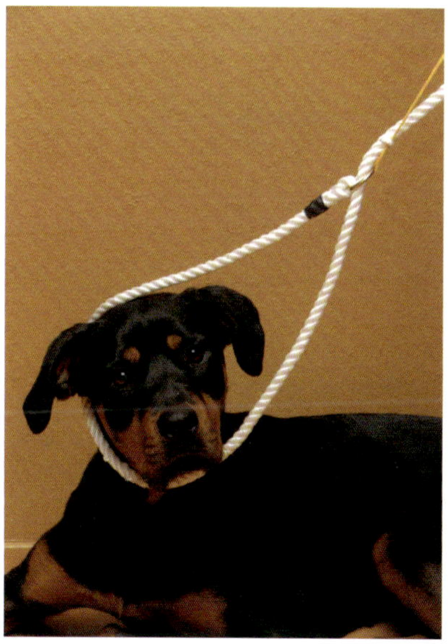

Figs. 9.2 O, P, Q: For dogs that exhibit fear or anxiety, connect a secondary leash or string to the O-ring of the slip lead. This configuration permits the handler to pull the leash off without using their hands while the door remains closed and stabilized with a foot.

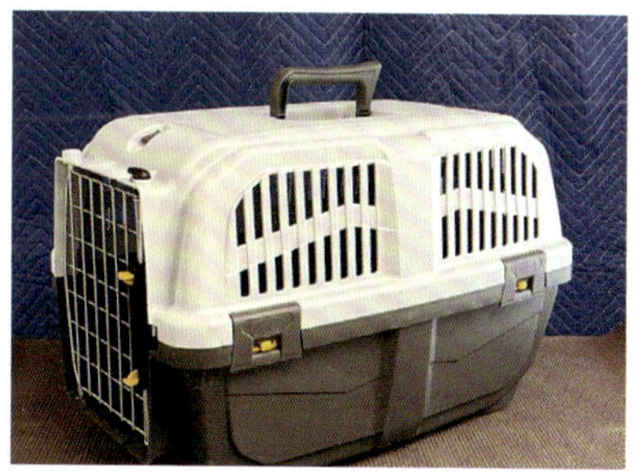

Fig. 9.2 R: A hard-sided carrier can be disassembled for easy access while allowing the cat to stay comfortable in the bottom of the carrier during examination.

The Ideal Carrier for Cats and Small Dogs

A cat or small dog carrier must be large enough for the animal to turn around and lie comfortably. A hard-sided carrier with clips and a removable top is preferred.

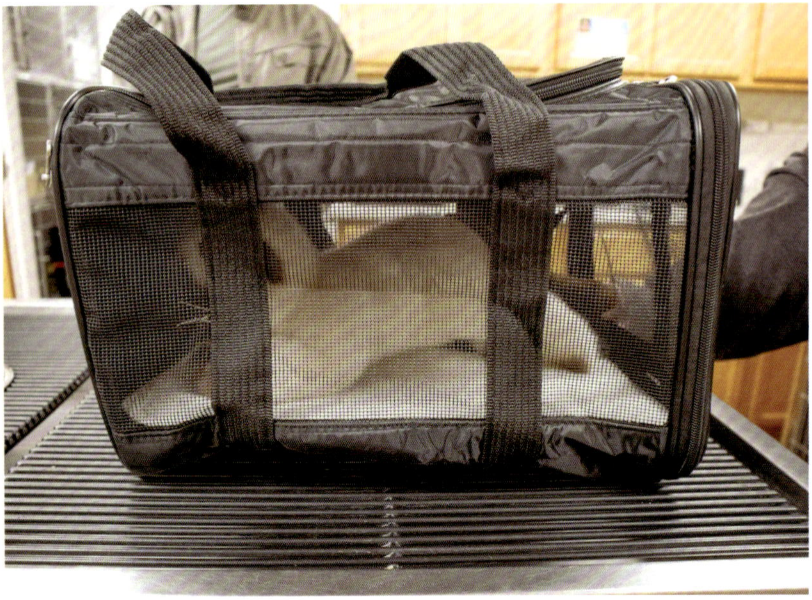

Fig. 9.2 S: A soft-sided carrier with an opening at the top provides easy access to a cat or dog and can be used during the sedation process by injecting through the mesh sides.

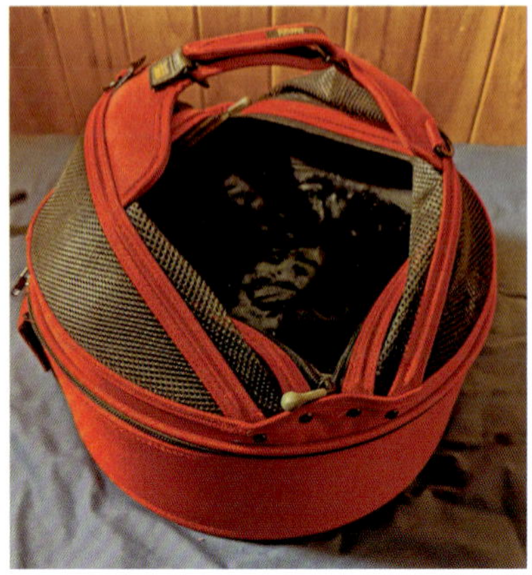

Fig. 9.2 T: A round open top carrier has many benefits including increased comfort for cats.

Choosing the Right Dog Muzzle for Low Stress Handling®

Basket muzzles, which allow dogs to pant, drink, and eat are preferred over other types of muzzles.[2] If a muzzle is used, dogs need to be conditioned to wear it rather than using it solely for the convenience of the procedure. This may require stopping the appointment and sending the dog home for muzzle training before

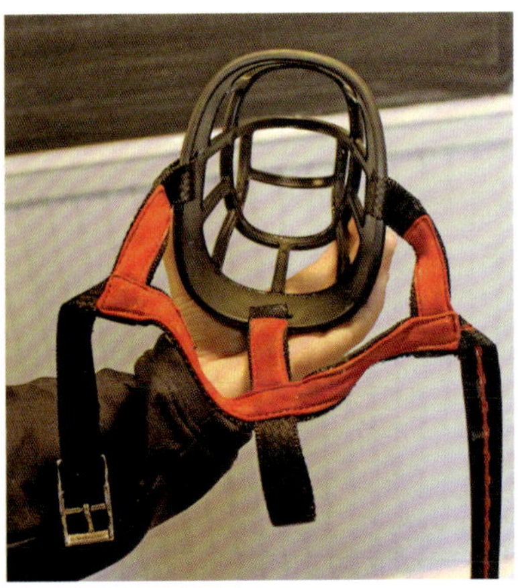

Fig. 9.2 U: Basket muzzles are preferred over sleeve muzzles. The muzzle should be large enough for a dog to eat, pant, and drink water.

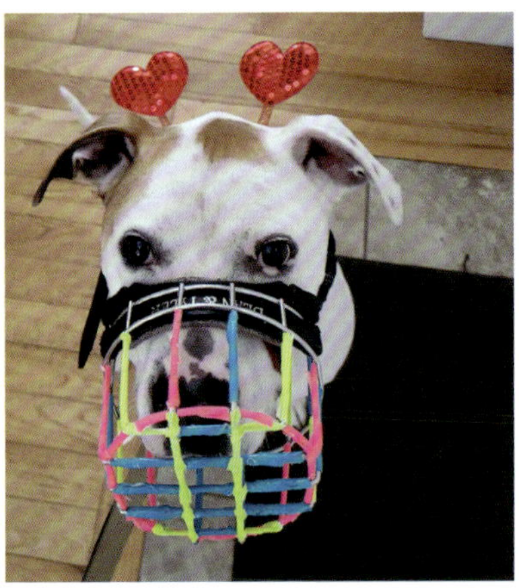

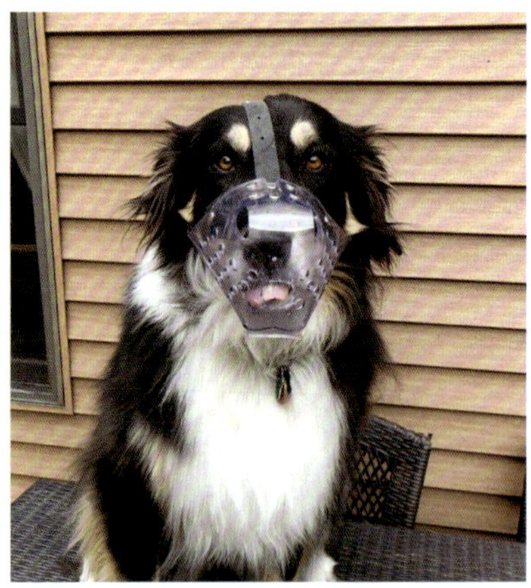

Figs. 9.2 V, W: Muzzles should never be used for punishment and dogs can learn to like wearing their muzzles. They can also be fun! Colored duct tape or vet wrap can add padding and flash. (Photo V courtesy of Casey Paul [Dean & Tyler brand muzzle] and photo W courtesy of Pat Koven [Jafco brand muzzle])

rescheduling. Once the dog is accustomed to wearing their own muzzle, a follow-up appointment can be scheduled, preferably with pre-visit medications on board. Sedation may still be needed and planned for accordingly.

For urgent procedures, a basket muzzle is still preferred before administering sedation. In contrast, nylon sleeve muzzles are restrictive and should only be applied for brief periods of time, (e.g., two to three minutes) during sedation or urgent catheter placement. Leash muzzles can be painful and should only be used in a life-threatening emergency when a basket or sleeve muzzle is not available.

Muzzling Cats and Low Stress Handling®

Muzzling a cat is never recommended, as muzzles can be painful on sensitive whiskers and tend to result in protective emotions and defensive behaviors. This includes cone, nylon, and air muzzles.[3–5] Instead, a warm, pheromone infused, loosely wrapped towel should be used.[3–5,9–12] While cats, like dogs, can be conditioned to wear a muzzle, if a muzzle is necessary, sedation and cooperative care training should be the preferred plan.[3–5]

Five Alternatives to Muzzling a Cat

1. Make sure the cat is in a quiet environment and preferred location.
2. Let the cat choose a comfortable position.
3. Use the least amount of restraint possible combined with distractions (food, toys, petting).
4. Lightly wrap the cat in a warm, pheromone infused towel, sheet, or blanket.
5. Utilize pre-visit medications, pain medications, sedation, and general anesthesia.

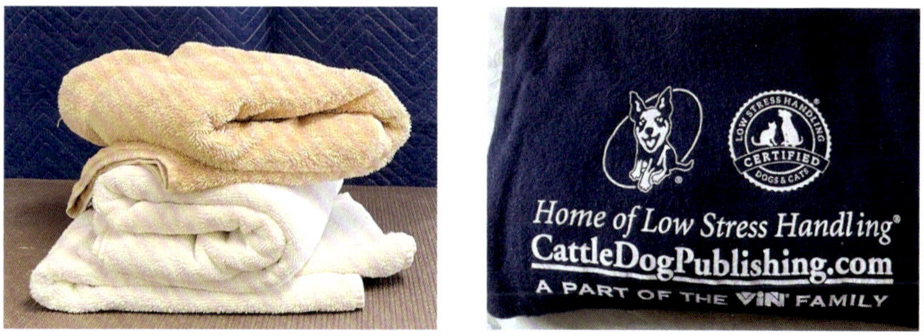

Figs. 9.2 X, Y: Towels and blankets are preferred handling tools over muzzles and restraint devices.

9.3 Picking Up Dogs

Picking up dogs may be necessary at times, but it is often stressful for them. Even if some dogs appear to tolerate being lifted, they are not truly relaxed. Luring and asking for familiar behaviors, such as stepping up or following a target, are preferred alternatives. If lifting is necessary, hand-feed the dog and closely monitor their body language throughout the process, making adjustments to enhance their comfort.[11]

Small Dog Football Hold

With one hand, gather the leash and hold the collar to stabilize the dog's head and neck. Slide the palm of the other hand against the dog's outer shoulder, gently sliding it down under the chest and between the front legs. Spread out the fingers and position the thumb on the outside surface of the dog's elbow. This prevents the dog from attempting to retreat from the hold. The handler should utilize their outer elbow to secure the dog against their body while lifting.

Alternatives to Lifting

Always allow dogs and cats the chance to jump onto benches or tables on their own, provided they are comfortable and it is safe to do so. To facilitate this safely and easily, consider the use of ramps and steps. Caregivers and team members should employ familiar cues like "step up" and "touch" to encourage this behavior. Engaging dogs in pattern games, such as the Up and Down Game, can be helpful before lifting them when necessary.[13] If a dog is stressed, pre-visit medications or sedation may be needed. With cooperative care training, dogs can learn to associate a specific cue with being picked up, making the lifting process more comfortable for them.

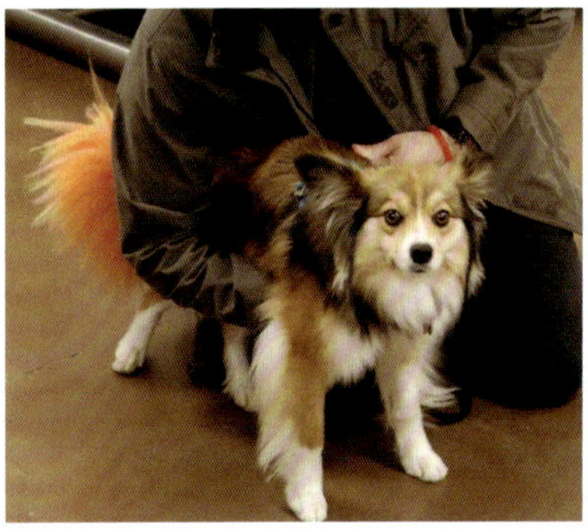

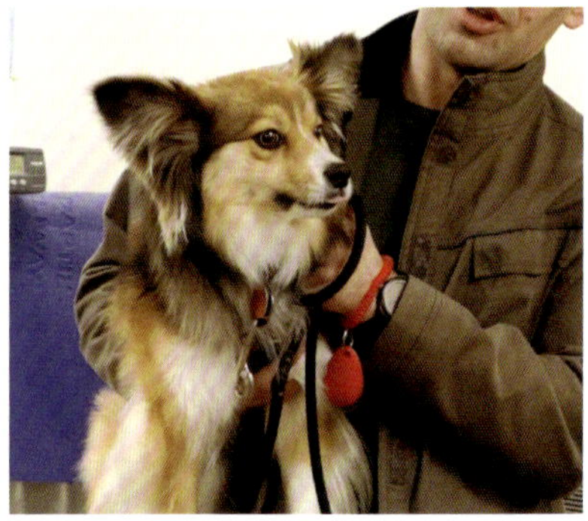

Figs. 9.3 A, B: Despite being adequately supported during the lifting process, this dog's body language indicated he is stressed. His ears are back, eyes wide with dilated pupils, his brow wrinkled, and mouth tight. In the second picture (B), you can observe him beginning to lick his lips, which is another sign of discomfort or anxiety.

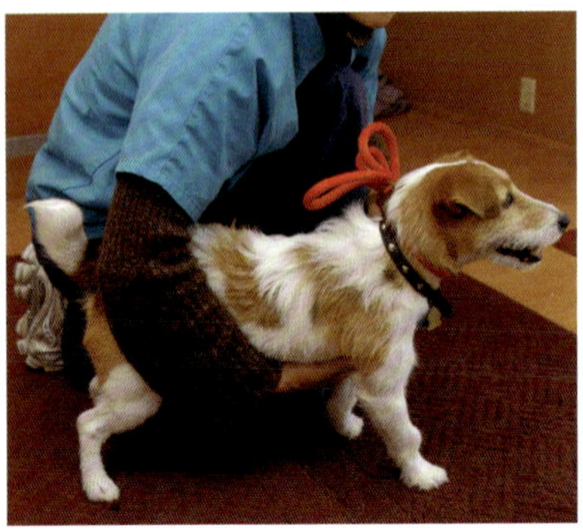

Fig. 9.3 C: To prevent startling, maintain continuous contact with the dog's body and provide support using both hands.

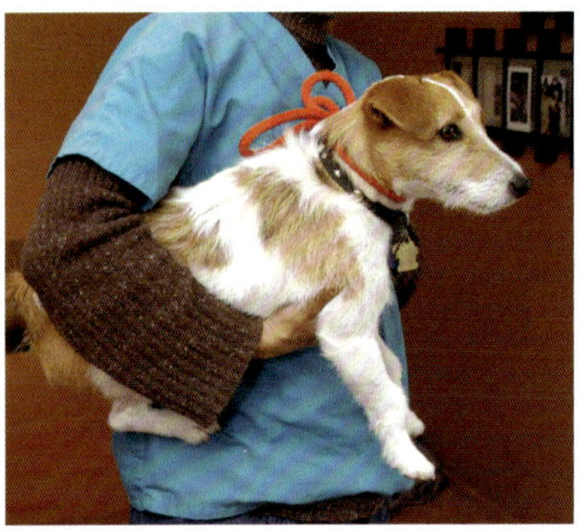

Fig. 9.3 D: While some dogs may be carried safely with a one-handed football hold, the other hand may be necessary to guide the dog's head for added safety.

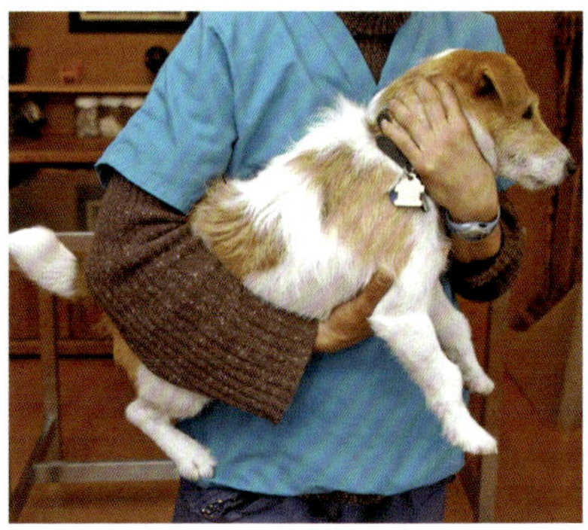

Fig. 9.3 E: An alternative method is to use a C-hold. With this hold, the dog's neck can be secured against the handler's body for added safety.

Rolled Towel

In emergency or urgent situations, when a muzzle cannot be safely applied, a rolled towel or a small blanket to cover and wrap the entire dog may be used when picking up a small dog. Food should be used as a distraction when possible. Once the towel is applied, the dog should be picked up in one fluid motion, but not so quickly that it frightens the dog.

This method is not appropriate for routine procedures such as examinations, nail trims, anal sac expressions, vaccinations, intravenous catheter placement, or subcutaneous fluid administration. In such cases, pre-visit medications, sedation, or general anesthesia would be more suitable options.

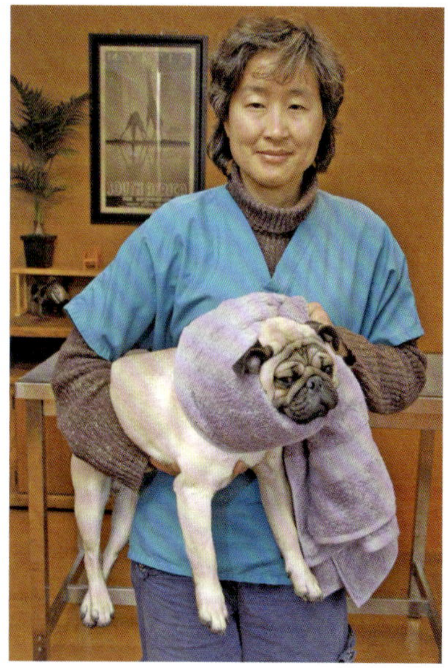

Fig. 9.3 F: A rolled towel should only be used in an emergency or urgent situation.

Receiving Small Dogs

Passing a small dog to an unfamiliar person can be challenging and frightening, potentially resulting in a bite. To prevent this, offer the hind end of the dog to the receiver or place the dog on the floor, allowing the handler to either walk the dog on a leash or pick up the dog without assistance.

Lifting Medium-Sized Dogs

Traditionally, picking up medium-sized dogs involved placing an arm under the abdomen in front of the hind legs, which provided minimal support to the spine and allowed the legs to dangle. Most dogs are uncomfortable with this type of handling, and lifting dogs in this manner is not recommended. Instead, two people should be used to lift a medium-sized dog. The incorrect and correct ways of lifting a medium-sized dog are shown below.

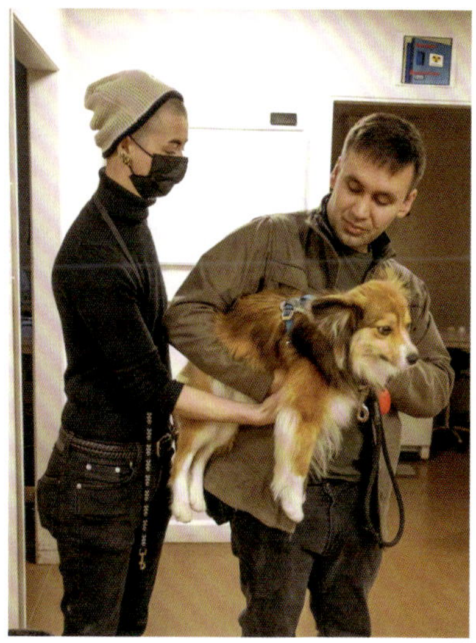

Fig. 9.3 G: When passing small dogs between handlers, face the dog away from the receiving handler before making the transfer.

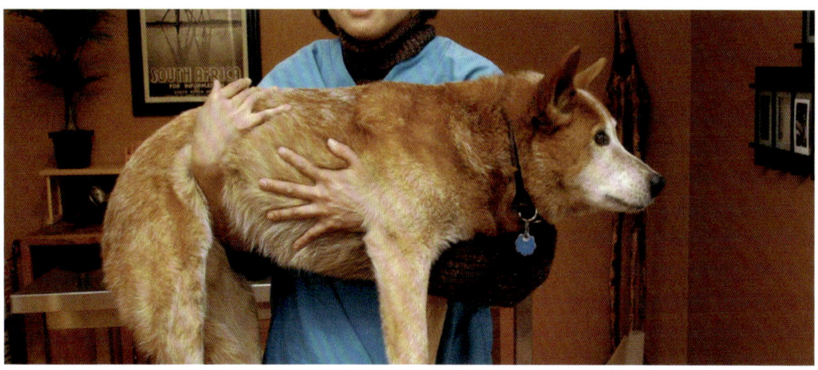

Fig. 9.3 H: Incorrect The handler has an arm in front of the hind legs and is applying too much pressure to the abdomen. This could be painful for an animal.

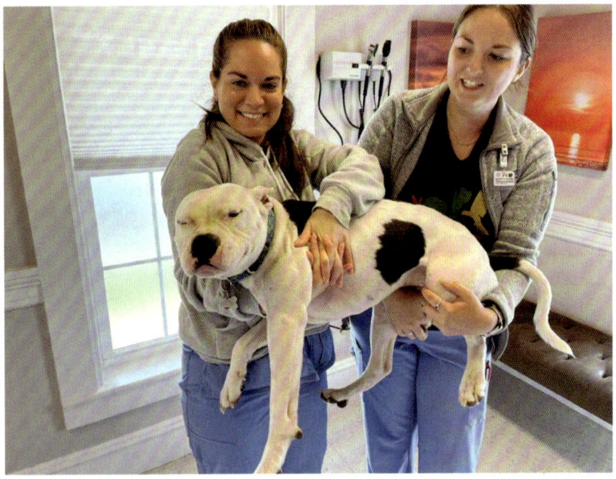

Fig. 9.3 I: Incorrect The handler in the front is placing both hands behind the front legs; This method does not provide adequate control of the head; and may be uncomfortable for the dog. The handler at the hind end is not providing adequate support for the spine or hips, and there is minimal control if the dog were to struggle. (Photo courtesy of Eliot Veterinary Hospital)

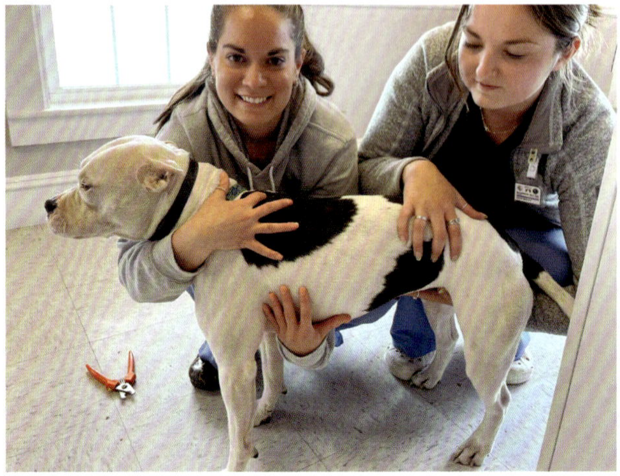

Fig. 9.3 J: Correct hand placement before lifting. Two people are preferred when lifting a medium-sized dog. Notice the second handler places her hands in preparation for a lift to keep the back straight and support the hind end. (Photo courtesy of Eliot Veterinary Hospital)

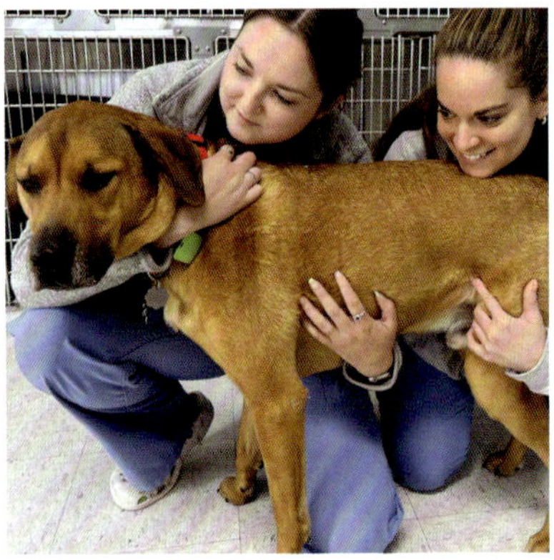

Fig. 9.3 K: In this image, the front handler is correctly stabilizing the front end of the dog by wrapping one arm around the dog's head and neck and the other under the chest, just behind the front legs. However, the second handler does not have adequate control of the dog's hind end, lacking lumbar spine stabilization for the pick-up, which can be problematic. (Photo courtesy of Eliot Veterinary Hospital)

Lifting Large Dogs

Refrain from lifting or picking up large dogs whenever possible. Lifting often causes them to feel unstable, leading to squirming and fidgeting. Instead of lifting, explore other options first, such as examining the dog on the floor, using a standing hold, luring the dog into position, or asking for familiar behaviors such as "step up", stationing, or following a target.

Front End Support: Head and Neck Restraint

When lifting a large dog, control the movement of their head and neck to reduce the risk of injury to both the dog and handlers. Since that the front end of a large dog is typically heavier than the hind end, stabilize the front end with both hands before attempting to lift the dog.

To lift a large dog safely and comfortably, stabilize both the front and hind end at the same time. Position one arm around the hind end or between the dog's legs for support. The handler's free hand should align along the lumbar spine to enhance hind end stabilization, ensuring the dog's safety and comfort during the lifting process.

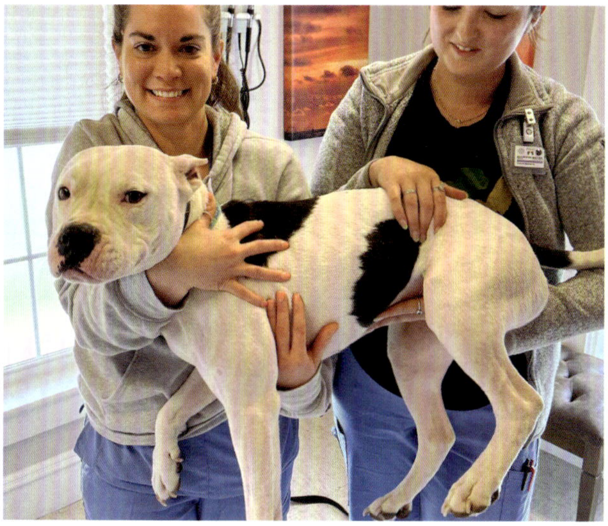

Fig. 9.3 L: Correct An alternative method, as shown in the picture, involves one handler stabilizing the hind end. Despite correct handling, the dog displays signs of distress—stiff body, tight mouth, ears back, and dilated pupils—suggesting discomfort and stress with this approach. (Photo courtesy of Eliot Veterinary Hospital)

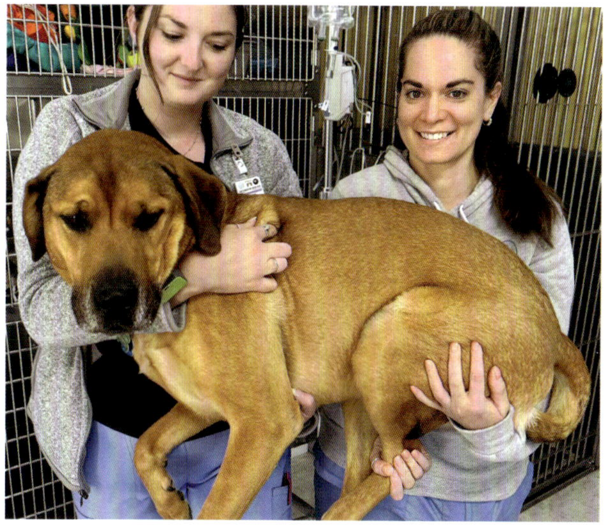

Fig. 9.3 M: Incorrect Lowering the left arm so that the hind-end rests in the bend of the elbow and placing the right hand along the lumbar spine would help improve this dog's comfort level and provide better stability. (Photo courtesy of Eliot Veterinary Hospital)

9.4 Alternatives to Lifting: Cueing, Luring, Lift Tables, and Stretchers

All examinations and procedures should be conducted where the animal feels most comfortable.[11,14] Providing choice and control helps reduce fear, anxiety, and frustration.[15–20] Dogs and cats should have the option to enter and exit cages or runs independently. After exiting, keeping the door open gives them the choice to return to their enclosure, enhancing their sense of control and safety.[15,16,18] Using steps, ramps, and mats makes this process both easier and safer.

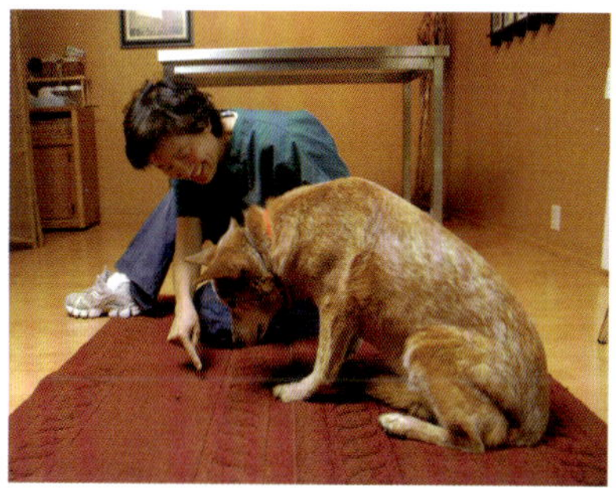

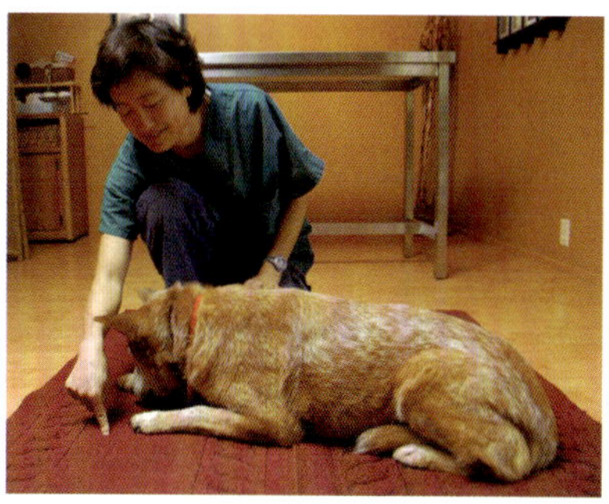

Figs. 9.4 A, B: A cue helps to position a dog without manual manipulation.

Using Familiar Cues

Before lifting larger dogs or those with medical needs such as arthritis or neurological conditions, use prompting and luring to encourage them to step onto and lie down on a cushioned stretcher. The dog should willingly get onto the stretcher, and force should never be used.[15–20] Familiar behaviors such as nose targeting, stepping onto a platform, and stationing can help with positioning and moving animals without lifting.[19]

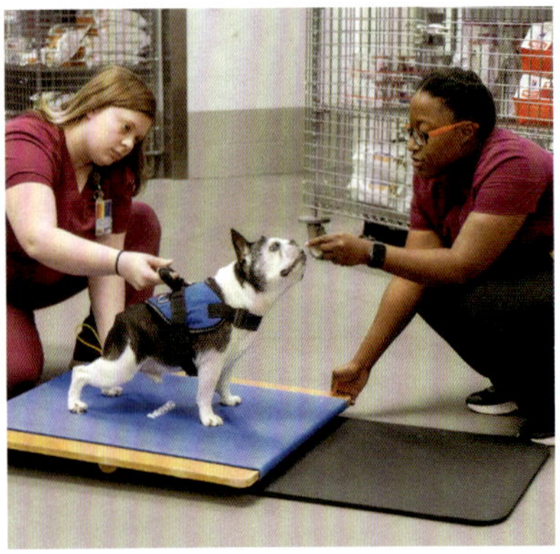

Fig. 9.4 C: A lure requires minimal handling and restraint. (Photo courtesy of Mississippi State University College of Veterinary Medicine, photography Tom Thompson)

Luring and Distractions

Luring and distractions minimize stress and eliminate the need for heavy restraint.[14] Luring involves using food or toys to guide animals into desired positions without physical manipulation. To effectively use a food lure, hold a high-value treat that the animal finds appealing where they can see and smell it. This treat can then guide the animal into the desired position or location. For example, to lure a dog into a sitting position, hold the treat slightly above the dog's nose and gradually raise it in an arc toward the top of their head. As the dog's nose follows the treat, their natural response will be to watch the treat, raise their head, and transition into a sitting posture. Once the dog is seated, mark the behavior and follow up with a reinforcer, such as a treat.

Luring with a toy follows a similar process. Many cats can be lured onto a scale using a wand toy. Using affection as a lure can vary in effectiveness. Some animals find affection highly reinforcing, while others may view it as aversive. If affection is used for recall, squatting and calling "come here" may prompt some animals to approach, while others might move away.

Although often confused with luring, distractions teach the animal to associate handling and other procedures with something engaging, such as food, play, or affection.[14] When using distractions, timing matters, and the distraction needs to be consistently present throughout the procedure. For example, during a puppy's examination, a lickable mat smeared with canned dog food can minimize fidgeting and movement. As a bonus, the puppy learns to associate the examination with food.

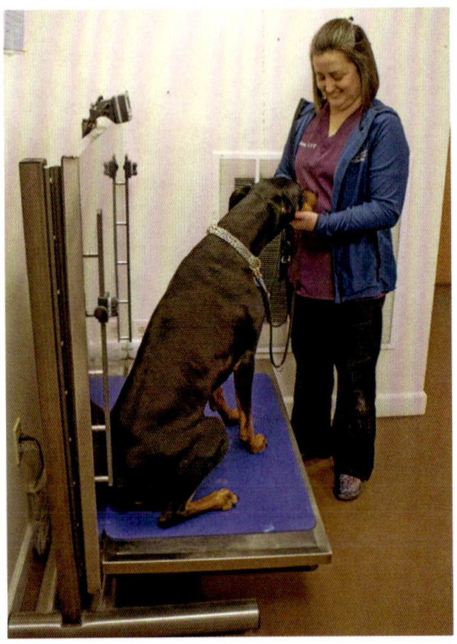

Fig. 9.4 D: Using targeting or a "step-up" cue is preferred over lifting the dog onto the table.

On the Table or Scale

Cues like "touch" and "feet up" (stepping up on an elevated surface) can help alleviate anxiety and reduce conflict by enabling the dog to position themselves on a table, scale, or other elevated surface without requiring lifting.[15–20] When working with tables, stairs or a ramp might be necessary but the use of a treat trail can be an effective way to encourage the dog.

Using a Stretcher

When walking a medium to large-sized dog onto a stretcher, it is more appropriate to cue a "sit" or "down" rather than resorting to lifting. Using this approach, the dog can then be sedated, if necessary, and subsequently lifted together by two handlers and gently slid onto the elevated surface. This method is particularly effective in emergency situations and for dogs experiencing orthopedic pain or neurological issues.

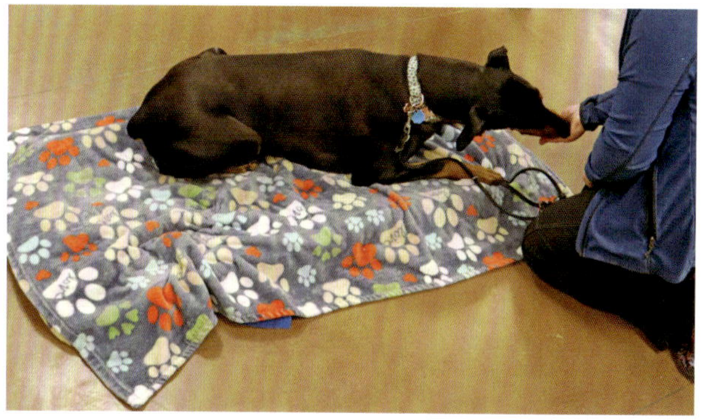

Fig. 9.4 E: For larger and mobility-impaired dogs, cue or lure them on to a stretcher before lifting.

9.5 Entering and Exiting Cages: Small to Medium-Sized Dogs

Whenever possible, house small to medium sized dogs in lower cages. Most of them will enter willingly if you drop treats into the cage or smear something spreadable on the interior wall. For upper cages, scatter treats on the bedding before placing the dogs inside.

When placing dogs and cats into cages, direct them away from the handler and gently place them on their bedding, allowing them to find and eat the treats. Once released, some animals might quickly turn around, attempting to flee or cling to the handler. Applying spreadable food to the back wall of the cage can help distract them as the door is closed. For animals that are reluctant to enter, continuously offering treats throughout the transition may be necessary.

Lower Level Cages

Never forcefully pull a dog out of a cage or reach in to pull them out. If a dog is unable to exit independently due to physical limitations or the height of the cage and resists assistance, consider alternative options such as using a run or placing a platform in front of the cage for an easier exit. A non-slip mat can improve traction and prevent injuries or fear of slipping. In some cases, sedation may be needed for safe handling.

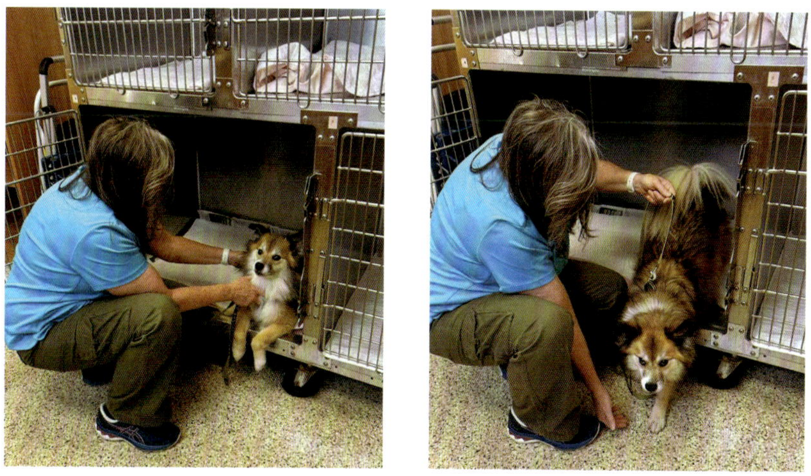

Figs. 9.5 A, B: Dogs should be given an opportunity to exit kennels on their own. (Photos courtesy of Colleen Koch)

Safe Lifting Techniques for Small Dogs in Upper-Level Cages

Small dogs in a top cage that cannot safely exit on their own will need to be lifted. When the door is opened, some dogs may jump up or reach with their front legs in anticipation of being lifted. To lift these dogs, slowly reach toward them, scoop them up, and be sure to support their hind end. Never pick up a dog by their front legs only, as this can be painful or aversive for some.

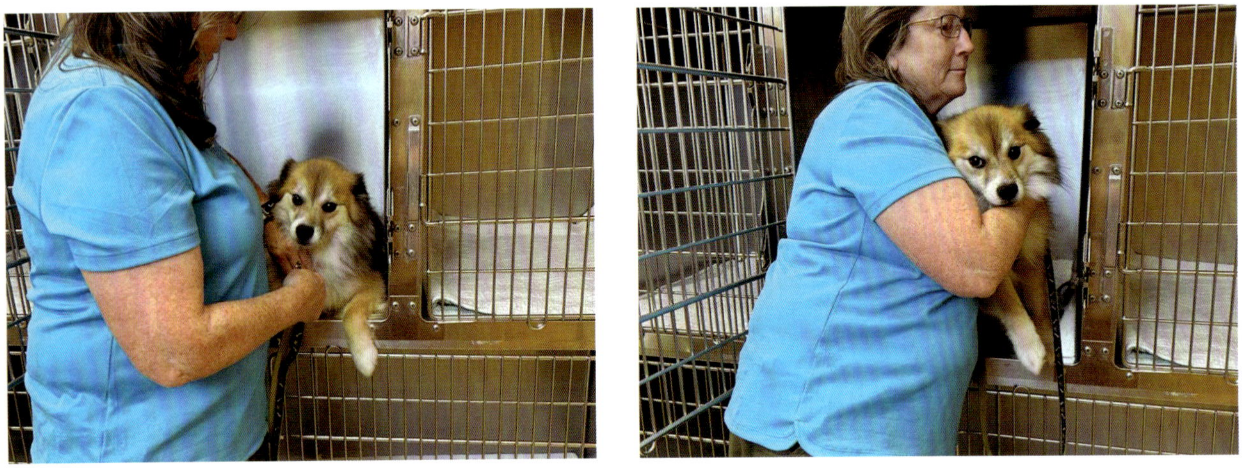

Figs. 9.5 C, D: When lifting a small dog from an upper cage, scoop them up and support their hind end. (Photos courtesy of Colleen Koch)

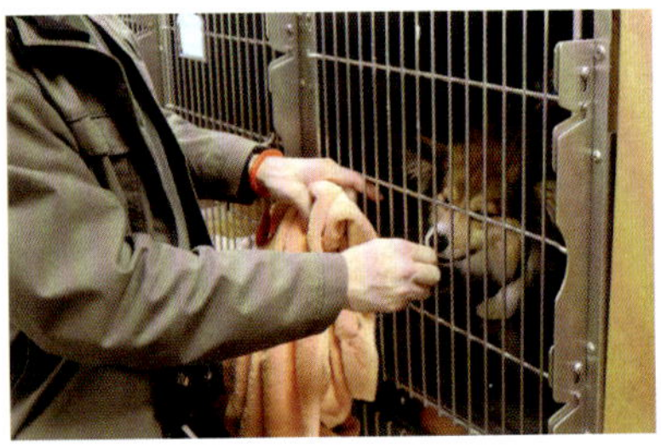

Fig. 9.5 E: When lures and high-value treats are offered, dogs are more likely to move closer to the handler for lifting.

Using Blankets for Safety

Use food distractions and place a blanket or towel over a fearful dog before lifting.

Fearful Dogs in Cages

Just as some dogs move to the front of the cage to be picked up when the door opens, others will move away or to the back of the cage out of reach. For these dogs, attempt to lure them to the front of the cage but never reach for them directly or try to forcefully extract them. Instead, cover them with a blanket or towel before lifting. If they will eat, scatter treats on the bottom of the cage or use a lickable mat for distraction as you place the towel over their head and body.

For dogs that bark and lunge at the cage door, keep the door covered with a towel when not directly interacting with them. Periodically toss high-value treats into the cage when people walk past or work with dogs in adjacent cages. This will help build a positive association with team members and create anticipation of something "yummy" when people are nearby.

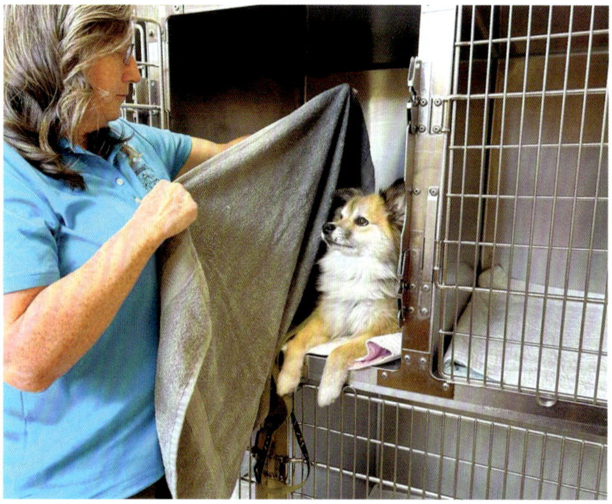
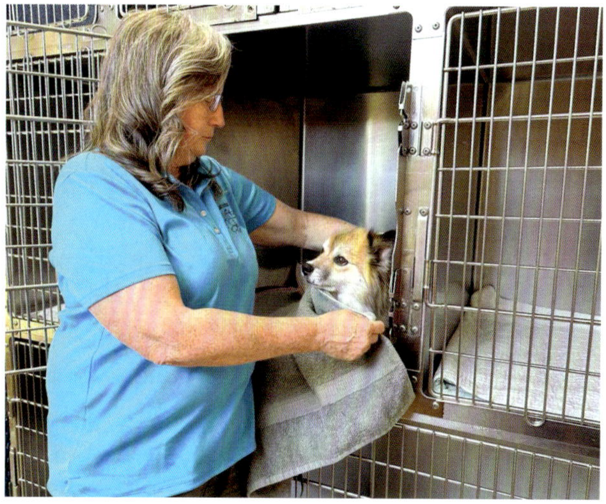

Figs. 9.5 F, G: Placing a towel around the dog's neck before lifting improves safety. (Photos courtesy of Colleen Koch)

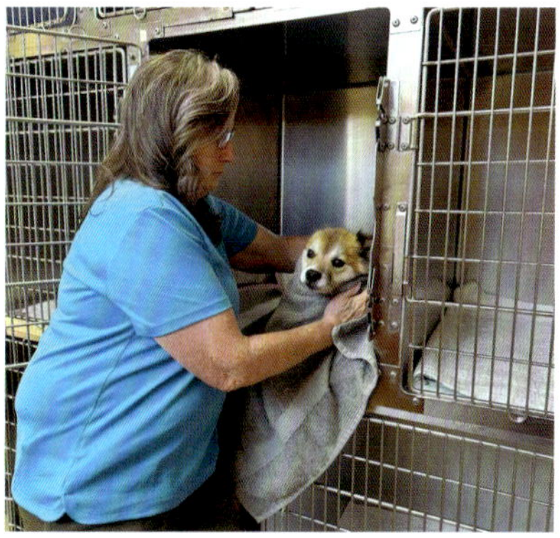
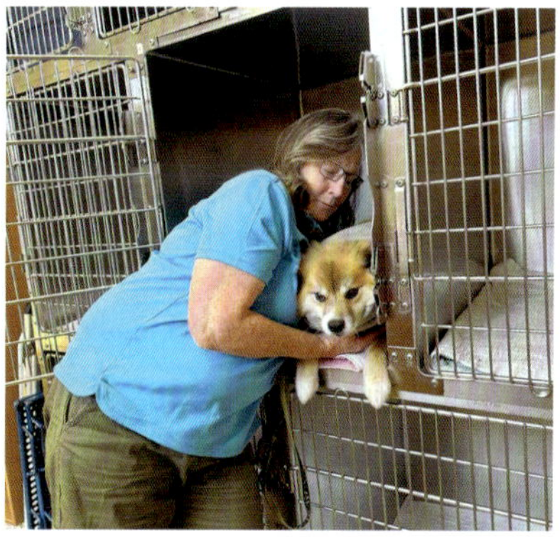
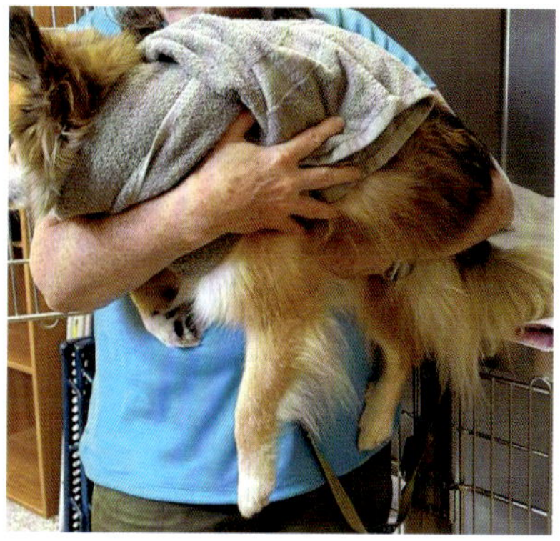

Figs. 9.5 H, I, J: A towel can be used for safety when removing a fearful or anxious dog from a cage. (Photos courtesy of Colleen Koch)

9.6 Entering and Exiting Kennel Runs: The Human

In animal care facilities, runs need to be entered and exited for various reasons, such as cleaning, feeding, treatments, or managing a dog's behavior. Animals should never be pulled or forced into or out of a run; they should always enter and exit of their own accord. To minimize the risk of escape during this process, manage the opening of the door, cue familiar behaviors such as stationing or sitting, and use food lures.

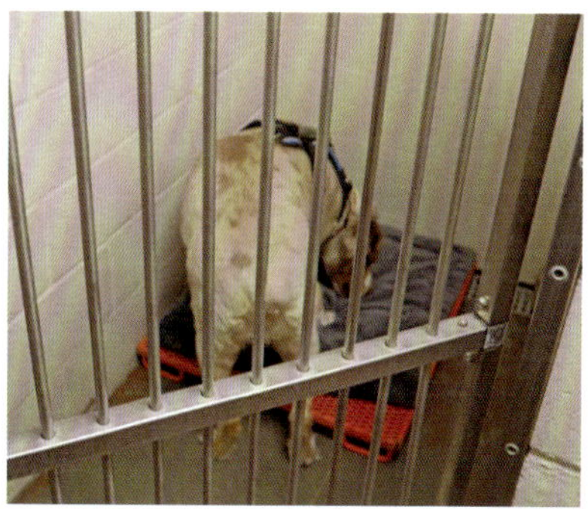

Fig. 9.6 A: Tossing treats into the run prior to entry can provide the handler an opportunity to enter without being jumped on.

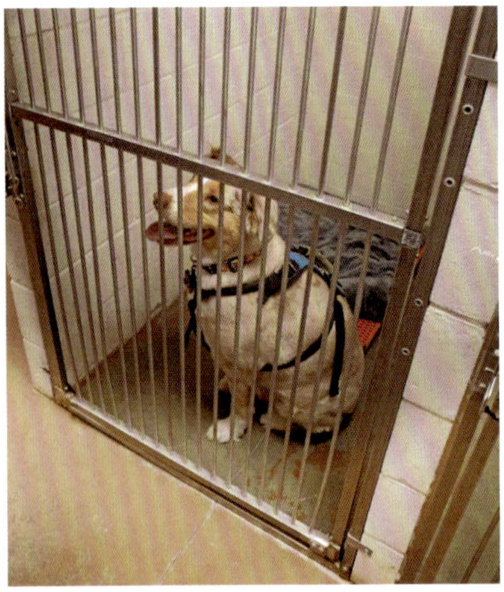

Fig. 9.6 B: Having a dog sit quietly on a mat before opening the door reinforces the dog for desirable behavior (sitting) instead of undesirable behavior (jumping).

Strategies for Entering a Dog's Space

Dogs may exhibit various behaviors when attempting to enter a run, such as sitting quietly at the door waiting for it to open, barking, nipping, or jumping on the door, retreating to the back of the kennel, or attempting to dash out the open door. Several strategies can reduce the risk of an animal bolting out the door and help the dog associate people entering their run with positive or engaging emotions.

Regardless of a dog's behavior, the goal when entering a dog's space is to do it safely. Entering a run with an excited or agitated dog can be challenging and risky. Tossing a handful of treats toward the back of the kennel as a lure and distraction before stepping into the run is an effective strategy to safely and quickly move a dog away from the door. Alternatively, to lure a dog to the front of the run, if the dog is fearful or moves away from the door when people are present, food lures in the form of spreadable food on pretzel rods, tongue depressors, lickable mats, or spoons can be used. Both strategies can help fearful dogs associate people entering their space with positive or engaging emotions and, for overly excitable or agitated dogs, provide an opportunity to reinforce more desirable and incompatible behaviors.

Before entering a run, the handler should position themselves sideways, not directly in front of the door, and place a foot at the bottom of the door for stabilization to minimize the risk of the dog slipping past and bolting. Once the door is stabilized, lift the latch and open the door just wide enough to fit through, entering the run sideways and leading with the run-side leg, before securing the door once inside. Directly facing the dog is unnecessary during latching, as the handler's legs and body should block the door, preventing the dog from slipping past and bolting. This process should take only one to two seconds and involve no more than two steps. If the dog crowds the door, slip through the opening and gently toss treats to guide the dog to the back of the run. Never use physical force or push the dog away. If the dog growls or has a known history of aggression, do not enter. Refer to the guidelines for handling fearful and anxious dogs below.

Guidelines for Entering a Kennel or Run

- Cue known behaviors before opening the door.
- Toss in food to move the dog away from the door.
- Do not open the door wider than needed when entering a run, as this might provide the dog with an opportunity to escape.
- Refrain from using force to keep the dog inside. Such actions could be perceived as threatening, prompting some dogs to snap or bite.
- Avoid using hands to hold back the dog when opening the door, as this can unintentionally make it easier for the dog to slip past the handler.

Leaving a Dog Run Safely

The procedure to safely and efficiently exit a run is the opposite of entering. The handler uses their outside hand (the hand nearest the run door) to open the door, while closely monitoring the dog's location. The door should open only enough for the handler to slide out sideways. Once outside, the handler can use a foot to secure the bottom while latching it.

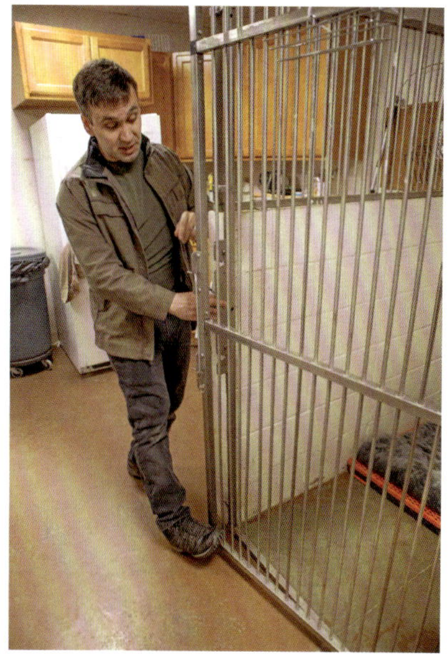

Fig. 9.6 C: A foot placed on the outside of the door helps to reduce bolting.

Preventing Escapes

Monitor the dog while exiting, leading with the foot closest to the run door first. Avoid crossing feet while stepping out, as this could cause the door to open wider than necessary, giving the dog an opportunity to push past and escape. If bolting is a concern, identify what motivates the dog (known behavioral cues, toys, or high-value food lures) and use them to keep the dog distracted and safely inside and close to the back of the run. Using a lickable mat suctioned to the back kennel wall or tossing a stuffed, food puzzle toy behind the dog helps to reduce the chances of the dog lunging at the handler's back, nipping at arms, hands, feet, and fingers, or lunging at the door as the handler exits and secures the latch.

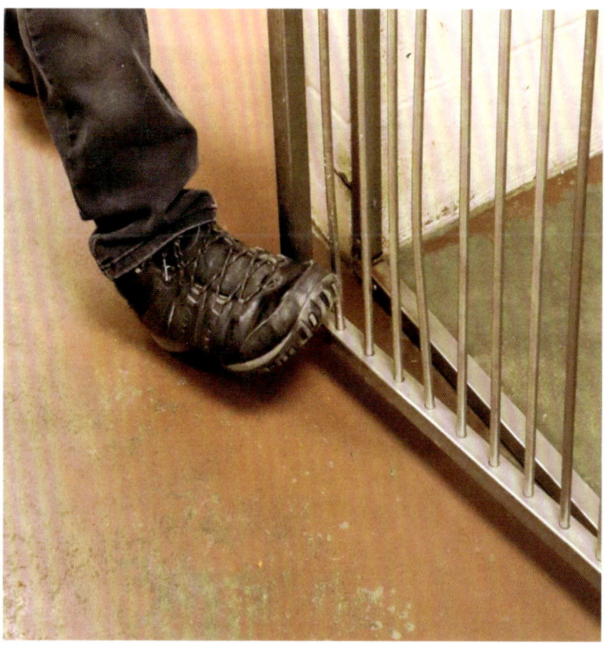

Fig. 9.6 D: Using a foot to secure the door while latching it can decrease the chance of the dog escaping.

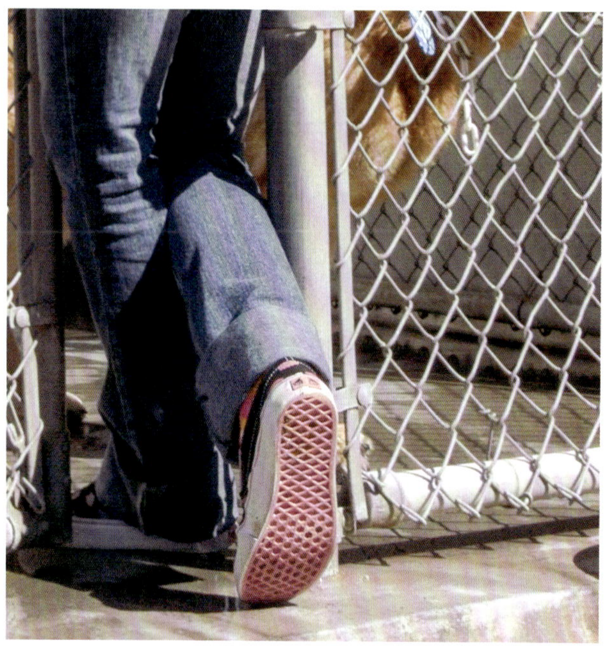

Fig. 9.6 E: Incorrect Crossing feet requires the door to open wider when exiting which creates an opportunity for the dog to escape.

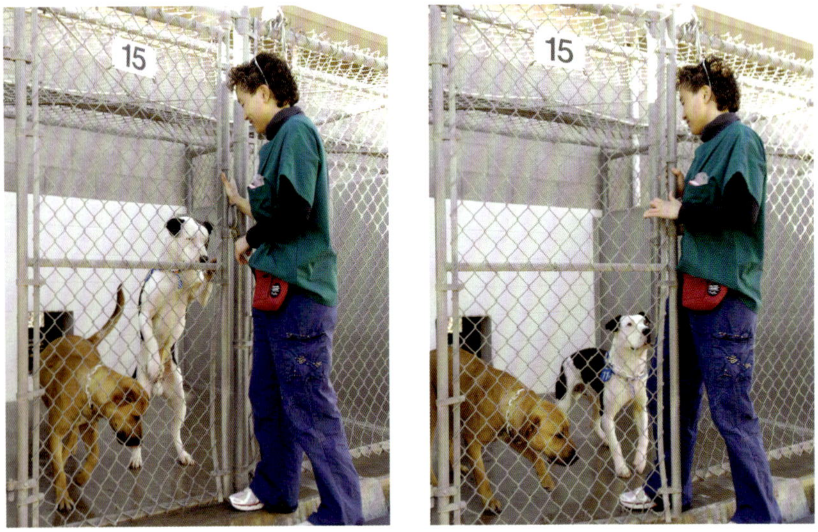

Figs. 9.7 A, B: If familiar cues are unknown, reinforce all four feet on the floor by waiting to open the door until the dog is standing still and not jumping.

9.7 Entering and Exiting Kennel Runs: The Dog

Dogs should always be encouraged to enter and exit kennel runs on their own. Familiar cues, food, and toy lures can all be used to encourage the dog to exit and enter. They should never be pulled or forced into or out of the run.

Using Familiar Cues

Familiar cues include behaviors such as "sit," "down," "place," and "touch," among others. When opening a kennel door, using these cues is more effective than telling a dog "no" or opening the door to push them out of the way. For dogs that lunge at or jump on the kennel door, using a familiar cue such as "sit" provides an opportunity for a reward, which is more effective than using positive punishment. This is why finding out what cues a dog already knows and documenting them in the medical record is beneficial. For extended stays, reinforcing alternative behaviors, such as having the dog stay in a specific location ("place") before opening the door, simplifies the process of attaching a leash before leaving the enclosure. Positive reinforcement, using a marker and treats, should be used to teach these behaviors.

> **Using Cues**
>
> Knowing what behaviors pets are familiar with can help facilitate handling and transitions during their stay at the animal care facility. Caregivers should be asked about the cues their pets know, and the answers should be documented in the pet's record.

Using Lures

When a dog does not have familiar behavioral cues, or if they are not known, a lure can be used. Tossing high-value treats into the run or smearing peanut butter on the floor or opposite wall can often work for food-motivated dogs. If they are not interested in food, alternatives such as petting, verbal praise, toys, or a play session might be effective. Engagement should begin with the dog outside the run to capture their interest and motivate them to follow the handler inside. Once inside, dropping treats at the back of the run can distract the dog while sliding out the door. This technique can also be effective in reverse.

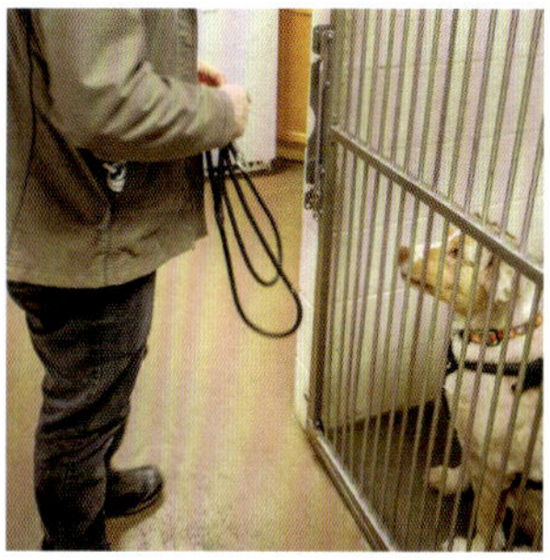

Fig. 9.7 C: Using a familiar cue such as "sit" before opening the door stops jumping and reduces the chance that the dog will bolt.

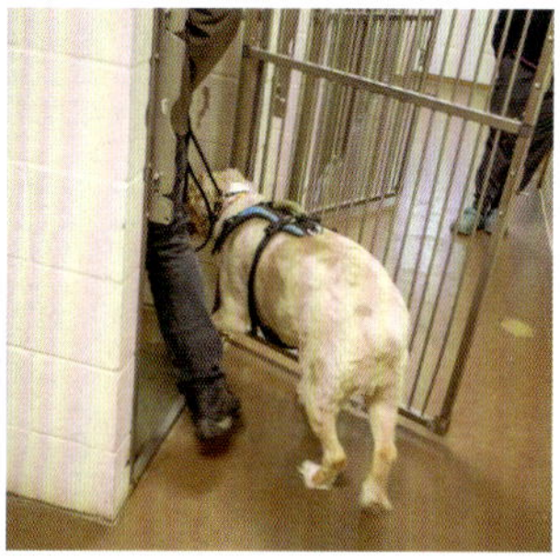

Fig. 9.7 D: Entering a run alongside the dog can encourage them to enter.

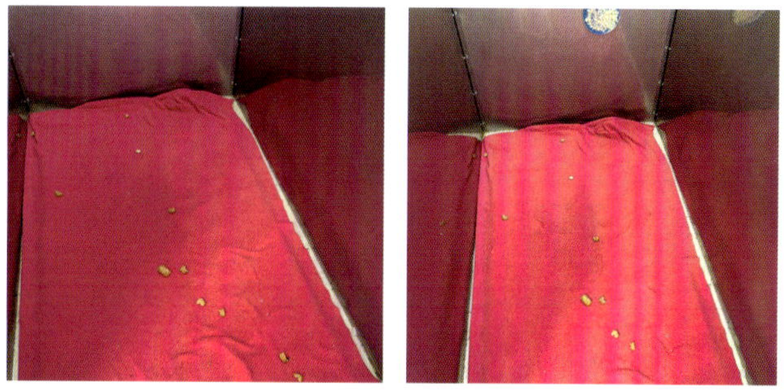

Figs. 9.7 E, F. A trail of treats makes a good lure to encourage a dog to walk into a kennel or cage. A lickable mat or smearing food on the wall of the run or cage can be used as an alternative. (Photos courtesy of Eliot Veterinary Hospital)

Reluctant Dogs

When a dog hesitates or refuses to enter or exit a run, it warrants an investigation of the surrounding area for potential causes. For instance, is there a dog in the next run that is barking and lunging at the front of their kennel or side wall? Is there an object in the walkway or on the wall that may be intimidating? If a cause can be identified, address it to help the dog feel more comfortable. Either move the object or relocate the dog to a quieter run.

Confinement Anxiety

Dogs with ***confinement anxiety*** might enter the run once with food but refuse the next time. Asking caregivers about potential confinement anxiety can help prepare for the possible need for medications.

Fearful and Anxious Dogs

Some dogs may hesitate to approach the front of a run or exit when an unfamiliar person is in their way. To encourage these dogs, step aside and slightly open the door, which may make them more likely to exit independently. Avoid extending a hand or leash into the run; instead, squat sideways near the door while using treats to lure them. If the dog refuses treats, move away and try again later.

Helpful Phrases

Helpful phrases to use when coaxing a dog into a run include: "with me" or "this way." For exiting, use "want to go for a walk" or, if they are being discharged, "want to go for a ride."

Positioning a Slip Lead

In certain situations, a slip lead may be the only leash available for moving dogs. These types of leashes are only appropriate for moving dogs a short distance (run to run) and should be replaced with a flat buckle collar or harness and standard leash as soon as possible. If a slip lead is used, always encourage the dog to willingly place their head through the leash rather than reaching over to place it directly on the dog. If the dog does not willingly place their head into the leash, a lure may be needed.

Non-Slip Mats

A non-slip mat placed over the run threshold and in front of the run provides traction, which can be helpful if the dog hesitates to exit or is recovering from surgery.

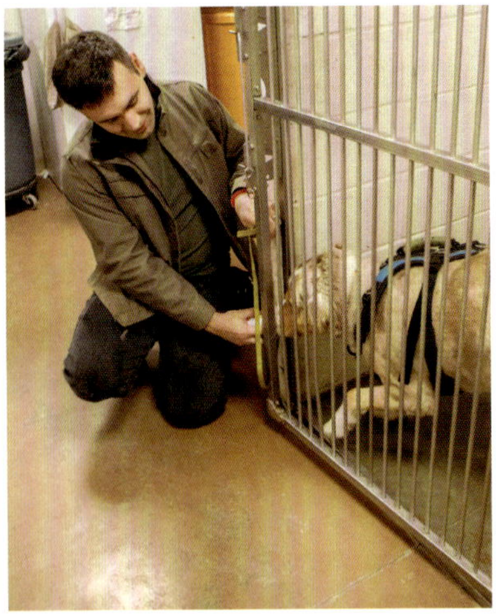

Fig. 9.7 G: Kneeling by the door gives an opportunity to assess a dog's behavioral response and make the individual appear less intimidating.

When exiting the run, position the slip lead between the wall and the slightly open door to motivate the dog to follow the treat into the lead as they exit. If the dog will not do this, use a long treat, such as cheese on a pretzel rod, while the handler stands outside the run door and holds the slip lead. If the dog hesitates, adjust the door opening to position the slip lead between the dog and the inside of the door, using a treat within the wires as an enticement. As the dog eats the treat, slide the leash over their head to secure the dog before opening the door. Once the dog is out of the run, switch to a flat buckle collar or harness using the same luring method as above.

Barking and Lunging Dogs

Fearful or anxious dogs may retreat to the back of the run or bark and lunge at the door when people and dogs pass. Tossing high-value treats, such as chicken, cheese, or hot dogs, into the run as people pass can help reduce this behavior. Though it might seem like this approach rewards barking and lunging, if the behavior decreases, counterconditioning has been effective.

> **Directing Traffic**
>
> One-way directional arrows placed on the floor or wall can help establish a one-way directional flow of traffic.

9.8 Walking Dogs and Transitions

When moving dogs throughout the facility, flat buckle collars and harnesses are the preferred walking equipment. Cue a known behavior, such as "sit," before placing this equipment on the dog in the run before exiting. Never forcibly apply the collar, harness, or leash and avoid leaning over the dog.

Walking dogs on a leash in the hospital and other animal care facilities can escalate their fear, anxiety, and frustration. There are many techniques, using both environmental modifications and training skills to improve the walking experience, reduce leash pulling, and decrease stress for both the dog and the handler.

Environmental

Identifying common bottlenecks or tight spaces within the facility helps avoid congestion and the congregation of animals in hallways, doorways, entryways, and exits. Wall-mounted mirrors can improve visibility around corners. Implementing one-way directional traffic flows and using "occupied" signage on doors leading to communal areas help reduce accidental encounters.

Leash Skills

All dogs should be walked on a six-foot leash with a front-clip harness whenever possible.[6,7] Slip leads should be used only for short distances and quick transfers. Carrying a toy or food lure during walks can help maintain engagement and minimize pulling.

When on leash, overstimulated dogs might bite or play tug-of-war with the leash. By using two leashes, the primary lead can be released while maintaining control of the dog with the secondary one. For dogs that are motivated by toys, a long tug toy can be used instead of the leash. While walking on a leash, using treats can be highly effective for managing a dog's behavior. Scattering a few treats on the ground encourages sniffing and foraging, which slows the dog down, reduces pulling, and provides enrichment. This tactic can also serve as an emergency distraction for reactive dogs when other dogs or people are passing by. In some instances, two people might be needed to walk a dog: one to hold the leash while the other clears the path ahead.

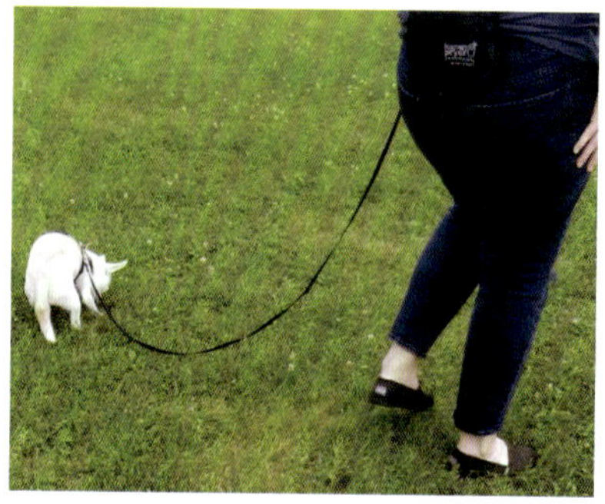

Fig. 9.8 A: Sniff walks are an effective way to slow dogs down and offer them enrichment. (Photo courtesy of Katharine Schwarz)

For an even more enriching experience, consider a sniff walk. Treats can be pre-hidden along the route, or an assistant can scatter them randomly to guide the dog. Using a longer leash can provide added freedom during these walks.

Lures and nose targeting can be used to keep dogs engaged and encourage forward movement, especially for those prone to freezing on walks. Additionally, the 1–2–3 Game introduces a predictable rhythm with engagement, which is particularly useful during transitions and leash walking around distractions.[13]

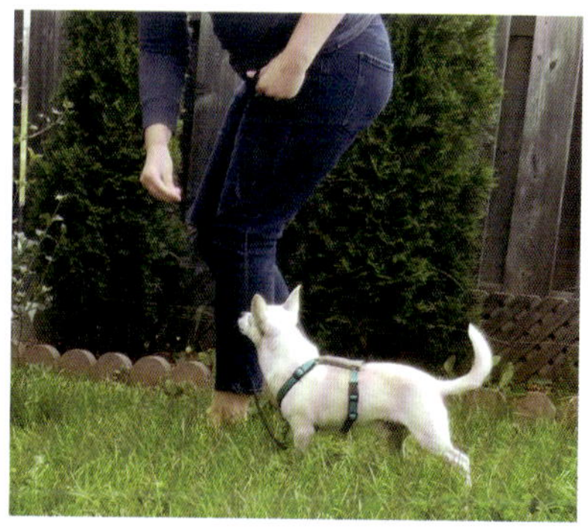

Fig. 9.8 B: Luring can be used to encourage a dog to move forward. (Photo courtesy of Katharine Schwarz)

Apollo: The Tale of a Shelter Dog

Apollo, an energetic young dog, found himself in a busy animal shelter. While he loved humans, he was reactive to other dogs. Whenever he passed other runs, he would sometimes bark and lunge at the dogs, creating a stressful environment for both him and the other residents.

Apollo's caretaker, Sarah, was determined to help him overcome his reactivity and make his shelter stay more comfortable. She had learned about the 1–2–3 Game; a technique designed to change behavior patterns, reduce reactivity, and encourage engagement in stressful situations.

Phase 1: Creating the Pattern Sarah started training in the large inside exercise area of the shelter, which was quiet and had few distractions. She did not use a leash at this stage, wanting Apollo to feel as relaxed as possible. She initiated the game with a pocket full of tasty treats and Apollo by her side.

"Walk with me, Apollo," Sarah said, and as they began to move, she counted softly, 1, 2, 3. She emphasized "3" in a slightly higher pitch. She kept her hands flat against her stomach so Apollo would not focus on her hand.

After "three," Sarah stopped and held a treat next to her thigh. Apollo, curious about the treat, positioned himself next to her and accepted the reward. They repeated this process five times. As they practiced, Apollo began to catch on, moving to be by Sarah's side with each repetition.

Phase 2: Picking Up the Speed Once Apollo reliably walked next to her after taking the treat, Sarah decided to challenge him a bit more. After Apollo received his treat, she did not stop after "three," but only paused briefly before resuming walking. They repeated this sequence five times.

Phase 3: Walking Patterns With Apollo's progress evident, Sarah introduced more fun into their training sessions. She guided him through turns, figure-eight patterns, and even walked around obstacles in the shelter. Apollo, now focused and engaged, handled these challenges with enthusiasm.

Phase 4: Adding Distractions It was now time to add the leash and start all over again. Apollo caught on quickly, so Sarah moved the game outside. Soon, Apollo was engaged both when on leash outside and when on or off leash inside as Sarah counted out the pattern. The real test came when they walked by the other dogs' runs. Sarah maintained the 1–2–3 pattern, and Apollo's reactivity began to decrease. Instead of barking and lunging, he started to walk past the other dogs focused on Sarah and the game.

Once they reached the exercise yard, Apollo had a blast, running and playing. However, the real challenge came when it was time to return to his run. A neighboring dog was particularly intimidating, barking and jumping aggressively whenever Apollo approached the door.

Sarah remained patient and started the 1–2–3 Game to guide Apollo past the barking neighbor. With each repetition, Apollo hesitated less and and eventually walked into his run without hesitation.

9.9 Transporting Cats

All cats should be placed in a carrier when transported throughout the facility.[3–5] For short distances within the same room, options such as a football hold (with or without a towel), a high-sided bed, carrier base, or baby scale might be appropriate.[3–5] Always observe the cat's body language during transportation and adjust accordingly for their comfort and safety.

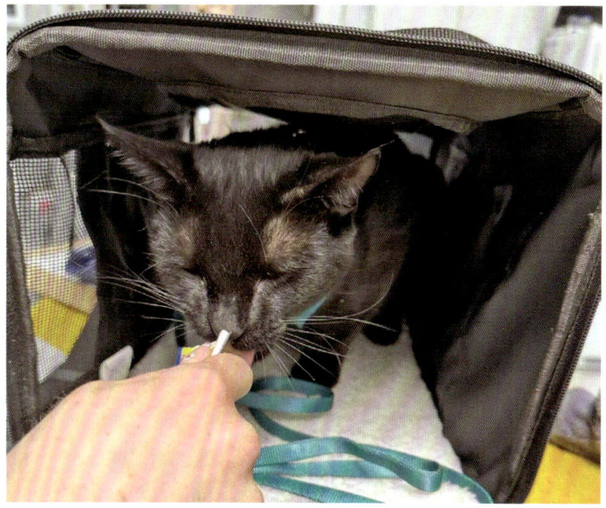

Fig. 9.9 A: It is important to let cats exit the carrier on their own. Food can be used to help with this. This cat is wearing a leash and harness, not a slip lead. (Photo courtesy of Eliot Veterinary Hospital)

Carriers

Carriers are not just for transportation but also a useful tool for removing cats from cages. Sliding a carrier into a cage often encourages the cat to enter it on their own. If the cat shows hesitation or appears stressed, the carrier should be removed, and a different method should be considered.

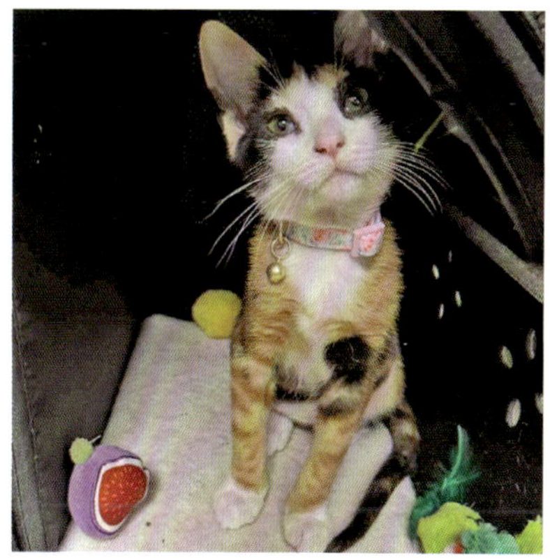

Fig. 9.9 B: The carrier should be welcoming, furnished with soft bedding and toys inside. (Photo courtesy of Louisiana State University School of Veterinary Medicine Community Practice)

Carrier Training

Carrier training can significantly reduce a cat's stress during car rides and veterinary examinations.[21,22] To help familiarize the cat with the carrier, it should be left out and accessible at all times. Encourage the cat to eat their food or enjoy tasty treats inside the carrier to motivate voluntary entry, creating positive associations. This way, the cat can enter and exit the carrier at their own will. Never force a cat into a carrier except in emergencies, and even then, the cat should ideally be already carrier trained.

Carrier Training Resource

For more information on carrier training, please see ***https://veterinarypartner.vin.com/doc/?id=10282561&pid=19239***

Working in Carriers

Exams, vaccines, and other procedures might be less stressful and more manageable for some pets if they remain in the carrier.[3–5,11,14] Placing a pheromone-infused towel over the carrier can help alleviate stress during car rides, entry into the building, movement within the facility, and before examinations.[3–5]

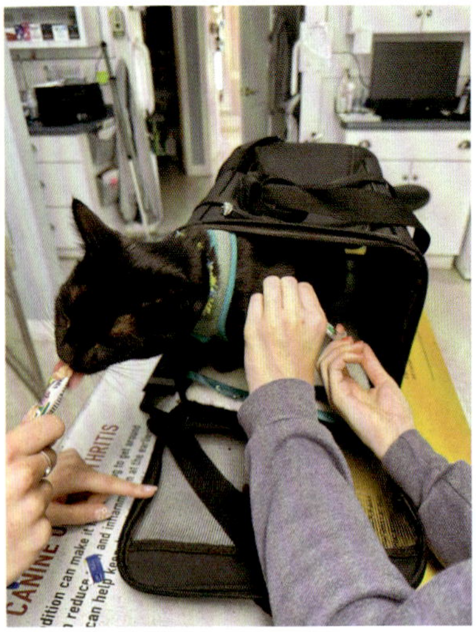

Fig. 9.9 C: Examinations and procedures within the carrier are preferred by some cats. (Photo courtesy of Eliot Veterinary Hospital)

Removing Cats from Carrier

Always give a cat an opportunity to exit the carrier on their own.[3–5] Do not tip or shake the carrier or pull the cat out, as this can escalate the cat's fear and anxiety and potentially cause injuries to both the cat and human. If needed, use a food or toy lure to encourage them to exit.

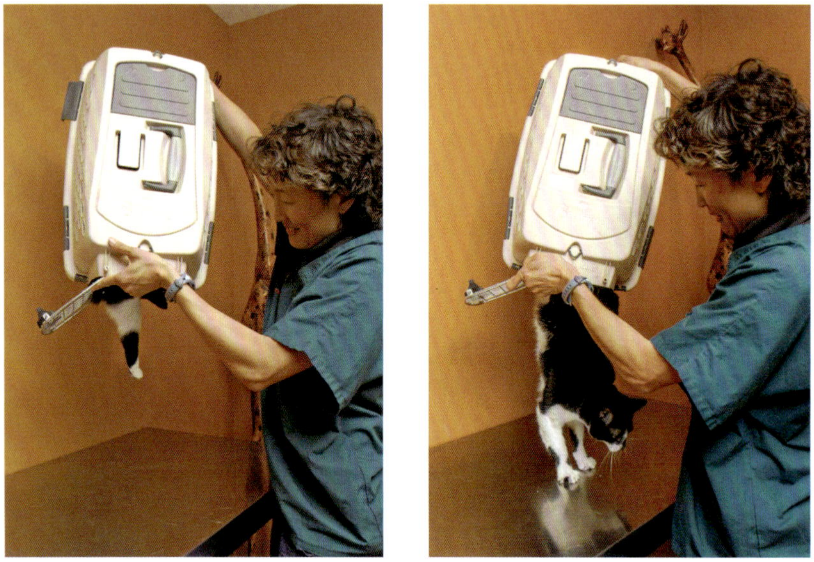

Figs. 9.9 D, E: Incorrect: Do not attempt to dump a cat out of their carrier.

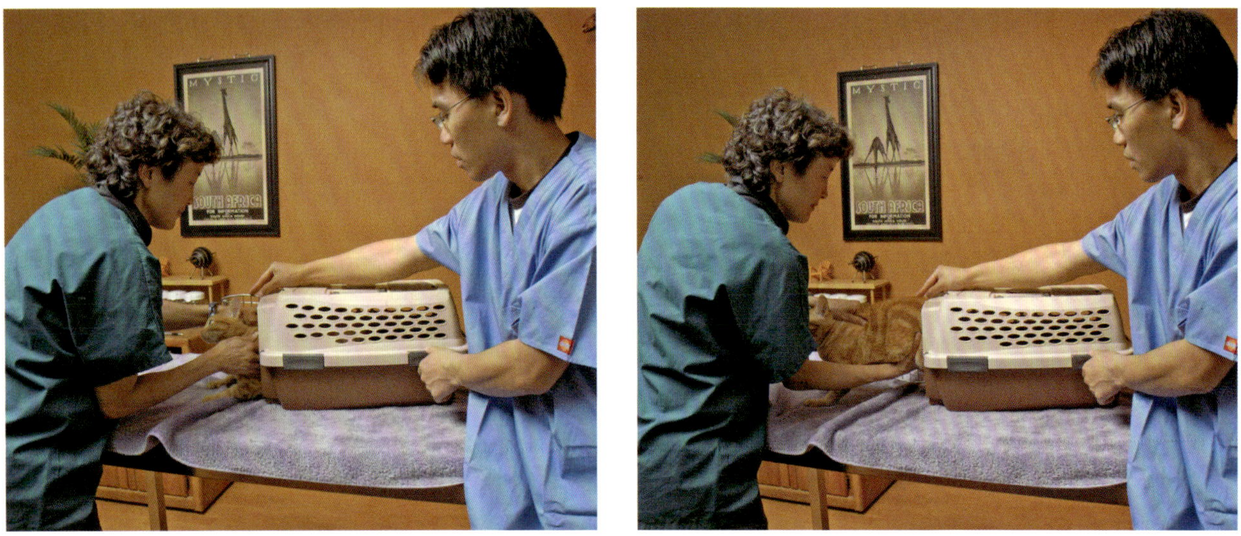

Figs. 9.9 F, G: Incorrect Physically pulling a cat out of their carrier is not an appropriate way to remove a cat from a carrier.

Some cats are more willing to exit the carrier when placed on the floor instead of a table or other elevated surface.[3–5] If the carrier contains a towel or bed, detach the lid and wrap the cat with the towel or bed while lifting. Keeping all four of the cat's feet in contact with a surface can help the cat feel more secure.[3–5]

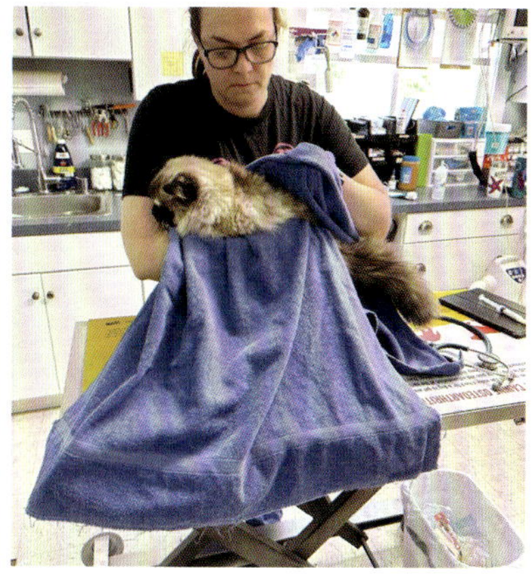

Fig. 9.9 H: Lightly wrapping a cat in a towel before lifting can be less stressful. (Photo courtesy of Eliot Veterinary Hospital)

9.10 Temporary Housing for Cats

Short Stays

For short stays, place the carrier in the cage with the cat inside it. Drape a pheromone-infused towel over the carrier, leaving the door open or the top section unzipped to create a familiar, scented hiding spot.[5,23–26] With this setup, the cat can hide, explore, use the litter box, and eat or drink at their own pace. For additional privacy and security, drape a towel over at least half of the cage door to provide more opportunities for the cat to hide.[5,23–26]

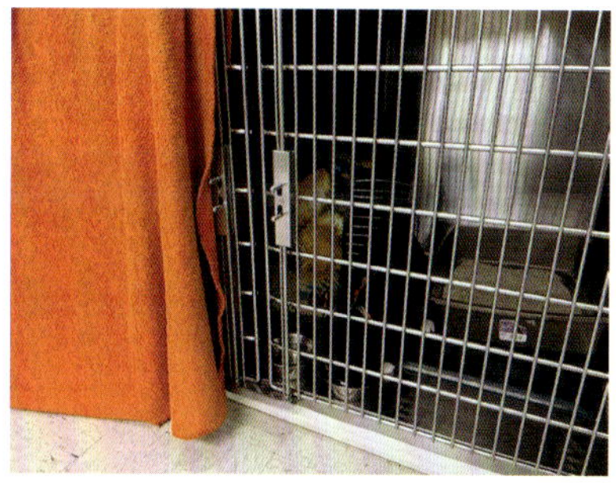

Fig. 9.10 A: A towel placed over the front of the cage door provides privacy. (Photo courtesy of Eliot Veterinary Hospital)

Long Stays

A welfare-friendly long-term cage setup for hospitalized or boarding cats involves selecting a spacious cage that allows ample room for comfortable movement, ideally with distinct areas for resting, eating, and using a litter box, along with a high-sided, soft, and comfortable bed. The litter box should be kept clean and easily accessible, with water and food dishes located away from the elimination area.[5,23–26]

Enrichment is essential for long stays. Provide toys, scratching posts, and opportunities for stretching and exercise. In addition to food-dispensing and puzzle toys for mental stimulation and problem-solving opportunities, regular positive human interactions, exposure to natural light, and access to fresh air are also necessary.

Greeting Cats

Like dogs, some cats may approach, vocalize, and paw in greeting when the cage door opens, indicating a desire to be picked up. For those that do not initially approach, offering food through the door or scattering it on the bedding can encourage engagement. After opening the door, do not instantly lift the cat and never scruff them.[3–5,11,27–31] Instead, move slowly, as cats can be sensitive to quick movements and may try to flee or freeze. They

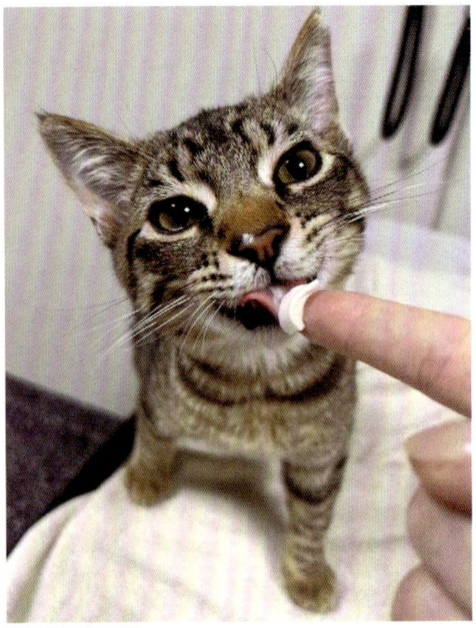

Fig. 9.10 B: Just like dogs, food can be used for cats to form positive associations with handling. (Photo courtesy of Louisiana State University School of Veterinary Medicine Community Practice)

may also feel trapped in a cage, which heightens their anxiety. Allowing them more freedom within the room can help them feel a greater sense of control over their surroundings, making them more relaxed before handling.

When it is time to lift the cat, open the door and, before lifting, turn sideways, avoid direct eye contact, and extend a non-threatening hand low along the bottom of the cage. Lift the cat securely but gently, providing proper support with or without a towel. Fearful cats should be swaddled in a warm, pheromone-infused towel or blanket before relocation.[3–5] Sedation may be necessary before subjecting them to additional handling for examination or procedures.

9.11 Removing Cats from Cages

Carriers are a safe and efficient tool for transporting fearful cats around the animal care facility or removing them from cages. Many cats will enter a carrier voluntarily when it is placed in their cage for transport. If lifting is required and the cat shows signs of distress, remove the carrier and use a different approach, such as a warm, pheromone-infused blanket or towel, or a high-sided cat bed.[3–5]

Using Cues

Many cats are uncomfortable being lifted or held, and their individual preferences need to be identified and respected. Using targeting techniques, such as following a target, the "touch" cue, or stationing to a mat or platform, can direct a cat in an efficient and non-confrontational way, maintaining the cat's sense of choice and control.[3–5,15–20]

Lifting Cats

Before lifting a cat, start by gently massaging the cat's head and ears to encourage relaxation.[32–33] Carefully observe their body language to assess their comfort level and willingness to engage before lifting them.[32]

To lift the cat, position one hand beneath their chest and the other under their hindquarters, lifting smoothly and slowly while supporting the cat's body. Avoid letting their legs to dangle or hang.[3–5] Cradle the cat close to the handler's body to deter squirming or attempts to jump.[3–5] Continually monitor the cat's body language while holding them. If they show signs of tension, gently place them down and either try again later or use an alternative method.

Many cats may find comfort perched on or draped over someone's shoulder. However, this is not a secure method for holding or carrying a cat through a clinic. Should the cat get startled by a loud noise or another animal's presence, they could easily flee, possibly scratching the handler in the process or injuring themselves.

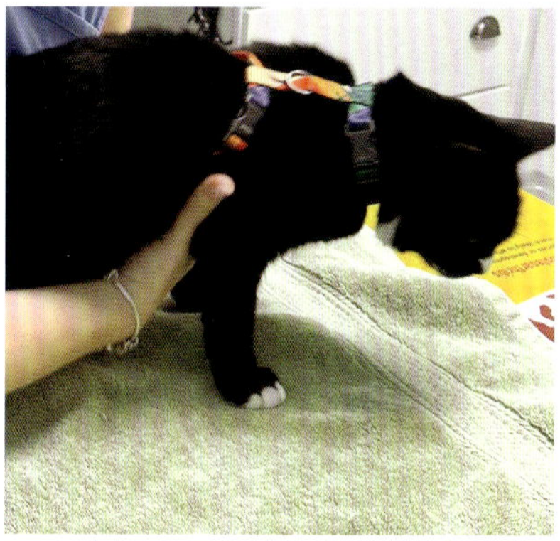

Fig. 9.11 A: The handler is providing support to the cat's chest with her forearm and her hand is fanned out beneath the cat's chest. (Photo courtesy of Eliot Veterinary Hospital)

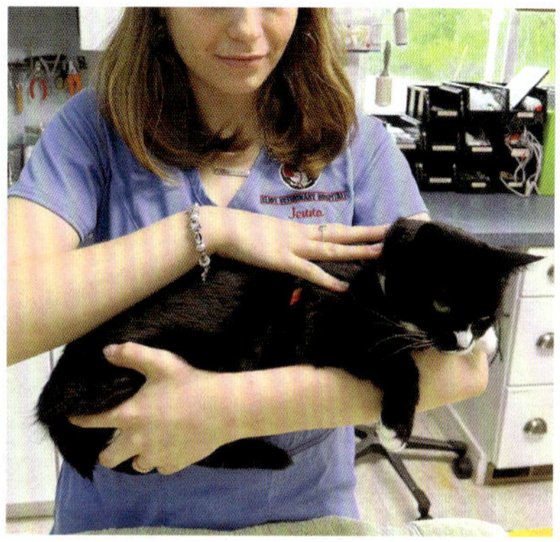

Fig. 9.11 B: While this cat is adequately supported, her front end remains insufficiently secure, creating a risk of bolting if startled. Positioning the right arm along the cat's spine, with the thumb and pinky finger over the dorsal neck and shoulders would enhance stability. The other three fingers could then be used to massage the cat's head and ears, encouraging relaxation. Given this cat's sideward ear position, offering a loose towel to hide within may improve the cat's comfort level before lifting. (Photo courtesy of Eliot Veterinary Hospital)

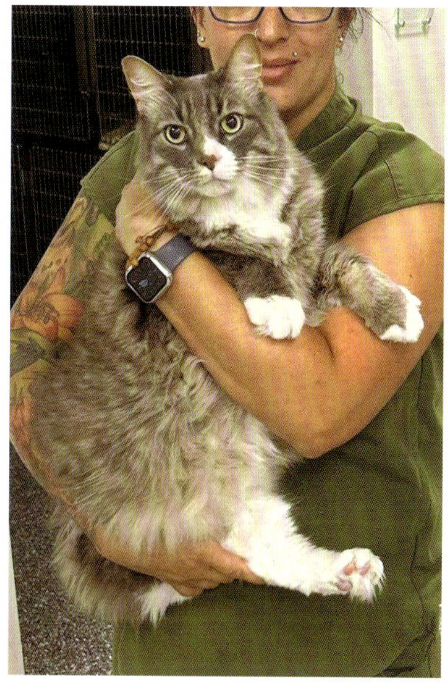

Fig. 9.11 C: Cats should be held close to the body with the handler supporting the chest and back end. (Photo courtesy of Louisiana State University School of Veterinary Medicine Community Practice)

Fearful Cats

Pheromone-infused towels can help create a sense of safety and aid in handling or transporting fearful cats.[3–5] However, cats might become more stressed when wrapped. Quick, unexpected movements with the towel can make a cat feel trapped, leading to defensive reactions. If a cat becomes agitated and swipes at the towel, this method might not be suitable for that individual and record these observations in the medical record.

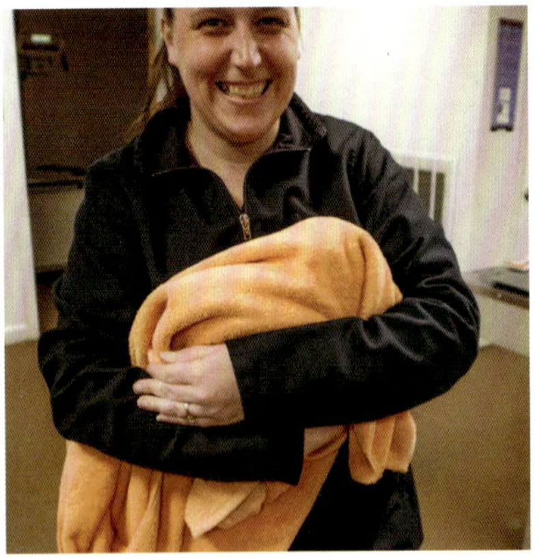

Fig. 9.11 D: A loose but securely placed towel over a cat, known as the blanket wrap method, can be employed for transport. However, it's important to note that if this method is used, the cat should be headed for sedation.

Instead of tightly wrapping, softly drape the towel over the cat and tuck the edges beneath, encompassing their body.[3–5] The handler should maintain consistent contact along the cat's sides, gently turning them and holding the cat close to the handler's abdomen. Before lifting, the handler should be aware of where the cat's head is and that the towel is snug but not overly restrictive. The cat should be able to breathe comfortably without a chance of escape. Some may be more comfortable with their head exposed.

9.12 Conclusion

Low Stress Handling® techniques offer a range of strategies for safely transporting animals within a an animal care facility. Animals should be given choice and control through the use of cues, lures, and distractions. Whenever possible, refrain from lifting both dogs and cats. Carriers are the most secure method of transport for cats. Dogs should be walked using a harness paired with a six-foot lead. Slip leads are never appropriate for cats and should only be used for dogs in specific circumstances, such as brief distances, transfers, or emergencies.

9.13 References

1. The Association of Shelter Veterinarians. (2022). The guidelines for standards of care in animal shelters: Second edition: Second Edition. *Journal of Shelter Medicine and Community Animal Health*, 1(2), 1–76. https://doi.org/10.56771/ASVguidelines.2022

2. Arhant, C., Schmied-Wagner, C., Aigner, U., & Affenzeller, N. (2021). Owner reports on the use of muzzles and their effects on dogs: An online survey. *Journal of Veterinary Behavior*, 41, 73–81.

3. Bessant, C., Dowgray, N., Ellis, S. L., Taylor, S., Collins, S., Ryan, L., & Halls, V. (2022). ISFM's Cat friendly principles for veterinary professionals. *Journal of Feline Medicine and Surgery*, 24(11), 1087–1092.

4. Rodan, I., Dowgray, N., Carney, H. C., et al. (2022). 2022 AAFP/ISFM Cat friendly veterinary interaction guidelines: Approach and handling techniques. *Journal of Feline Medicine and Surgery*, 24(11), 1093–1132.

5. Taylor, S., St Denis, K., Collins, S., Dowgray, N., Ellis, S. L. H., Heath, S., Rodan, I., & Ryan, L. (2022). ISFM/AAFP Cat friendly veterinary environment guidelines. *Journal of Feline Medicine and Surgery*, 24(11), 1133–1163.

6. Hunter, A., Blake, S., & De Godoy, R. F. (2019). Pressure and force on the canine neck when exercised using a collar and leash. *Veterinary Animal Science*, 8, 100082. https://doi.org/10.1016/j.vas.2019.100082

7. Pauli, A. M., Bentley, E., Diehl, K. A., & Miller, P. E. (2006). Effects of the application of neck pressure by a collar or harness on intraocular pressure in dogs. *Journal of the American Animal Hospital Association*, 42(3), 207–211. https://doi.org/10.5326/0420207

8. Haug, L. I., Beaver, B. V., & Longnecker, M. T. (2002). Comparison of dogs' reactions to four different head collars. *Applied Animal Behaviour Science*, 79(1), 53–61.

9. Anseeuw, E., Apker, C., Ayscue, C., Barker, L., Blair, D., Brennan, J., Brooks, S., Case-Pall, D., Caspersen, H., Clark, J., & Colson, L. (2006). Handling cats humanely in the veterinary hospital. *Journal of Veterinary Behavior*, 1(2), 84–88.

10. Couture, M., Stellato, A. C., Moody, C. M., & Niel, L. (2022). Owner perspectives of cat handling techniques used in the veterinary clinic. *Journal of Applied Animal Welfare Science*, 1–11.

11. Herron, M. E., & Shreyer, T. (2014). The pet-friendly veterinary practice: a guide for practitioners. *Veterinary Clinics: Small Animal Practice*, 44(3), 451–481.

12. Riemer, S., Heritier, C., Windschnurer, I., Pratsch, L., Arhant, C., & Affenzeller, N. (2021). A review on mitigating fear and aggression in dogs and cats in a veterinary setting. *Animals*, 11(1), 158.

13. McDevitt, L. (2007). *Control unleashed: Creating a focused and confident dog*. Clean Run Productions LLC.

14. Yin, S. A. (2009). *Low Stress Handling, Restraint, and Behavior Modification of Dogs and Cats.* CattleDog Publishing.

15. Englund, M. D., & Cronin, K. A. (2023). Choice, control, and animal welfare: definitions and essential inquiries to advance animal welfare science. *Frontiers in Veterinary Science*, 10.

16. Horowitz, A. (2021). Considering the "dog" in dog–human interaction. *Frontiers in Veterinary Science*, 8, 642821.

17. Jones, E. (2023). Cooperative care for companion dogs: emotional health and wellness. *Companion Animal*, 28(7), 1–6.

18. Littlewood, K. E., Heslop, M. V., & Cobb, M. L. The agency domain and behavioural interactions: Assessing positive animal welfare using the Five Domains Model. *Frontiers in Veterinary Science*, 10, 1284869.

19. Sydänheimo, A., Freeman, M., & Hunt, K. (2023). Cooperative care does not scare-use if cooperative care training in routine husbandry in dogs. *Animal Behaviour and Welfare Cases*, doi.org/10.1079/abwcases.2023.0010.

20. Wess, L., Böhm, A., Schützinger, M., Riemer, S., Yee, J. R., Affenzeller, N., & Arhant, C. (2022). Effect of cooperative care training on physiological parameters and compliance in dogs undergoing a veterinary examination–A pilot study. *Applied Animal Behaviour Science*, 250, 105615.

21. Gruen, M. E., Thomson, A. E., Clary, G. P., et al. (2013). Conditioning laboratory cats to handling and transport. *Lab Animal*, 42(10), 385–389.

22. Pratsch, L., Mohr, N., Palme, R., Rost, J., Troxler, J., & Arhant, C. (2018). Carrier training cats reduces stress on transport to a veterinary practice. *Applied Animal Behaviour Science*, 206, 64–74.

23. Arrandale, L., & Buckley, L. (2017). Towels versus hides: which are best at reducing acute stress in the newly hospitalised domestic cat (Felis sylvestris catus)? *Veterinary Nursing Journal*, 32(10), 285–288.

24. Buckley, L. A., & Arrandale, L. (2017). The use of hides to reduce acute stress in the newly hospitalised domestic cat (Felis sylvestris catus). *Veterinary Nursing Journal*, 32(5), 129–132.

25. Vinke, C. M., Godijn, L. M., & Van der Leij, W. J. R. (2014). Will a hiding box provide stress reduction for shelter cats? *Applied Animal Behaviour Science*, 160, 86–93.

26. Williams, T., Carroll, A., & Montrose, V. T. (2019). Environmental methods used by veterinary centres to reduce stress of cats and dogs during practice visits. *The Veterinary Nurse,* 10(1), 47–52.

27. Moody, C. M. (2018). Improving the welfare of cats during handling and restraint (Doctoral dissertation, University of Guelph).

28. Moody, C. M., Dewey, C. E., & Niel, L. (2020). Cross-sectional survey of cat handling practices in veterinary clinics throughout Canada and the United States. *Journal of the American Veterinary Medical Association*, 256(9), 1020–1033.

29. Moody, C. M., Mason, G. J., Dewey, C. E., & Niel, L. (2020). Getting a grip: cats respond negatively to scruffing and clips. *Veterinary Record*, 186(12), 385–385.

30. Moody, C. M., Mason, G. J., Dewey, C. E., Landsberg, G. M., & Niel, L. (2019). Testing two behavioural paradigms for measuring post-handling cat aversion behaviour. *Applied Animal Behaviour Science*, 210, 73–80.

31. Moody, C. M., Picketts, V. A., Mason, G. J., Dewey, C. E., & Niel, L. (2018). Can you handle it? Validating negative responses to restraint in cats. *Applied Animal Behavior Science*, 204, 94–100.

32. Haywood, C., Ripari, L., Puzzo, J., Foreman-Worsley, R., & Finka, L. R. (2021). Providing humans with practical, best practice handling guidelines during human-cat interactions increases cats' affiliative behaviour and reduces aggression and signs of conflict. *Frontiers in Veterinary Science*, 8, 835.

33. Soennichsen, S., & Chamove, A. S. (2002). Responses of cats to petting by humans. *Anthrozoös*, 15(3), 258–265. https://doi.org/10.2752/089279302786992577

Contributing Authors:
Sandra Robbins BS, CVT, VTS (Anesthesia and Analgesia), CPDT-KSA, KPA-CTP
Christine D. Calder DVM, DACVB
Pat Koven BA/Journalism, LVT, KPA-CTP

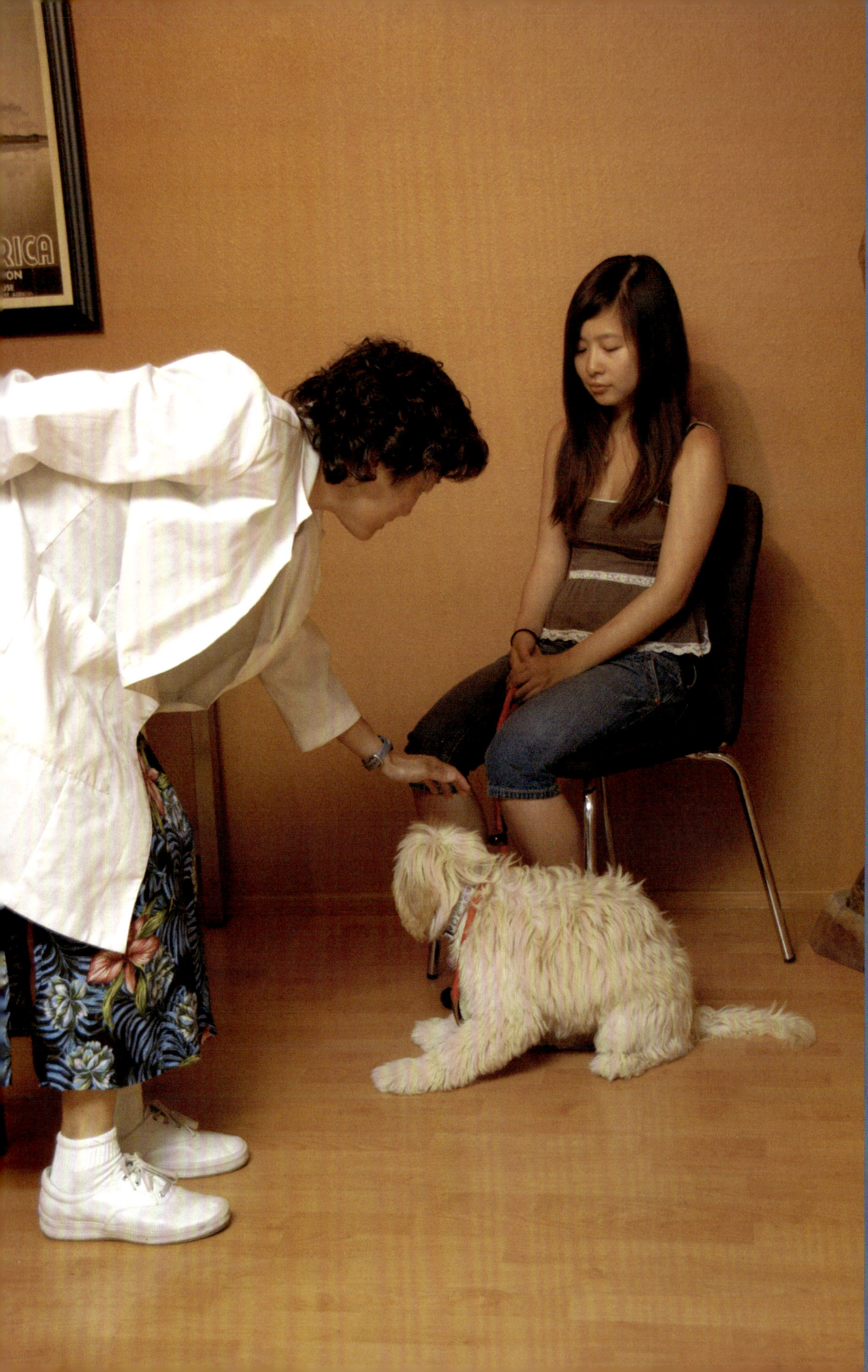

CHAPTER 10

Canine Low Stress Handling®

10.1 Introduction

Historically, handlers have been trained to tightly restrain dogs during examinations and diagnostic procedures, a practice that is not without risks. Forceful or unskilled handling can cause pain, discomfort, frustration, and fear in dogs, negatively impacting their welfare and safety.[1] Additionally, these techniques can affect the results of a physical examination, altering physiological parameters like heart rate, respiratory rate, temperature, blood glucose levels, and blood pressure.[2–4] These effects make it difficult to differentiate between illness and distress. Over time, a dog's response to handling may escalate, leading to heightened protective emotions and defensive behaviors, including aggression.

10.2 Examination

When examining and performing procedures on dogs, choose locations that are comfortable for both the dog and the examiner, such as the floor, a chair, or a bench. If an examination table is utilized, placing a non-slip mat on it can help reduce slipping and increase the dog's comfort. Similarly, a mat on the floor can provide a sense of security for the dog. Should the dog prefer a chair or bench, encourage them to hop up.

Avoid forcing interactions and give the dog time to acclimate to the environment. Toss treats behind the dog, allowing them the choice to move away before deciding to return for more. Refrain from reaching out to dogs, grabbing their collars, or pulling them out of hiding spaces. Instead, gently invite them to come closer. Utilize familiar cues, such as "touch," "sit," "down" to encourage their approach and prepare for handling. Offer distractions and rewards to improve their comfort level during examinations or

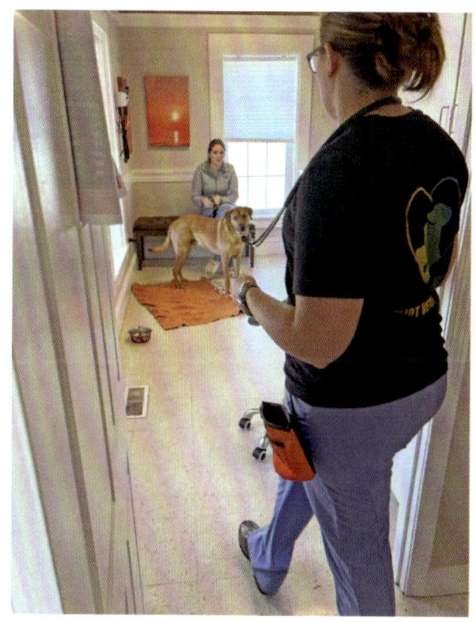

Fig. 10.2 A: Benches or a non-slip mat on the floor might be the most comfortable locations for examinations. Provide a water dish in each room and keep treats on hand. (Photo courtesy of Eliot Veterinary Hospital)

procedures. Always document each dog's individual preferences in their medical record for future reference.[5]

When managing reactive dogs in a clinical or hospital setting, adopt a strategy to minimize their stress and arousal. For most reactive dogs, the sound of knocking on the door can increase their arousal levels, so it is generally better to avoid this. Instead, alert the client of your entrance by slowly opening the door just a few inches and softly greeting the caregiver with a "hello." Take a moment to pause and assess the situation before fully entering the room. For patients with a history of aggression or those who have exhibited aggressive behavior in the hospital, ensure the caregiver has a secure hold on the leash before entering the room. For added safety, use a tether bolted to the wall or floor, an exercise pen (ex-pen) stretched across the room, or another barrier. Before fully opening the door, begin tossing treats behind the dog to distract them, encourage them to turn away, and move away from the door. Continue gently tossing treats on the floor behind the dog while transitioning into the room and taking a seat. Apply this technique in reverse when leaving the room and during all transitions, such as standing or moving around the room.

Engagement

When team members enter examination rooms, caregivers can engage their dog with interactive activities like "touch," the Up and Down Game, or the 1-2-3 Game to manage their pet's behavior and keep them focused during the visit.

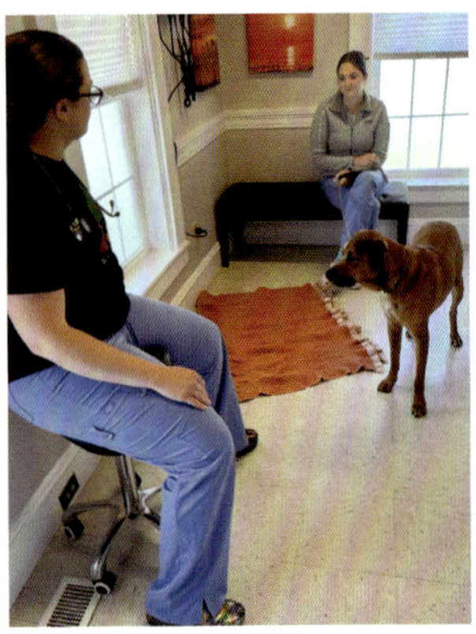

Fig. 10.2 B: The veterinarian is positioned to give the dog time to acclimate and to allow for voluntary interaction if the dog chooses. (Photo courtesy of Eliot Veterinary Hospital)

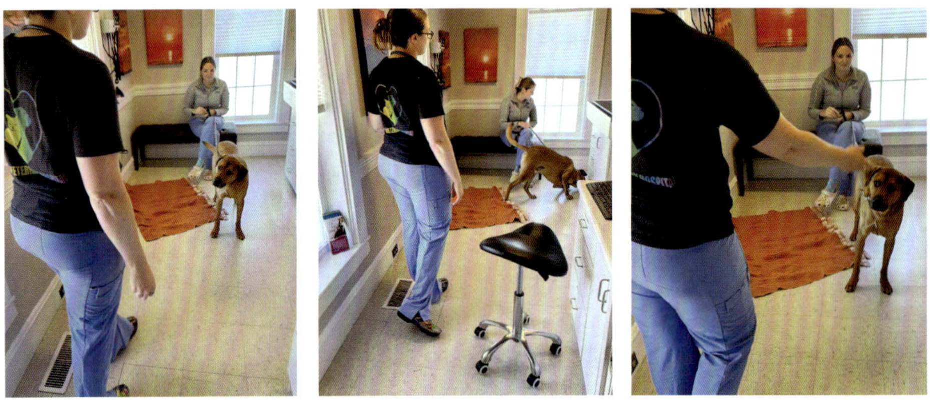

Figs. 10.2 C-E: By using cues the dog recognizes, such as 'find it' when tossing treats away, gives the dog an opportunity to move away and make a choice to return for more. (Photos courtesy of Eliot Veterinary Hospital)

Physical Examination

During a physical examination of a dog, understand that various factors can influence their behavior. These factors range from daily events to the dog's health status and level of pain. Typically, dogs experiencing pain tend to exhibit more protective emotions and defensive behaviors compared to those dogs that are healthy and pain free. Thus, continuous observation of the animal's body language is essential. By closely monitoring the dog's reactions, the examiner can make necessary adjustments keeping the examination process as low stress and complete as possible.

Distant Observations

Conducting a comprehensive examination while minimizing stress and discomfort for the dog starts with observing from a distance before initiating physical contact. Begin by watching the dog move around the room, paying close attention to the symmetry of their muscles and gait. These observations can provide valuable insights into the dog's physical health. Additionally, from a safe distance observe the size and symmetry of the dog's pupils; asymmetrical pupils may indicate neurological issues or other health concerns. Look for external signs of disease such as hair loss, skin redness, or inflammation. Also, note any abnormalities or discharge in the eyes and ears.

Assessing Pain at Home

Video footage provided by the caregiver showing their dog rising from a resting position, climbing stairs, and moving around the house and yard can be instrumental in identifying subtle lameness that might not be apparent during the physical examination.

Temperature and Stool Samples

In order to minimize stress, avoid taking the dog's temperature at the start of the appointment.[4,6] If a temperature reading is necessary, consider using an aural (in the ear) or axillary (under the arm) method, which tends to be less invasive.[6–8] For healthy animals, temperature readings are not a necessity and can sometimes be artificially elevated due to stress. Additionally, procedures involving venipuncture, such as heartworm tests, should be delayed until the end of the examination. Encourage caregivers to bring a stool sample to the appointment or return later with one. This practice eliminates the need for in-house collection using a fecal loop extraction which is often aversive to the dog.

Yellow Dogs

For a dog that will not come out from behind their caregiver's legs or has retreated under a table or bench, give them time to emerge on their own, rather than cornering them in a confined space. This approach helps to reduce their anxiety and prevent an escalation of fear. Alternative strategies include having the caregiver walk away while offering a treat or calling the dog over in a gentle, inviting manner. Using a touch cue then engaging the dog in alternative activities, such as the 1-2-3 Game, can also effectively encourage the dog to leave their hiding place.

Examination Location

Conduct the examination in a setting where the dog is most comfortable and avoid taking the dog out of this environment to minimize anxiety.[1,5,9–13] Involve the caregiver in tasks such as offering treats to the dog. If additional team members are needed for certain procedures, ask the caregiver to step outside temporarily rather than removing the dog.

> **Engagement During Examinations**
>
> A study on anxiety levels during physical examinations revealed that dogs exhibited fewer signs of anxiety when their caregivers actively engaged in petting and reassuring them throughout the process. In contrast, when caregivers were present but refrained from comforting their pets, the dogs showed more signs of anxiety. These findings suggest that encouraging caregivers to interact with and reassure their dogs during examinations can effectively help the animals feel more comfortable.[13]

Table 10.2.1: Green Dogs Ok to Proceed

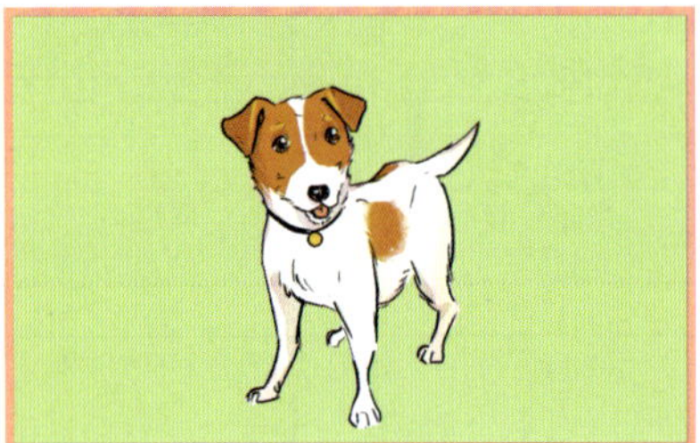

Relaxed, comfortable, and eating.

Low Stress Handling® Plan

- Monitor the dog closely throughout the procedure.
- Ensure the dog continues to eat or play, remains relaxed, continues to approach, and stays interactive.
- Stop the procedure if the dog starts taking treats roughly, begins to chew more slowly, or stops eating.
- Halt activities if signs of escalating emotional arousal appear, such as fidgeting, avoidance, looking away, staring, or if the dog becomes slow-moving and frozen.

The Hands-on Examination

When conducting a physical examination on a dog, it is more important to follow a systematic approach rather than examining from nose to tail. Always start with the less invasive areas of the body and gradually progress to the more sensitive ones. Begin with regions that are less likely to cause discomfort and save the potentially painful areas for last. This strategy involves starting the hands-on examination from the tail end, as areas around the dog's head, face, ears, eyes, and feet are typically more sensitive.

When examining potentially painful areas, such as an injured limb, start with the non-injured regions and leave the sensitive or painful areas for the final stages. This method allows for ongoing monitoring of the dog's emotional state, providing the opportunity to adjust the examination technique as needed. Maintain a consistent touch throughout the examination, avoiding abrupt movements that might startle the dog.[12] After examining the hind end, transition smoothly to the front, and reserve the examination of the ears, eyes, and mouth for the end.

> **Initial Touch**
>
> Initiating physical contact on the chest during a dog's examination may be beneficial, as this approach is less likely to increase heart rate compared to petting them on other body areas.[14]

Three-Second Rule

Continuously monitor the dog's emotional state during all interactions and adjust the approach as necessary. While handling, avoid letting the dog struggle for more than three seconds.[5,12] If the dog struggles, **STOP**, reposition, and then attempt again. If the dog continues to struggle, introduce a second person, but maintain the three-second rule.[5,12] After three attempts at repositioning, discontinue handling and consider alternative methods, such as rescheduling or sedation.[5,12]

Eating as an Indicator of Stress

A dog's willingness to eat can be a significant indicator of their stress level. If they stop eating, refuse food, or begin to take treats roughly at any point, an adjustment in positioning or approach may be necessary. Always allow the dog a break before attempting to handle them again. If they continue to refuse food, determine if the procedure is urgent. If it is, sedation may be required before continuing. If is not urgent, consider rescheduling the appointment for another date and prescribing pre-visit medications. For added comfort and safety, initiate basket muzzle training before the next visit.

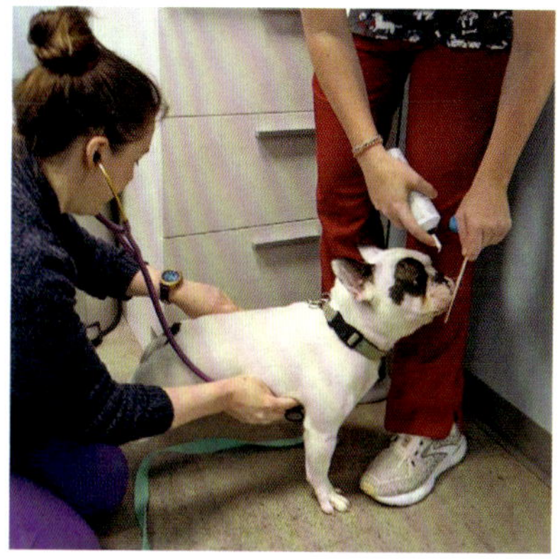

Fig.10.2 F: Food distractions have several benefits during examinations and can reduce struggling, the need for restraint, and help for create positive associations. (Photo courtesy of Ralphie the Demon Dog)

10.3 Neck Holds

During physical examinations, dogs often prefer standing. If a dog chooses to sit, the examiner should first examine the front half of the dog's body. When it is time for abdominal palpation or the hind-end examination, use a familiar cue or lure to encourage the dog to stand. Avoid physically manipulating the dog into a standing position, as it may cause discomfort or startle the dog.

In certain cases, an examination can be completed while the caregiver holds the dog on a loose leash. This approach provides an opportunity for the caregiver to comfort their dog by petting or offering treats. However, the dog should always have the ability to move away, and holding the collar should be avoided.

When examining a dog on a table, place a hand gently on the front of their chest to prevent them from jumping off. Distractions can be used as needed to maintain the dog's position during the examination without using heavy restraint.[12]

Toy Distractions

Some dogs may prefer toys over treats, or enjoy them in addition to treats. Observe how the dog interacts with their toy during handling. If the dog drops the toy or becomes disinterested, implement the three-second rule. Just as refusing food, this behavior may indicate increasing emotional arousal and stress.

Ring Hold

A ring hold helps to prevent the dog from jumping up or moving forward.[12] Use thumbs to stabilize the dog's head and form a ring around their neck with both hands. Once the dog relaxes, gradually release pressure.[12] This holding technique is appropriate only for small dogs and cats.[12]

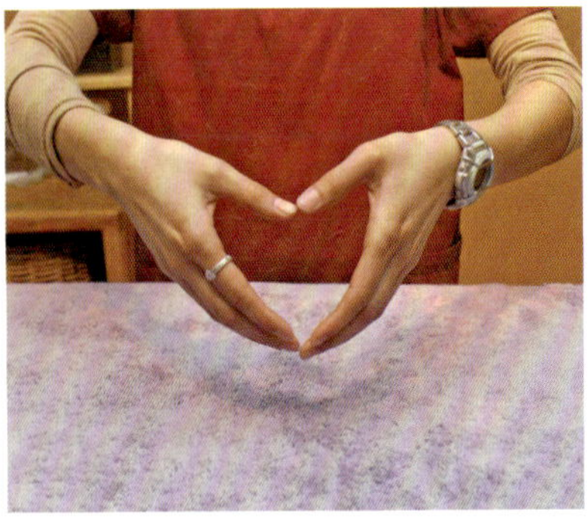
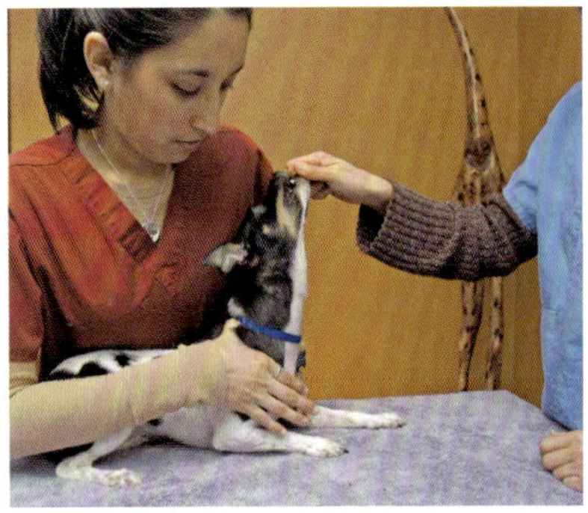

Figs. 10.3 A, B: A Ring Hold involves the use of both hands to make a ring around the neck reducing upward, lateral, and forward movements.

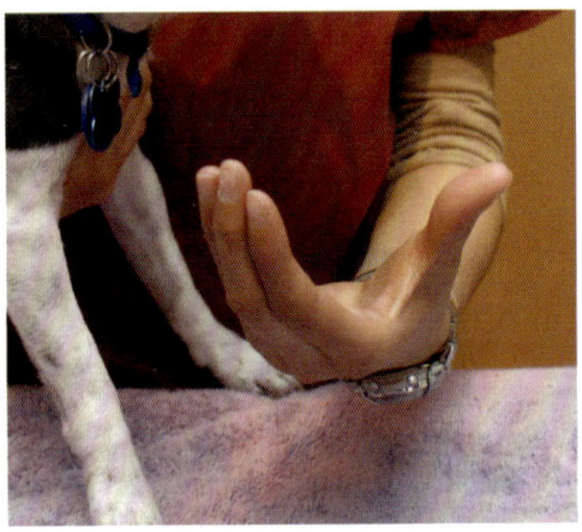
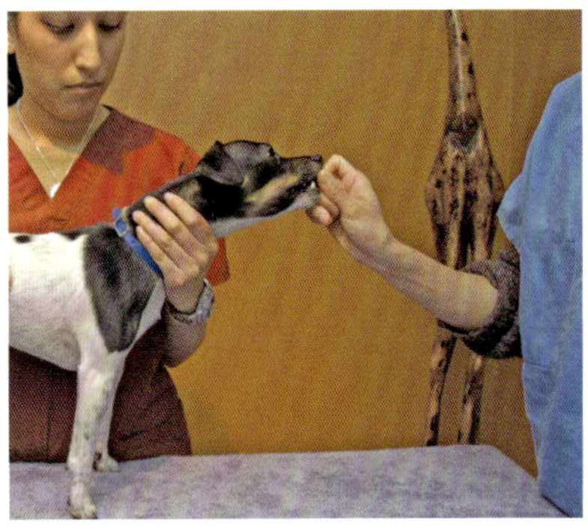

Figs. 10.3 C, D: U-Hold: This hold cradles the neck, effectively preventing forward and lateral movements of the dog.

U-Hold

Shape the hand into a "U" around the dog's neck to restrict forward and lateral movements.[12] This hand should provide support only, avoiding any forceful pressure on the neck. If the dog attempts to move away, smoothly transition the hand into a C-hold.[12]

C-Hold

Similar to the U-hold, the C-hold involves a slight variation in hand placement.[12] Rather than cradling the ventral part of the neck, move the hand to the outside of the neck, guiding the dog's head against the handler's shoulder.[12]

Avoid Excessive Pressure

When practicing the ***U- and C-holds***, use the wing of the atlas (the first cervical vertebra) as a reference point. This helps prevent excessive pressure on the neck area.

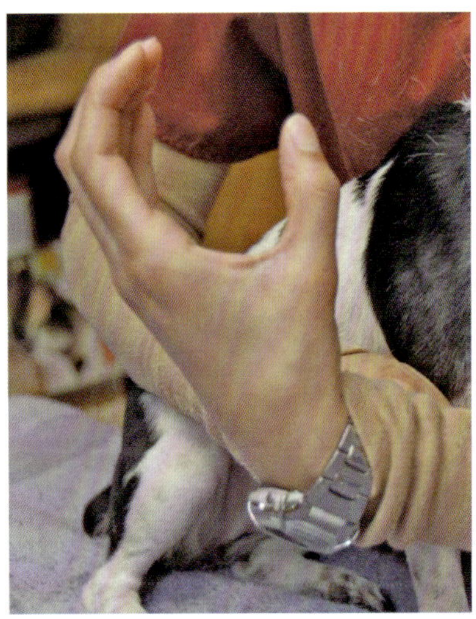
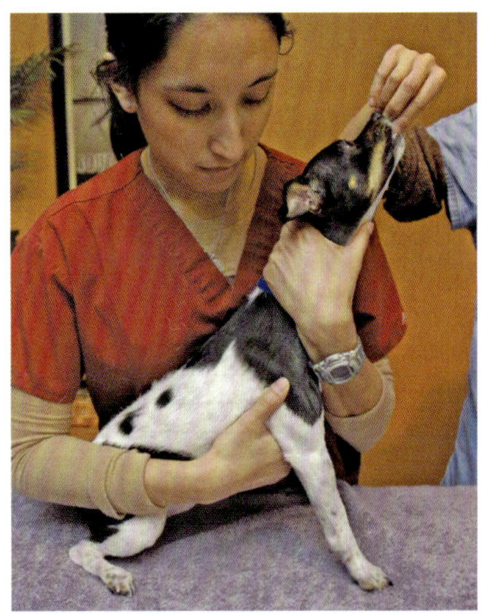

Figs. 10.3 E, F: The C-hold is designed to restrict upward, lateral, and forward movements of the dog. To prevent backward motion, securely wrap an arm around the dog's hind end.

Medium to Large Dogs

For medium and larger dogs, encircle the neck and head with the entire arm, ensuring the neck is positioned in the bend of the handler's elbow.[12] This maximizes the contact surface area with the neck and effectively prevents upward, lateral, and forward movements.[12]

The handler can draw the dog's head closer to their shoulder by turning their palm outward and resting the back of their hand on the dog's neck.[12] Positioning this hand behind the dog's skull minimizes backward movement.[12]

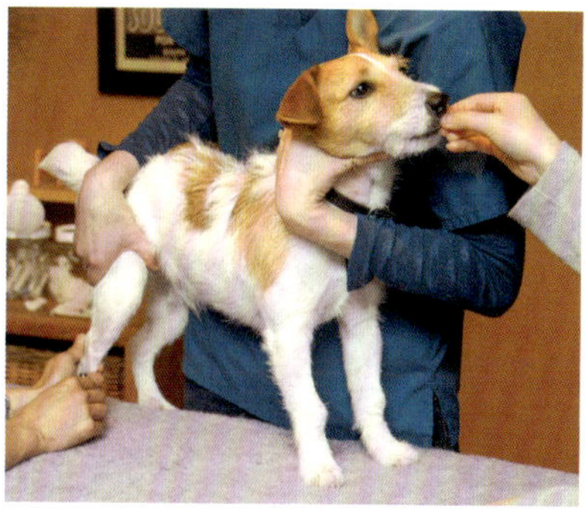

Fig. 10.3 G: The C-hold, designed to prevent upward, lateral, and forward movements, is suitable for securely positioning a small dog during a saphenous blood draw.

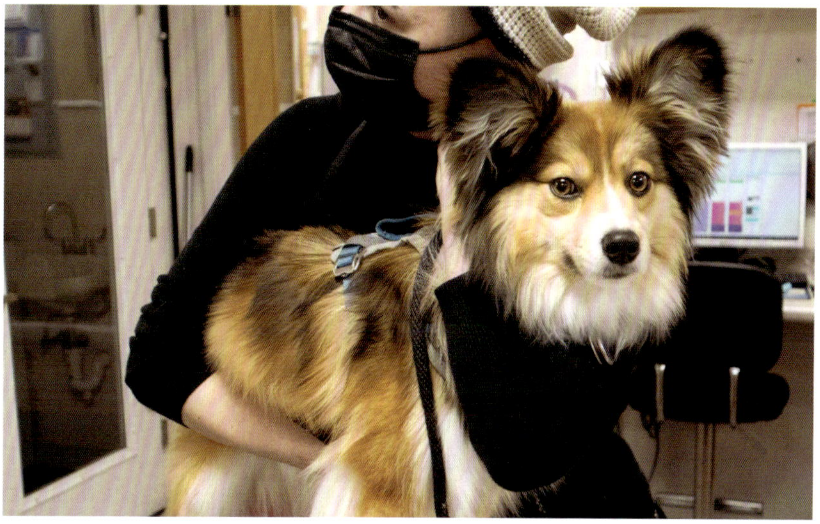

Fig. 10.3 H: The handler's left arm wraps around the dog's neck and chest, positioning the arm slightly higher beneath the dog's neck so that the dog's head rests in the crook of the elbow. For small or medium-sized dogs, position the handler's right arm over the dog's right hip, using an elbow hold to minimize lateral and backward movements.

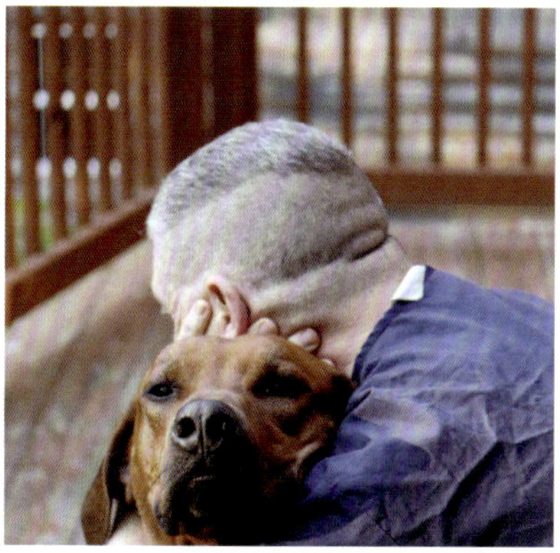

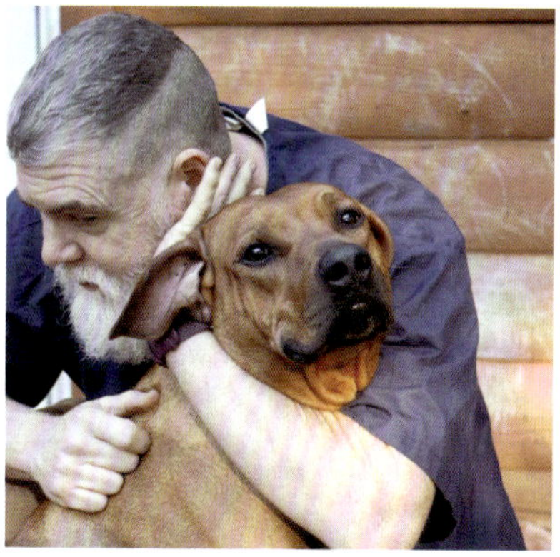

Figs. 10.3 I, J: For a more secure hold, the handler can place their hand with the palm facing up, resting it against their own neck.

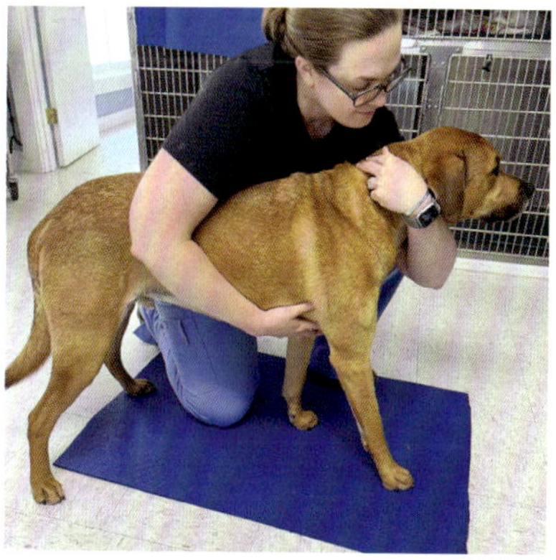

Fig. 10.3 K: For some dogs, simply positioning the entire arm across the dog's chest, without securing the head more tightly, is sufficient. (Photo courtesy of Eliot Veterinary Hospital)

10.4 Front Leg Holds

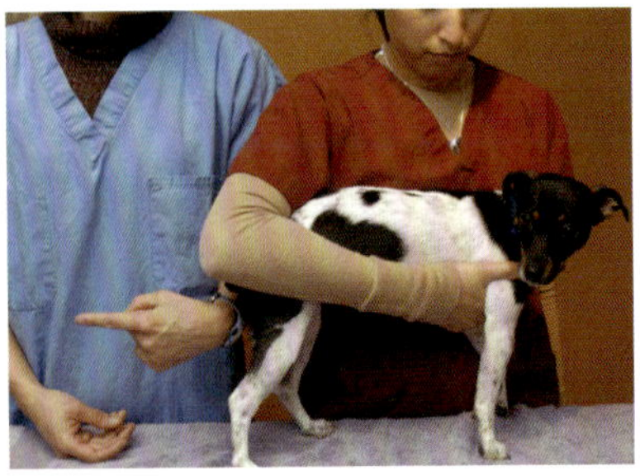

Fig. 10.4 A: A front leg hold reduces movement backward and laterally.

For dogs of any size, positioning the outside hand behind their elbow minimizes backward and lateral movements.[12] In this elbow hold, the palm is kept downwards, and fingers are open and flat to maximize contact with the axillary region.[12] The thumb rests on the lateral aspect of the upper leg to further limit backward and lateral movement.[12] If the dog starts to move backward, the handler can gently draw the dog against their body.

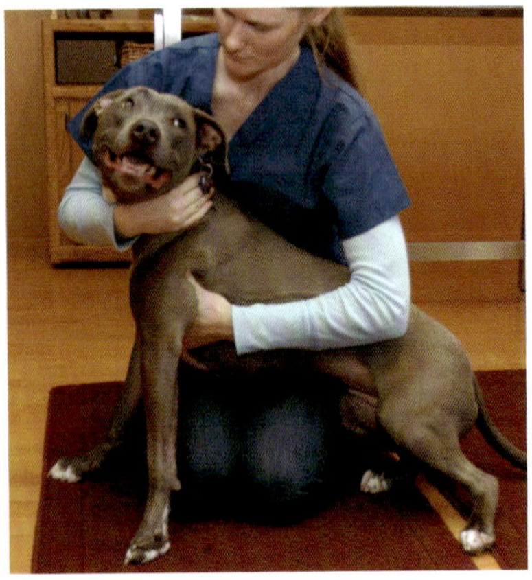

Fig. 10.4 B: For large dogs, placing a hand behind the elbow helps to reduce backward movement. The dog may need to be drawn closer to the handler's body using the elbow to reduce lateral movement with this hold.

Upper Leg Hold

Place the hand of the outside arm around the proximal aspect of the front leg to reduce upward movement.[12] The thumb and index finger should be above the elbow.[12]

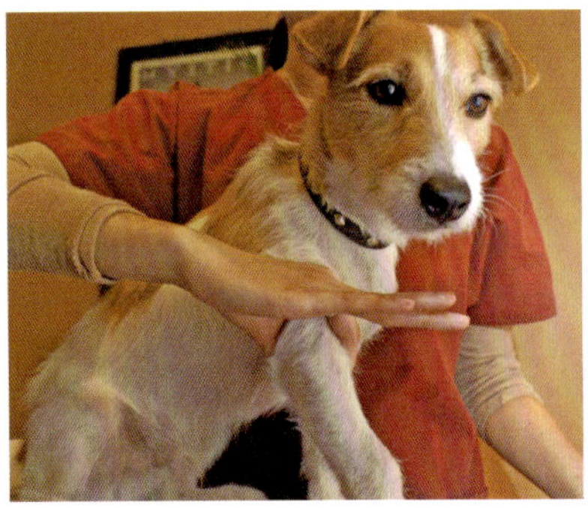

Fig. 10.4 C: The upper leg hold reduces upward movement.

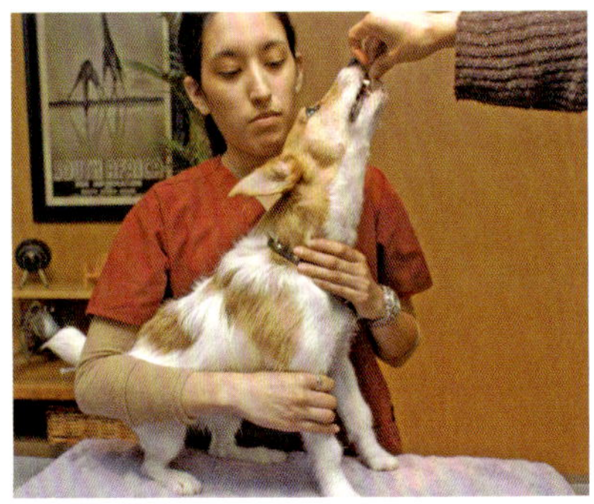

Fig. 10.4 D: Combining a U-hold, upper leg hold, and elbow hold minimizes forward, upward, lateral, and backward movements.

10.5 Hind End Holds

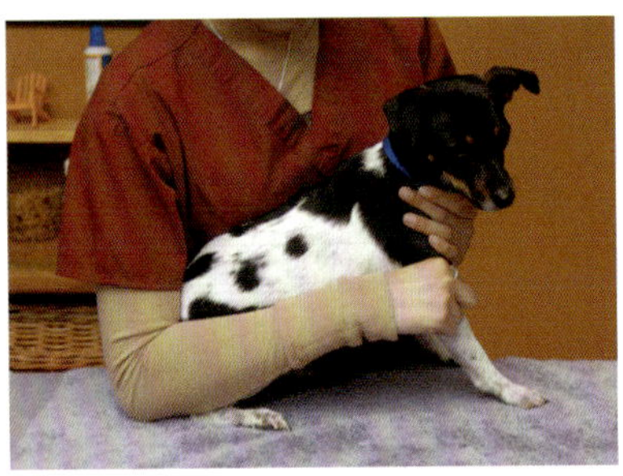

Fig. 10.5 A: In a small dog, securing the hind end and using an upper leg hold minimizes upward, lateral, forward, and backward movements.

Wrapping one arm around the dog's hind end prevents the dog from backing up. The addition of an upper leg hold on the outside front leg further restricts upward, lateral, and forward movements.[12] An elbow can then be used to secure the outside hip to further reduce lateral and backward movements.[12]

Hip Hold Technique

Positioning a hand on a dog's hip restricts lateral movement.[12] Gentle pressure applied when the dog attempts to move is eased once the dog settles.[12] Wrap a hand from around the back to prevent backing up.[12] Concurrent use of a U- or C-hold on the front end, combined with cupping the hand around the front part of the leg above the stifle, effectively prevents forward, backward, and lateral movements.[12]

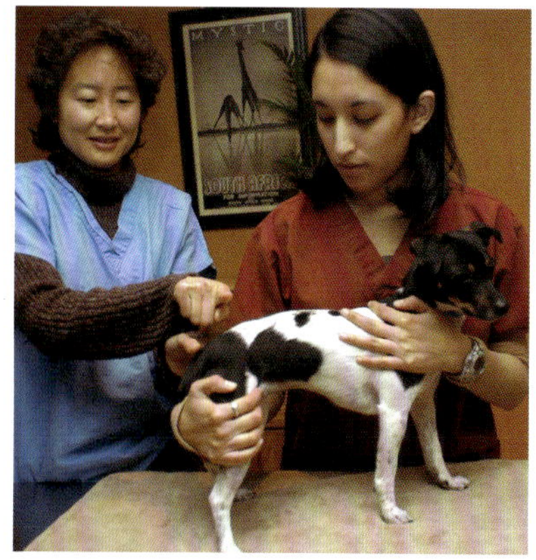

Fig. 10.5 B: Cupping the hand around the dog's thigh restricts forward, backward, and lateral movements. Positioning behind the dog prevents them from backing up.

Positioning Behind A Large Dog

When positioning behind a large dog, the handler's body can serve as a barrier to reduce backward and upward movement.[12] Both of the handler's legs should be positioned behind the dog to support their hind end, further limiting upward, backward, and lateral movements.[12] Incorporating a neck hold additionally reduces forward movement.[12]

10.6 Body Holds

Physically manipulating a dog into lateral, sternal, or dorsal recumbency is not recommended except in emergencies or when the dog is sedated. For orthopedic and neurological examinations, observing the dog from a distance can help localize lesions before sedation. Use familiar cues, lures, and distractions to guide and maintain the dog's position as needed.[12] Cooperative care training teaches dogs to assume these positions with minimal or no restraint.[15–17] In this approach, dogs should never be forcibly held in place and should always have the option to get up and move away.[15–19]

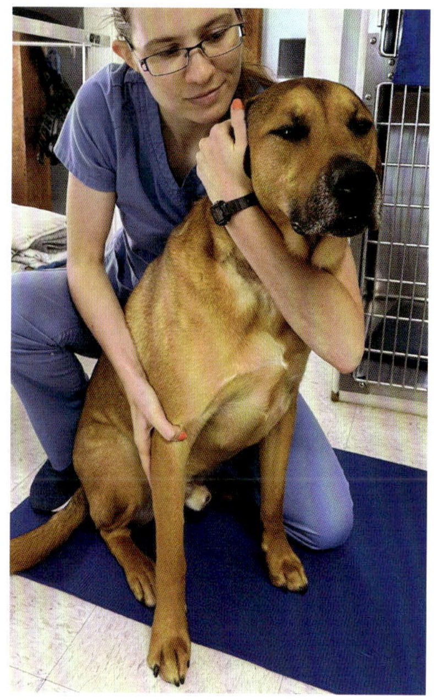

Fig. 10.5 C: Using the handler's body as a wall reduces backward, upward, and lateral movements. (Photo courtesy of Eliot Veterinary Hospital)

Ranking Holds

Restraint holds can be ranked from least to most aversive as follows:

1. Standing hold
2. Sternal recumbency
3. Lateral recumbency
4. Dorsal recumbency

Standing Hold

When handling a dog in a standing position for medical procedures such as injections, examinations, and venipuncture, prioritizing the dog's comfort is essential.[20] Although this position is often the least stressful for dogs, they should always have the option to change their position, such as to sitting or move away.[15–19] Forcing a dog to remain standing is not recommended.

The standing hold involves stabilizing the dog's hind end by placing one hand on the dog's flank or hip and using the other hand to stabilize the head, positioned just behind the skull. The handler's legs can create a barrier to prevent the dog from moving forward or sideways. Keeping the knees slightly bent helps prevent injuries to both the dog and the handler while effectively restricting forward and lateral movement.[5,12]

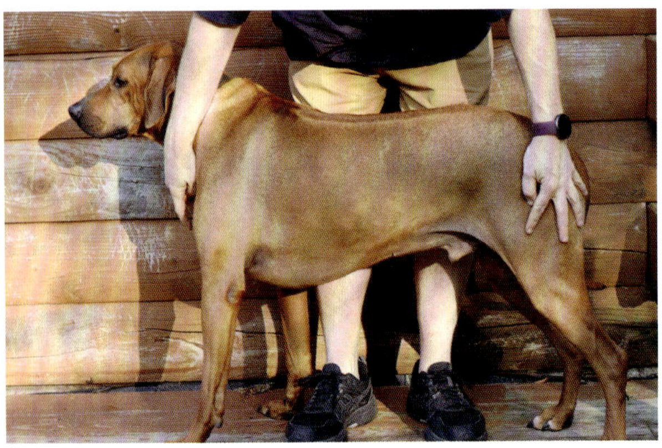

Fig. 10.6 A: In this position, one hand is on the outside of the hip to stabilize the hind-end.

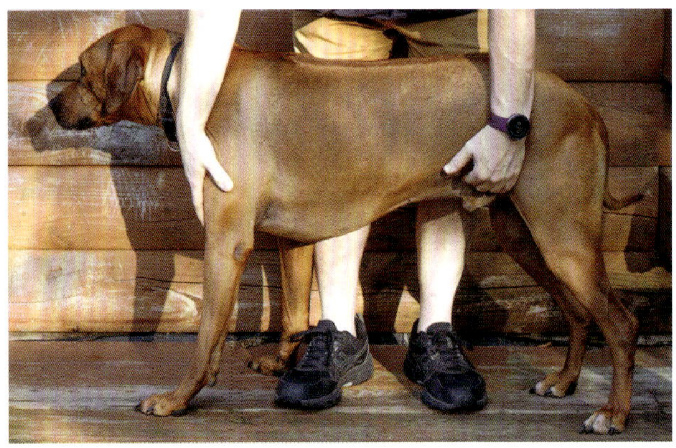

Fig. 10.6 B: For this standing hold, place one hand on the flank to stabilize the hind-end.

Fig. 10.6 C: In the described picture, minimal handling is used while maintaining safety measures. One handler has her hand on the dog's collar and is positioned to transition to an elbow hold if necessary. Her knee serves to limit the dog's forward motion. Additionally, the use of distractions offers an opportunity to utilize minimal handling effectively. (Photo courtesy of Eliot Veterinary Hospital)

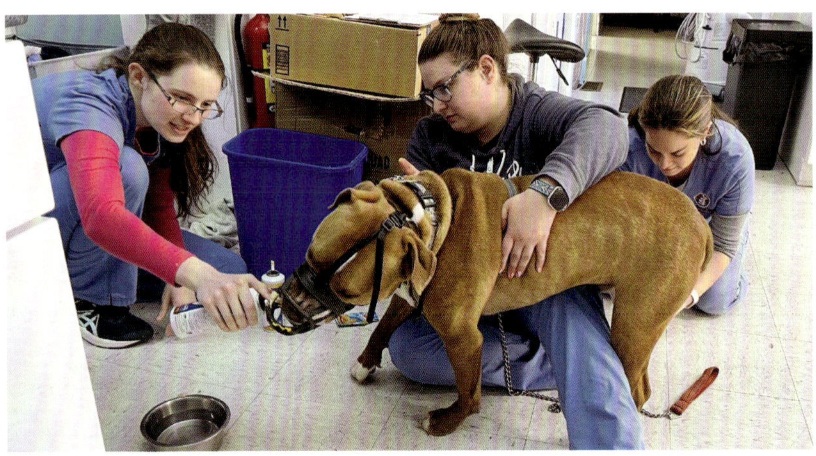

Sternal Recumbency

Sternal recumbency is often more comfortable and preferred by dogs when compared to the lateral or dorsal recumbent positions. Instead of manually manipulating a dog into position, use the down cue or lure the dog into position instead. Use distractions to encourage the dog to voluntarily remain in place, and provide a non-slip mat to increase traction and a sense of security.[5,12]

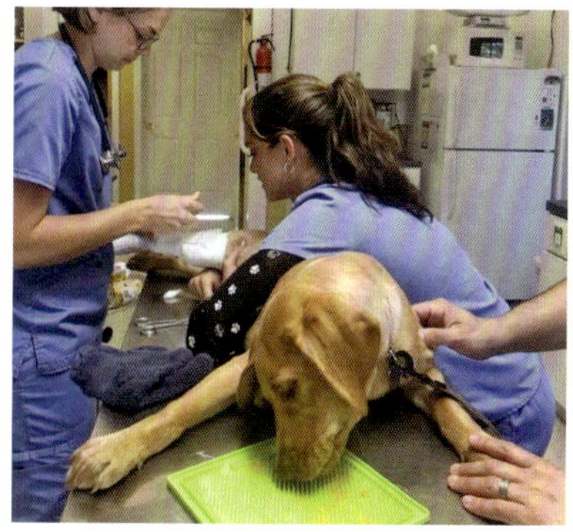

Fig. 10.6 D: In sternal recumbency, the use of distractions encourages the dog to remain in place with minimal handling. (Photo courtesy of Eliot Veterinary Hospital)

Table 10.6.2: Yield on Yellow

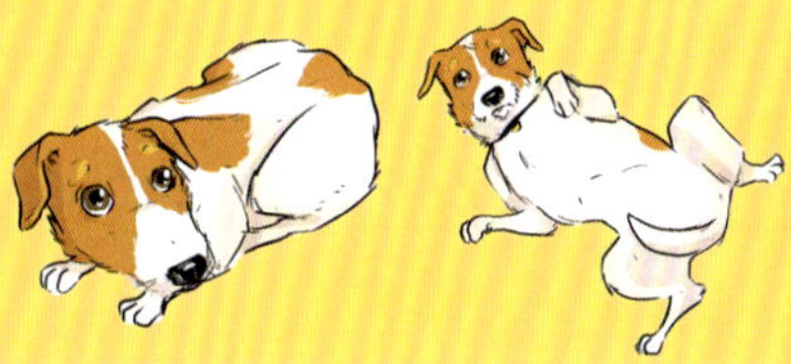

In this category, dogs may display different signs of increasing arousal:

- Increased activity (fidget and flight)
- For example: Hypervigilance, pacing, jumping, mouthing, actively avoiding

OR

- Decreased activity (freeze)
- For example: Slow cautious movements, frozen, still, stiff, tense, not relaxed, avoiding eye contact, head down, curled up on the floor, under the bench or chair behind the client, panting heavily, with a "worried" look

Both increased and decreased activity patterns are serious welfare concerns and need intervention.

Low Stress Handling® Plan

- This animal is stressed and needs to be monitored closely.
  - **CONTINUE** if the dog remains engaged, eating, playing, and interacting freely.
  - **STOP** if the dog's behavior worsens, leading to increased stress (e.g., refusal to eat, fidgeting, or freezing).
- Avoid letting the dog struggle >3 seconds before repositioning.
  - Limit repositioning to 2–3 times.
- Muzzle training should be a priority.
- Consider referral for cooperative care training and behavior modification.
  - Pre-visit medications +/- sedation.
  - Serious welfare concerns exist, and intervention is needed.

Lateral Recumbency

Prioritizing choice reduces fear, anxiety, frustration, and panic in dogs, which are considered protective emotions.[15–19,21–22] Regardless of the technique used, forcing a dog into lateral recumbency does not align with Low Stress Handling® principles. When lateral recumbency is necessary, using familiar cues such as "down" or lures for positioning should be tried first. In cases where this approach is not possible, sedation may be needed. Cooperative care training teaches dogs to voluntarily assume this position on cue, thereby increasing predictability and comfort for the dog.[15–17]

Dorsal Recumbency

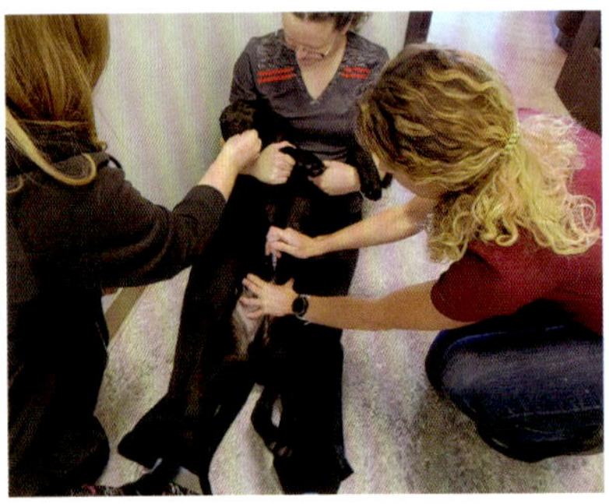

Fig. 10.6 E: The handler uses their legs to form a trough, supporting the dog during cystocentesis. Despite this support, few dogs are comfortable in this position. Therefore, the utilization of sedation and cooperative care training is necessary to maintain the dog's comfort and reduce stress during the procedure. (Photo courtesy of Anneliese Heinrich)

Traditionally used for diagnostic imaging and procedures such as cystocentesis, placing dogs in dorsal recumbency is a common but often unnecessary. This position can cause discomfort for many dogs, even when specially designed commercial troughs are used to support and hold the animal in place. If needed, the dog can be taught to voluntarily assume this position through cooperative care training. If a dog must be placed in dorsal recumbency, pre-visit medication and sedation should be administered first.

10.7 Eye, Ear, and Oral Examinations

Examinations of the eyes (ophthalmic), ears (otoscopic), and mouth (oral) can be particularly stressful for animals. To minimize this stress, make these examinations the last steps in the process. Cooperative care training and behavior modification techniques, such as desensitization and counterconditioning, help make these procedures more predictable and less stressful. In situations where these examinations might cause discomfort, due to conditions like corneal ulcers, ear infections, dental diseases, or abscessed teeth, sedation may be necessary to ensure the safety and comfort of both the animal and the examiner.[15–17]

Eye Examination

All ophthalmologic examinations should begin from a distance, as dogs may perceive prolonged direct eye contact as aversive, complicating the examination. When using an ophthalmoscope, turn on the light at a distance and avoid shining it directly into the dog's eye at first. Depending on the dog's comfort level, gradually approach while looking through the scope. To make this process more comfortable, use a lure or strategically placed treat, such as a lickable mat, squeeze cheese, or peanut butter tube, to help maintain the dog's position with minimal handling.

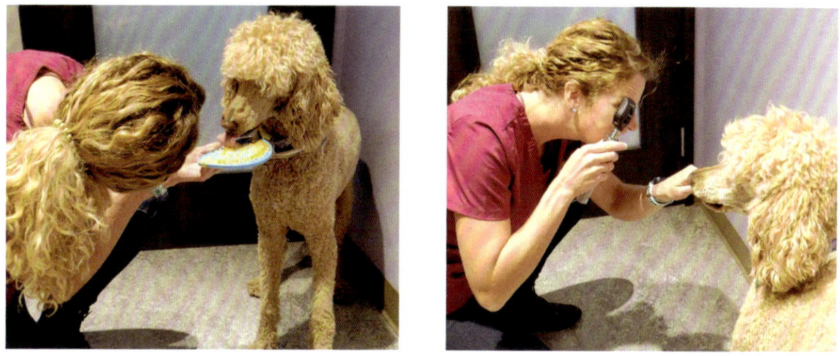

Figs. 10.7 A, B: Ophthalmologic examination should start at a distance. Offering strategically held treats can be effective in keeping the examination process smooth and less stressful for the dog. (Photos courtesy of Anneliese Heinrich)

The Painful Eye

When fluorescein staining is necessary, first apply a local anesthetic like proparacaine to the eye. Approach the dog from the side and behind their head. Place a hand gently on top of their head, carefully lift the upper eyelid, and apply a drop of the anesthetic from above before proceeding with the exam. For long-term eye medication, cooperative care training is essential.

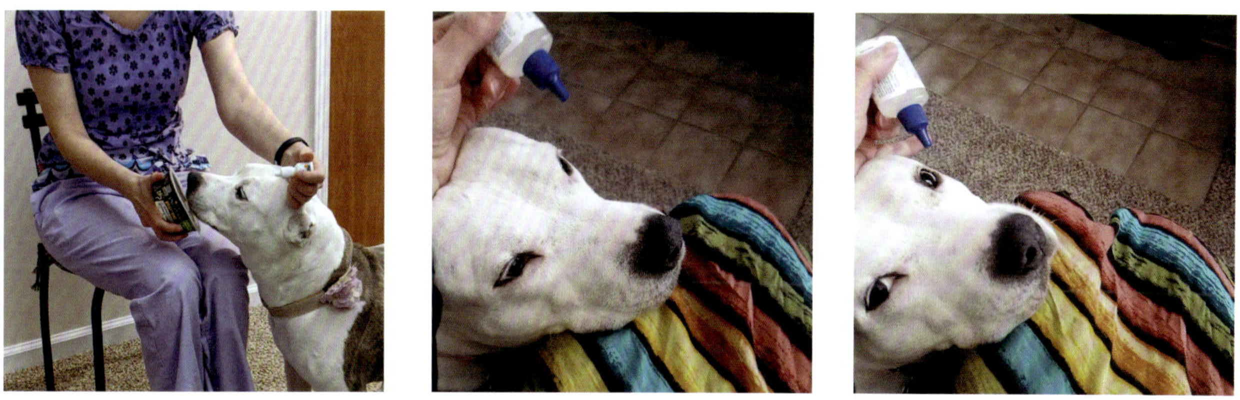

Figs. 10.7 C, D, E: Effective methods for applying eye drops include using a food lure to encourage the dog to approach the examiner (C) and approaching the dog from the side and behind. An alternative method is the chin rest behavior (D and E), which involves training the dog to rest their chin in the handler's or caregiver's hand or on a stable surface. This technique provides a secure position for administering eye drops comfortably and safely. (Photos courtesy of Leanne Lilly)

Ear Examination

Examining a dog's ears can be painful when they are inflamed or infected. Avoid conducting deep ear exams during these times to prevent escalating fear and anxiety and to reduce the risk of the dog generalizing this fear to all ear and head handling procedures, including the use of an otoscope. Distraction techniques during ear examinations, cleaning, and treatment significantly enhance a dog's comfort with the procedure. For chronic otitis requiring regular cleanings and treatment, cooperative care training is essential.[15–17,21,22]

Painful Ears

Chronic ear infections in dogs are often caused by allergies and can be very painful. Instead of sedation, veterinarians may send the dog home with topical otic medications, NSAIDs (non-steroidal anti-inflammatory drugs), or corticosteroids when appropriate to reduce inflammation. If rescheduling the otoscopic examination, pre-visit medication should be prescribed and the examination rescheduled for 24–48 hours later.

Initial Visual Inspection

An ear examination should start with a visual inspection from a distance to identify any signs of disease such as discharge, swelling, scabbing, hair loss, or head shaking. Before physically manipulating the pinna (ear flap) for a closer examination, consider asking the caregiver to lift the pinna, which can be less stressful for some dogs. Once the pinna is raised, evaluate the external ear canal for signs of discharge, erythema (redness), and swelling.

Using the Otoscope

If a deeper examination with an otoscope is needed, first attach the cone to the scope at a distance to allow for a gradual introduction of the instrument. If the dog remains relaxed, gently insert the scope into the ear and then lean in to look through it. However, if the dog shows signs of stress at any point, stop the examination and consider an alternative plan, such as sedation.

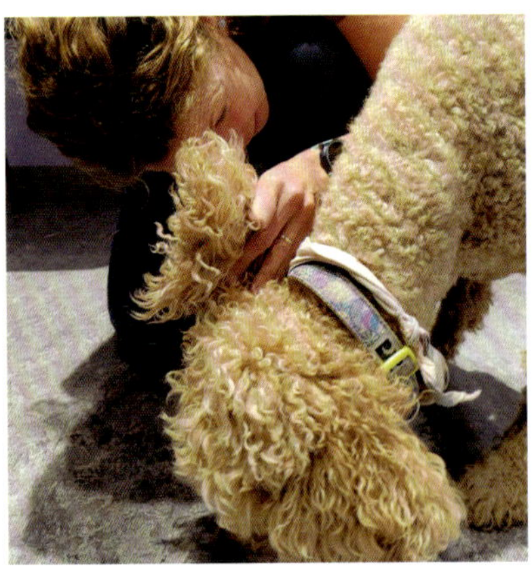

Fig. 10.7 F: Every ear examination, cleaning, and treatment should include high-value treats. (Photo courtesy of Anneliese Heinrich)

Painful Ears

When a dog's ears are painful, a useful distraction technique involves scratching the opposite ear while swabbing the affected one. However, if the ears are swollen and painful, cleaning should not be attempted without sedation. Caregivers should refrain from cleaning the affected ear until after two to three days of treatment, depending on the medication used.

Oral Examination

Just as with all examinations, oral examinations should start from a distance to observe for signs such as matting, drooling, swelling, or hair loss on the muzzle, lips, and neck. When the dog is panting, the tongue, lingual surface of the teeth, and mucous membranes can be easily assessed.

A useful technique for performing oral examinations involves using a thick, hard, crunchy treat. As the dog bites down on this treat, their dentition, including the symmetry and occlusions, can be evaluated. While the dog is nibbling, gently lifting the lip on either side allows for the examination of the buccal surface of the teeth and gums. If the dog is muzzled or the mouth is too painful, a more comprehensive examination will require sedation. Cooperative care training improves a dog's comfort level with oral examinations, tooth brushing, and medication administrations.[15–17]

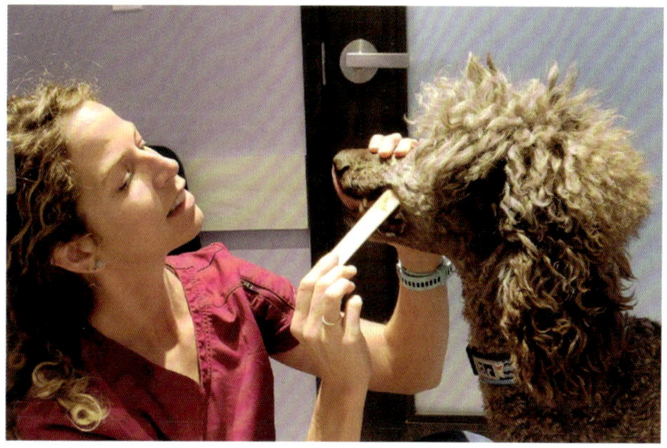

Fig. 10.7 G: Use a tongue depressor or pretzel rod to visualize the mouth. Some dogs may be more comfortable with this method, especially if treats or soft food have been smeared on these items. (Photo courtesy of Anneliese Heinrich)

Muzzle Hold

Grasping the dog's muzzle, using a leash to wrap around it, or employing any similar hold with hands is discouraged. These types of restraints can be uncomfortable for many dogs and increase the risk of biting. If this type of hold is unavoidable, the procedure should be stopped, and basket muzzle training should be initiated. For urgent procedures where this type of restraint is considered, sedation is preferred.

> **Oral Examination**
>
> When conducting an oral examination with a tongue depressor, caution is necessary as some dogs may bite and swallow pieces of it. A safer alternative is a pretzel rod coated with cheese or other lickable food. For those dogs with resource guarding tendencies, or if there is a concern regarding safety, a basket muzzle or sedation may be needed.

10.8 Venipuncture and Injections

Low Stress Handling® promotes minimal handling and restraint during diagnostic procedures such as injections and venipuncture.[12] Distractions are a key part of this approach, though some dogs may still require physical restraint.[12,20] With cooperative care training, dogs can learn to communicate their consent to participate in these procedures, making the process more effective and humane by giving them choices.[15–18]

Behavior modification techniques, including desensitization and counterconditioning, help minimize stress during the handling process. These techniques are designed to gradually acclimate dogs to the procedures and associated handling, making these experiences less stressful. In situations where specific positioning is required for diagnostic procedures such as orthopedic examinations, or when the patient is in pain, sedation increases safety and comfort for both the dog and the veterinary team. Using sedation reduces anxiety and discomfort for the patient and facilitates a safer, more efficient procedure for the team.

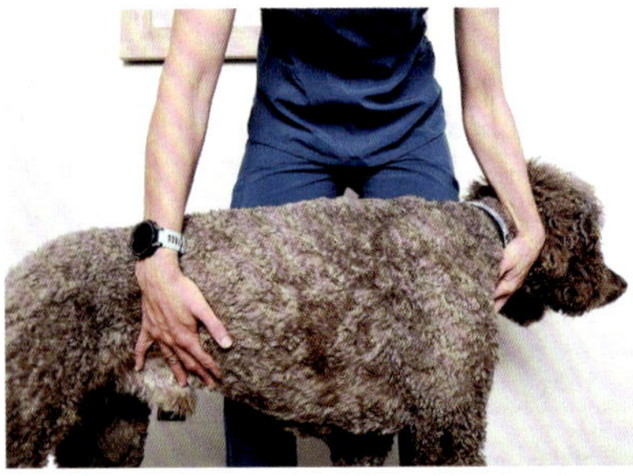

Fig. 10.8 A: The proper technique for administering subcutaneous (SQ) or intramuscular (IM) injections to a standing dog involves the handler stabilizing the dog's hind end by placing one hand on the flank or hip and the other hand just behind the skull on the neck. For added support, the neck should be gently pressed against the handler's leg. (Photo courtesy of Anneliese Heinrich)

Subcutaneous (SQ) and Intramuscular (IM) Injections

When administering SQ or IM injections, using a decisive, quick poke rather than slowly inching the needle through the skin skin tends to be less stressful and painful for the dog. A new needle should always be used for each injection and replaced after drawing up vaccines or other medications from a vial, as it can become dull after passing through the vial's stopper, making the injection more uncomfortable.[23,24]

Before proceeding with the injection, gently pinch the skin first to gauge the dog's reaction and make any necessary adjustments for a less stressful experience. Administering injections while the dog is standing with both their front and hind-ends stabilized is generally the best practice.

Needle Size

The size of the needle may not significantly impact the pain experienced during the injection. However, smaller needles can prolong the duration of the administration which might increase discomfort.[23]

Topical Anesthetic

Protective emotions may trigger the release of epinephrine prior to a blood draw or catherization, which can lead to hyperglycemia or changes in white blood cell counts.[2–4,20–22] To minimize pain and reduce this risk, apply a topical anesthetic cream at least 10–30 minutes before the procedure.

Venipuncture

Venipuncture intravenous injections, and catheterization often require some level of restraint to minimize movement and effectively isolate the vein for the procedure. Positioning the dog using luring techniques or familiar cues, such as "touch," "sit," or "down," is recommended, rather than manual manipulation.[12] To reduce stress during the procedure, applying topical anesthetics, like a cream containing lidocaine (2.5%) and prilocaine (2.5%), is advisable.[25–30]

The choice of vein for venipuncture typically depends on the handler's comfort and experience. However, accommodating the dog's preferred position is equally important. For routine venipuncture and intravenous injections, a butterfly catheter and the saphenous vein is commonly chosen because it is generally the least invasive option and poses less stress to the dog.[5,12,20,31,32] However, using a butterfly catheter in this vein poses a risk of positional occlusion during catheterization.[31,32] When a larger volume of blood is required, the jugular vein provides consistent blood flow and minimizes hemolysis.[33,34] Venipuncture in the cephalic and jugular veins may trigger protective emotions in some dogs due to the higher level of handling and restraint required.[1,21,22] Additionally, jugular venipuncture may cause less discomfort due to the anatomical positioning of the nerves, which are less likely to be touched or affected compared to other venous sites.

Lateral Saphenous Venipuncture or Catheterization

Accessing the lateral saphenous vein for venipuncture with the dog in a standing position tends to be more comfortable for the dog and safer for the team.[5,12] However, if a dog prefers a sternal (chest down) or lateral recumbent position, prompt or lure the dog into a "down" position on a mat or a soft, non-slip surface.

Venipuncture Site

Blood collection from the saphenous and jugular veins helps preserve the cephalic veins for future catheterizations, accommodating the dog's preferred position and reducing potential stress.

Venipuncture and Cooperative Care

Cooperative care training, which includes teaching positioning, desensitization, and counter-conditioning to handling and equipment, is beneficial for dogs requiring frequent venipuncture or those who find this process stressful.

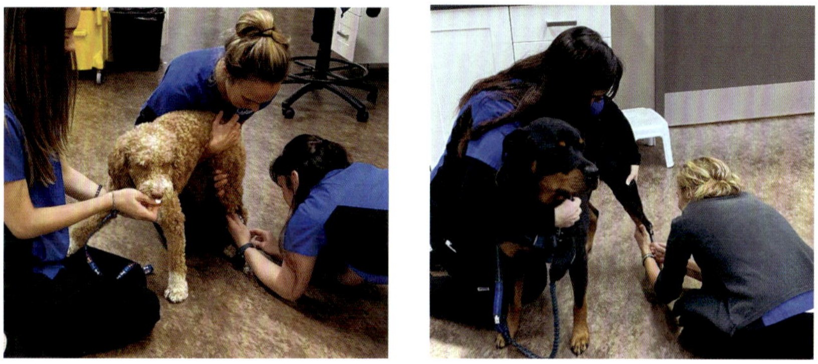

Figs. 10.8 B, C: Most dogs prefer to stand for this procedure. Using high-value treats as a distraction can allow for minimal restraint, making the process smoother and less stressful for the dog. (Photos courtesy of Anneliese Heinrich)

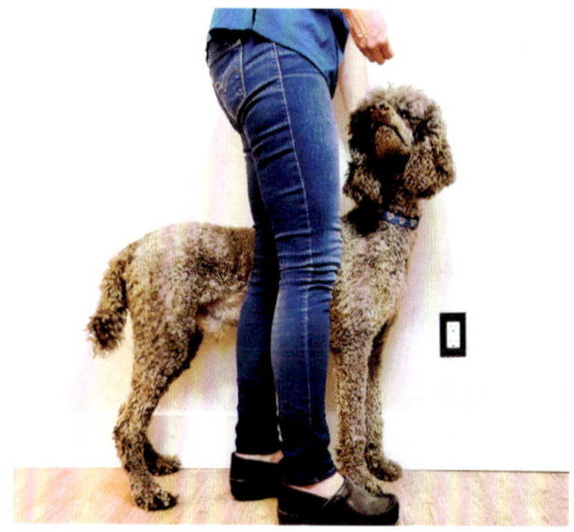

Fig. 10.8 D: The handler positions their leg against the dog's shoulder and uses a wall as support to keep the dog in place. This reduces lateral movement and allows for minimal handling and restraint. A lickable mat or smearing food on the wall helps to distract the dog while in position. (Photo courtesy of Anneliese Heinrich)

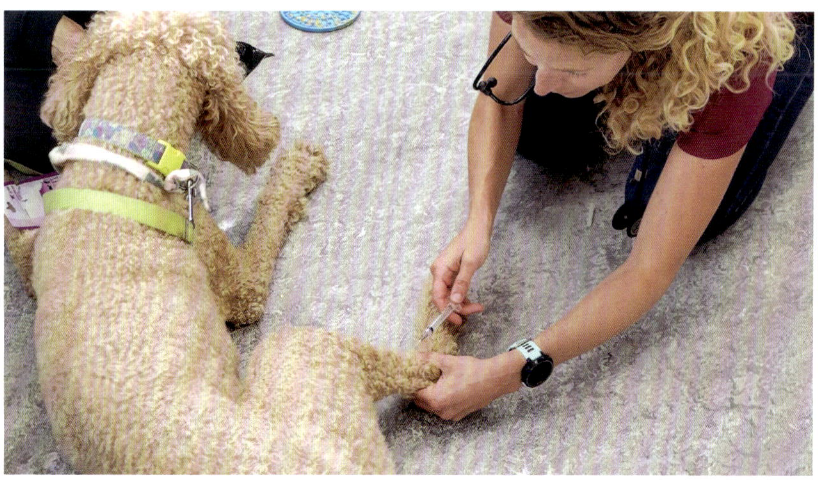

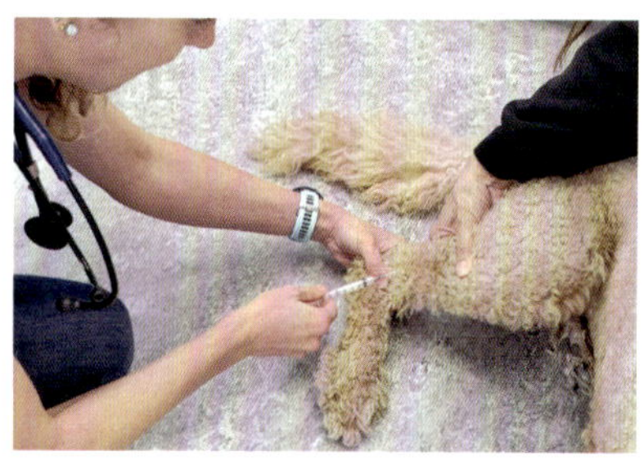

Figs. 10.8 E, F: These images depict scenarios where dogs undergoing venipuncture from the lateral saphenous vein prefer sternal recumbency, rather than lateral recumbency. This position allows for comfort and access to the vein. (Photos courtesy of Anneliese Heinrich)

Jugular Venipuncture in Small and Medium Dogs

For small and medium-sized dogs, jugular venipuncture requires a careful approach to positioning and handling. Cue or lure the dog into position.[12] The handler should hold the dog's head up slightly placing and arm on each side of the dog's body to provide support and prevent lateral movement.[12] The handler can then use their body to gently press against the dog's back, neck, and head for additional stability.[12]

Once the dog is comfortably positioned and appears relaxed, the venipuncture procedure can begin.[12] Avoid excessive stretching of the dog's neck or positioning the dog in a way that their body hangs over the edge of the table, since this can cause discomfort and fear.[12] Follow the three second rule and avoid struggling.[12]

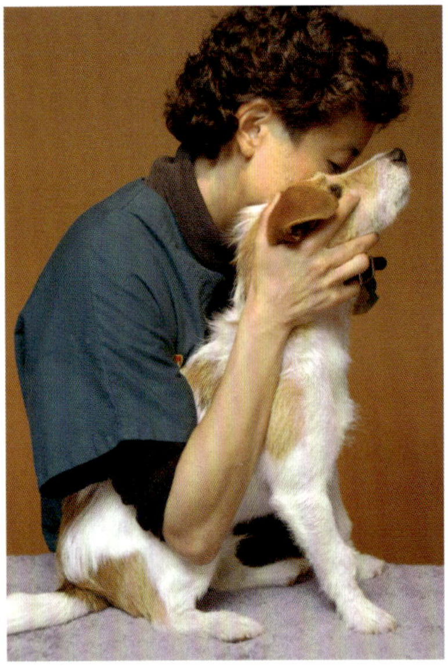

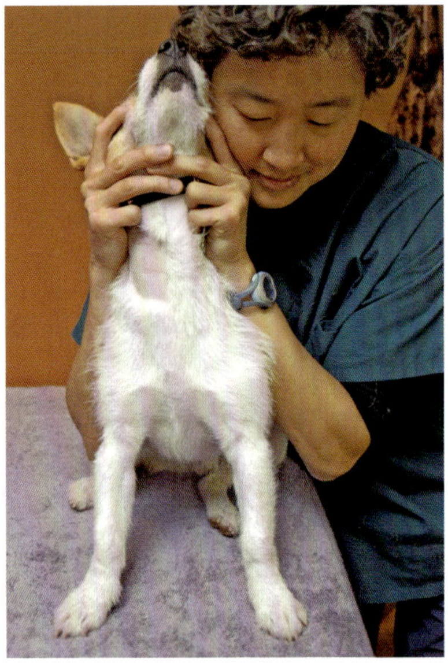

Figs. 10.8 G, H: With the dog sitting, hold the head up slightly, placing arms on both sides of the body to support the dog and prevent lateral and backward movements.

Jugular Venipuncture in Large Dogs

To perform jugular venipuncture in large dogs, the dog should be positioned perpendicular to the handler, which helps minimize lateral movement.[12] A wall or other solid barrier behind the dog prevents backward movement.[12] Alternatively, placing one leg behind the dog is also effective.[12]

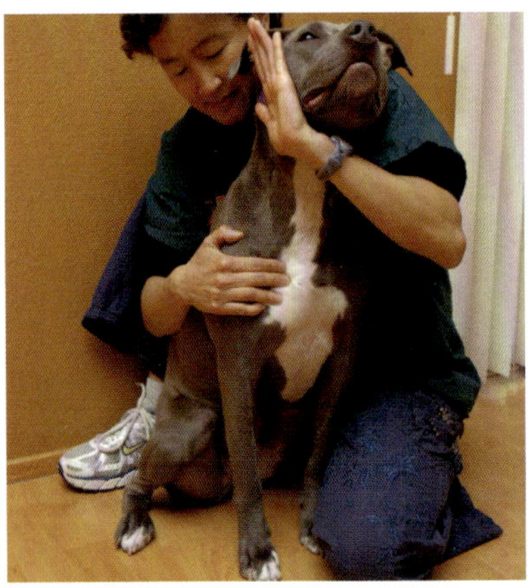

Fig. 10.8 I: The leg positioned behind the dog to reduce lateral and backward movements. The handler's hand is turned outward to secure the dog's head closer to the shoulder, ensuring stability.

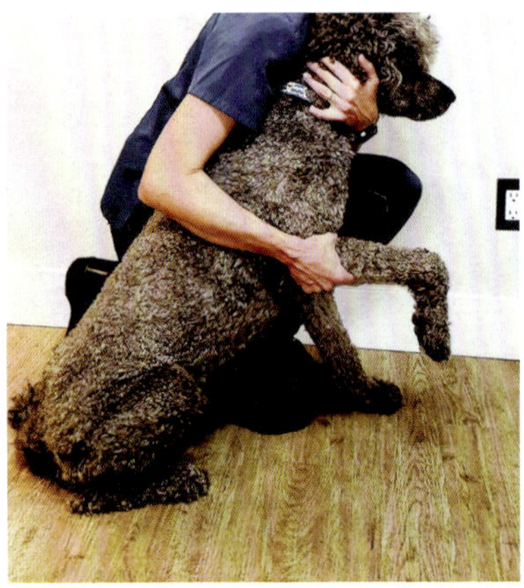

Fig. 10.8 J: For large dogs, the handler controls the dog's head with a modified neck hold while using an upper leg hold for venipuncture or catheter placement. (Photo courtesy of Anneliese Heinrich)

Cephalic Venipuncture and Catheterization

Handling during cephalic venipuncture and catheterization

can be stressful for the dog. To minimize this stress, different holds are recommended based on the size of the dog. For medium and large dogs, use neck and upper leg holds.[12] For smaller dogs, a C- or U-hold is more suitable.[12]

Modified Upper Leg Hold for Venipuncture and Catheterization

For cephalic venipuncture and catheterization, the thumb is used to occlude the vein. The remaining fingers should be positioned behind the elbow and to the inside of the leg.[12] Placing the dog's triceps in the webbing between the thumb and index finger helps prevent the leg from moving backward.[12]

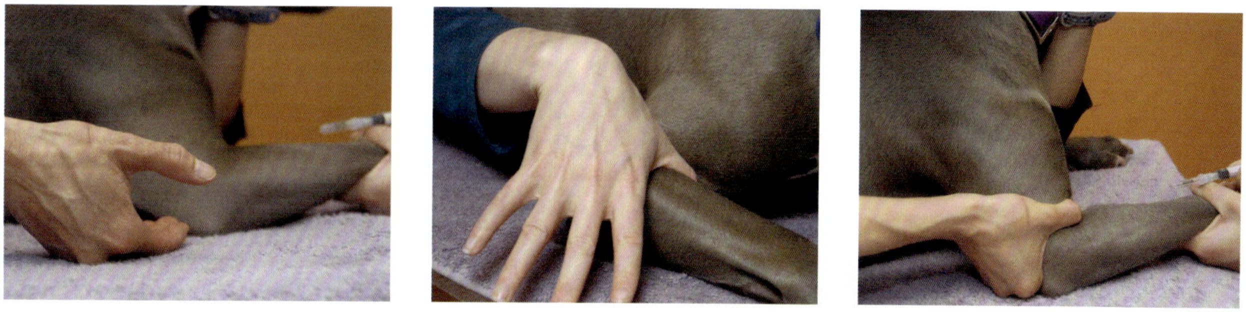

Figs. 10.8 K-M: These images illustrate the correct positioning of the thumb to occlude the vein, with the fingers behind and to the inside of the leg.

Depending on the angle and the dog's anatomy, it may be easier to occlude the vein using the index and third finger.[12] Keeping the dog's triceps in the webbing between the thumb and index finger is important to reduce backward movement.[12] An alternative method is to cup the elbow in the palm of the hand, as shown in Figures 10.8 N, O, and P.[12] This technique provides stability and control during the procedure.[12]

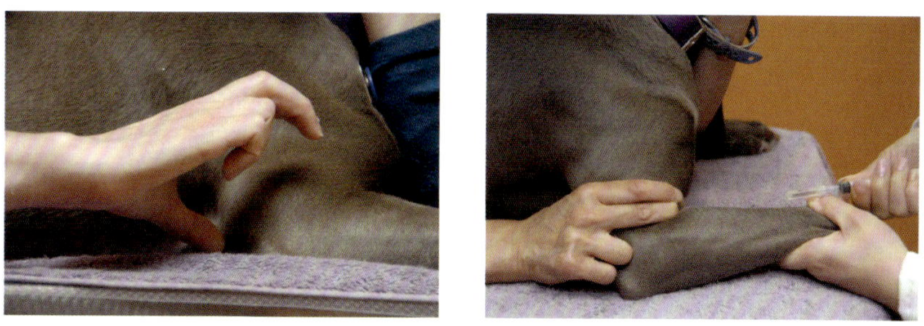

Figs. 10.8 N, O: An alternate method of occlusion involves using the index and third finger.

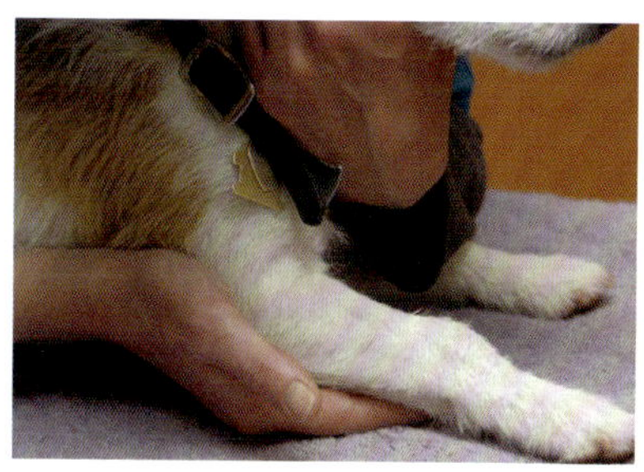

Fig. 10.8 P: Cup the elbow in the palm of the hand as an alternative.

10.9 Note About Fasting, Lipemia, and Reflux

Research indicates that giving dogs a small amount of food during venipuncture, catheter placement before surgery, and sedation does not increase the risk of gastroesophageal reflux.[35,36] In fact, fasting may increase this risk.[35,36] Additionally, administering maropitant (Cerenia®) on the day of surgery can further reduce the likelihood of perioperative nausea and vomiting. This practice has become standard in many veterinary practices, especially for elective procedures.[37]

Regarding the concern of lipemia affecting blood tests, giving treats just before a blood draw is unlikely to cause this issue. Postprandial triglyceride levels peak two to six hours after eating. Therefore, feeding a dog shortly before a blood draw will have minimal impact on test results.[38] Furthermore, if triglyceride levels are not a primary concern for the blood test, any lipids present in the sample can be removed through centrifugation, thus eliminating their potential to interfere with the results.

10.10 Advanced Procedures

Advanced imaging techniques, such as computed tomography (CT) and magnetic resonance imaging (MRI), typically require sedation or general anesthesia. In contrast, for radiographs and abdominal ultrasounds, it is common practice to physically restrain animals on tables and manipulate them into uncomfortable positions. This can lead to struggling, pain, potential injury, defensive aggression, and fear-related associations. These struggles often result in poor-quality images, necessitating additional handling and restraint, which increases radiation exposure risks for both humans and animals and the risk of a misdiagnosis. Therefore, sedation should be the standard approach for imaging patients who are fearful or in pain.

In certain cases, alternative positions such as standing, sternal, lateral, or dorsal recumbency can be used diagnosis without sedation. For example, placing a dog in a dorsoventral (DV) position for radiographs may cause less stress than a ventrodorsal (VD) position. Similarly, performing an abdominal ultrasound in lateral recumbency can yield diagnostic results comparable to those obtained in a dorsal position.

If handling causes pain or if minimal handling is possible, maintaining the dog in a single position for the procedure may be less stressful than adjusting their position for different image angles. As with positioning for examination, venipuncture, and injections,using cooperative care training is preferable. Desensitization and counterconditioning may be necessary to minimize stress and improve comfort for the dog.

Diagnostic Imaging

Sedation during diagnostic imaging is a common practice in many veterinary school teaching hospitals, offering several benefits. By minimizing protective emotions and defensive behaviors, sedation enhances the safety and comfort of both the patient and the veterinary team. Additionally, reducing the patient's anxiety and movement leads to higher-quality imaging and more accurate diagnoses, while also decreasing radiation exposure for humans.

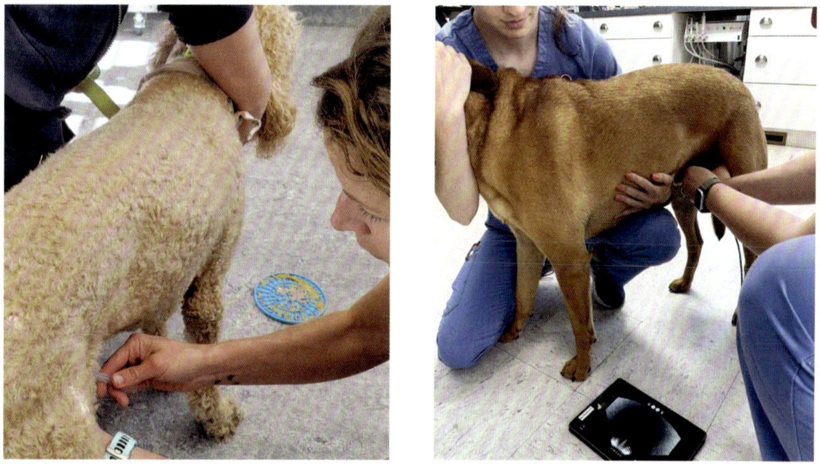

Figs. 10.10 A, B: Performing a cystocentesis in a standing position eliminates the need for dorsal recumbency. (Photo courtesy of Anneliese Heinrich). **Fig. B.** When standing, a neck hold helps reduce forward and lateral movement. (Photo courtesy of Eliot Veterinary Hospital)

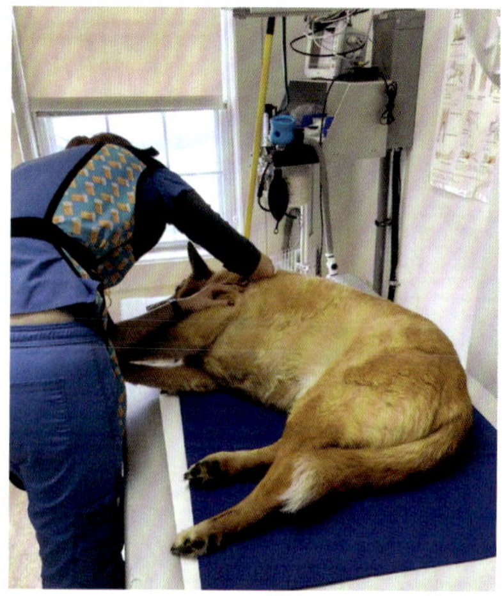

Fig. 10.10 C: When positioning the dog in lateral recumbency, it is essential to adhere to Low Stress Handling® principles. This means using minimal or no restraint at all. Avoid manipulating the dog into position or holding them in place. Always allow the dog the choice to sit up, stand, or move away as needed. (Photo courtesy of Eliot Veterinary Hospital)

10.11 Canine Ninja Sedation

Ninja Sedation or "drive-by" sedation techniques are useful for patients that are difficult to approach and safely handle.[5] The primary objective of these methods is to reduce protective emotions and defensive behaviors while maintaining safety for the patient, caregiver, and the veterinary team. These sedation techniques foster engagement, making the overall process less stressful and significantly improving the welfare of animals that are resistant to handling.

Table 10.11.3: Stop on Red

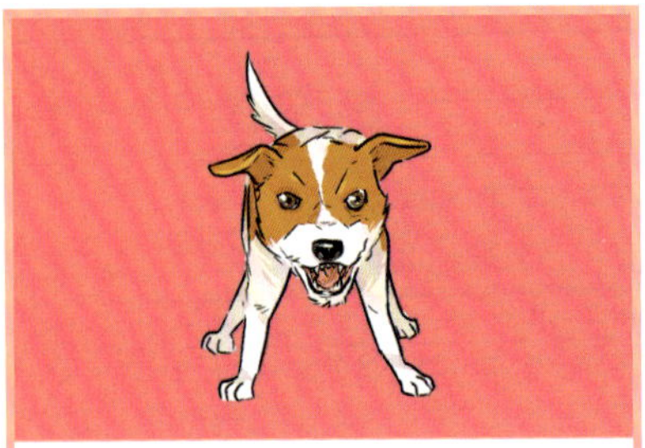

As with yellow dogs, there may be signs of:

- Flight
- Freeze
- Fidget
- Fight
- Pre-visit medications alone are often insufficient for these animals.
- Add IV or IM sedation in addition to pre-visit medications.

Low Stress Handling® Plan

- Pre-visit medications and sedation will be needed.
- Refer for cooperative care training and behavior modification.

Escalation of Fear at The Veterinary Hospital

In the brightly lit examination room, Razz, a mixed-breed Labrador Retriever, showed clear signs of anxiety with her ears flat, tail tucked, and eyes constantly scanning the room for an escape. As the veterinarian approached to give a rabies shot, Razz's anxiety turned into overt fear and panic, the whites of her eyes became pronounced, her body stiffened, and her panting intensified.

Food was offered to distract her, but Razz, in survival mode, refused. Her anxiety increased as more team members entered to assist, heightening her stress. When someone tried to muzzle her, Razz snapped in fear and frustration. Although the rabies vaccination was administered quickly, Razz's continued struggle making it impossible to draw blood for a heartworm test. Recognizing her distress, the team decided to stop and reschedule the procedure.

To better prepare for the next visit, an individualized handling plan was created. Razz was sent home with pre-visit medications to reduce her anxiety for her next visit. Instructions for muzzle training were also provided. This training involved conditioning Razz to voluntarily place her nose into the muzzle and to practice wearing it during activities she enjoyed such as walks. This strategy would help improve her comfort level with the muzzle, preventing her from associating it with only stressful events. She would arrive at her next appointment already wearing the muzzle.

On the rescheduled visit day, the veterinarian discreetly administered a sedative to Razz using a syringe and extension set as she entered the examination room, allowing the needle to safely detach after the injection without her noticing. In the dimly lit, quiet room, Razz was given time to relax on a soft blanket, letting the sedative take effect. This Low Stress Handling® approach facilitated a thorough physical examination and simplified the collection of samples for the heartworm test. This example highlights the value of an individualized handling plan and advanced preparations for a pet's overall well-being.

The Procedure

When employing the Ninja Sedation technique with dogs, the first step is to properly fit the animal with a muzzle for safety. Distractions such as lickable or snuffle mats help alleviate anxiety. For those that display fear or anxiety in response to unfamiliar people or medical instruments (like syringes, thermometers, or stethoscopes), creating a visual barrier is helpful. This can be achieved with the assistance of a caregiver or handler, or by using a wall or another object to block the dog's view of potential stressors. Avoid cornering the dog; instead, allow them the option to turn away from any approaching team members.

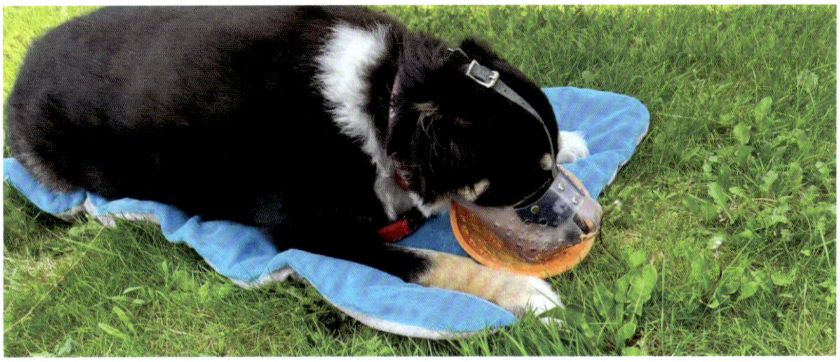

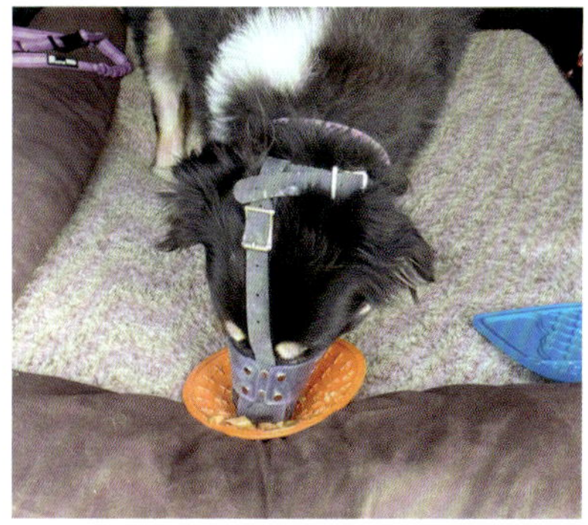

Figs. 10.11 A, B: Use of a lickable mat suctioned to the wall or floor can provide a distraction during the sedation process.

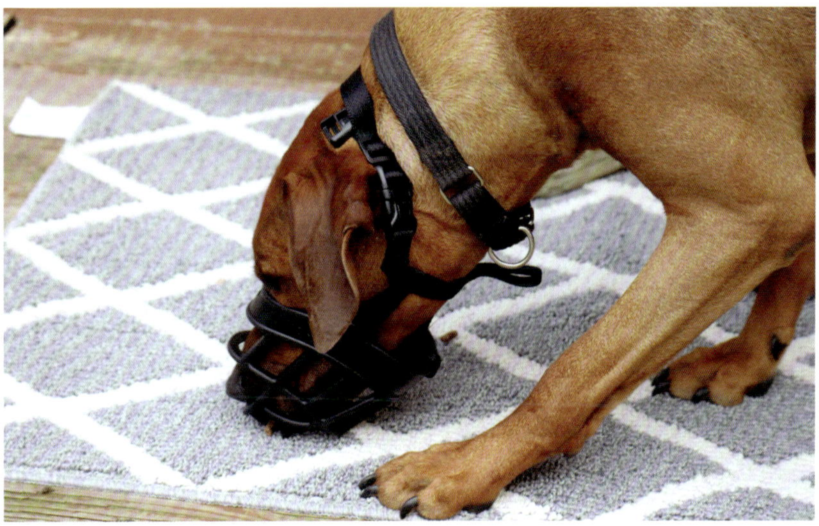

Fig. 10.11 C: Picking up treats off a mat while wearing a basket muzzle.

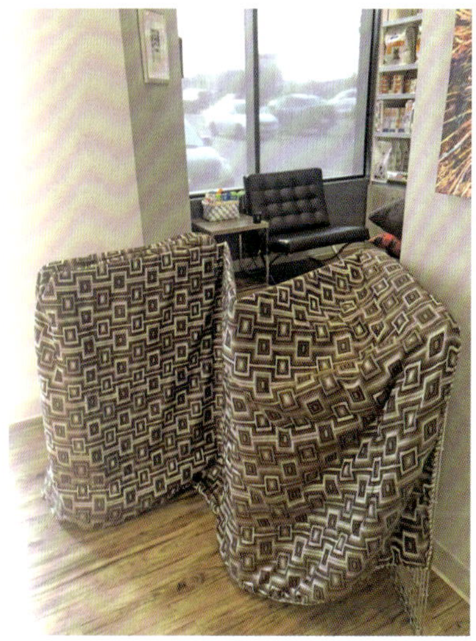

Fig. 10.11 D: A makeshift visual barrier can help block fearful or arousing stimuli during the sedation process. (Photo courtesy of Jessica Benoit)

Using a Blanket

In cases where a dog is lying down, appears disoriented, in pain, or is resistant to handling, covering their head and body loosely with a blanket prior to sedation can be effective. This method reduces visual stimuli for the dog and increases safety for the veterinary team. Minimizing handling during this process reduces stress, and ensures the sedation is as effective as possible.

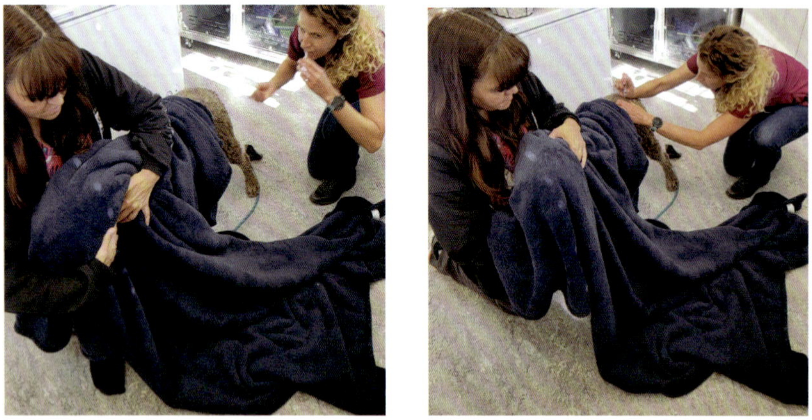

Figs. 10.11 E, F: Demonstrating the use of a large blanket, quilt, or comforter in the restraint of medium to large dogs, these images illustrate how draping the fabric over the dog's head and mid-section can effectively facilitate head control and provide quick access for injections. This method can be more successful if the caregiver covers the dog with the blanket before the veterinary staff approach for the injection. The technique shown ensures a safer and more efficient process for both the dog and the handler. (Photos courtesy of Anneliese Heinrich)

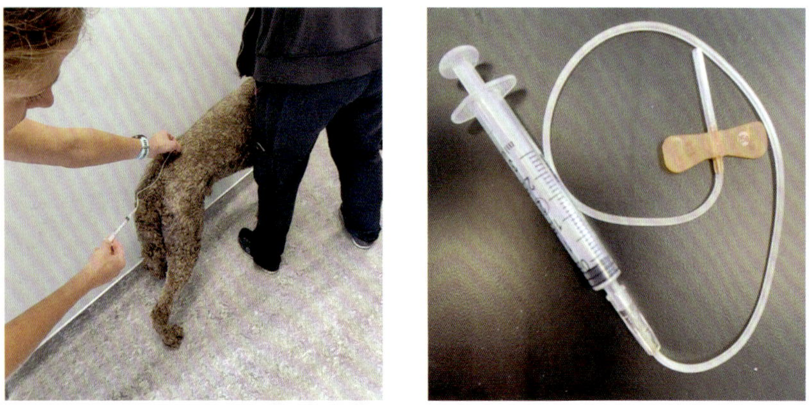

Figs. 10.11 G, H: A team member gives an injection from behind as a second team member creates a visual barrier. A preloaded butterfly catheter is attached to a syringe filled with saline. (Photos courtesy of Anneliese Heinrich)

During the injection procedure for standing dogs, one team member should position themselves between the dog and the person administering the injection, acting as a visual barrier. The dog should be securely placed against a wall or similar solid structure. Another team member or the caregiver should remain near the dog's head, offering treats and distractions to maintain the dog's engagement and focus away from the injection site.

Moving Sedation Technique

Another Ninja Sedation technique is the moving injection. This involves walking the dog past a team member who is prepared to administer the sedation. As the dog passes by, the team member swiftly and discreetly delivers the injection into the epaxial muscles. For this, an extension set connected to a needle is used, allowing for a smoother and less noticeable injection.

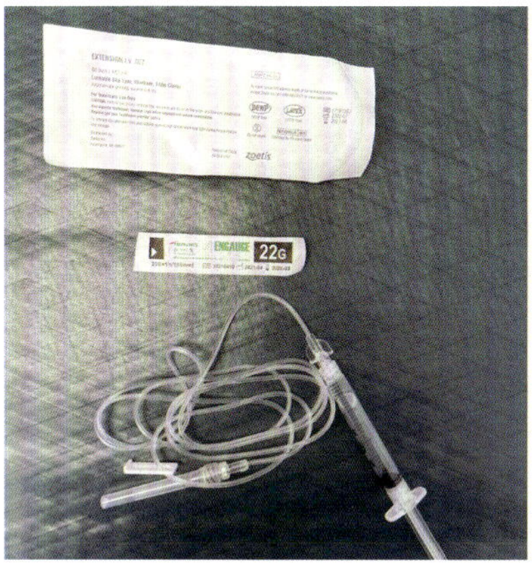

Fig. 10.11 I: This image demonstrates demonstrates preloading an extension set with sedation and attaching it to a syringe of saline. (Photo courtesy of Eliot Veterinary Hospital)

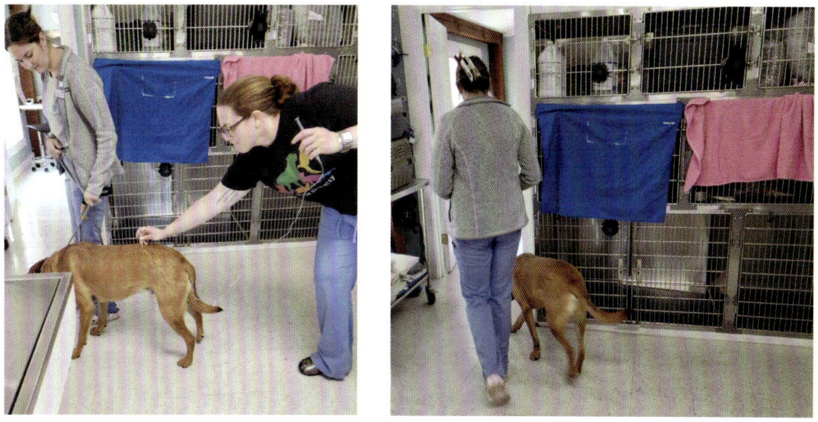

Figs. 10.11 J, K: These figures show how the extension set allows the injector to quickly move away from the dog for safety, while the handler continues to walk the dog forward towards an examination room or a quiet area. (Photos courtesy of Eliot Veterinary Hospital)

10.12 Conclusion

Many Low Stress Handling® options are available when handling and positioning animals for veterinary examinations and procedures. Always begin with the least aversive method for each individual dog and sedate when necessary. For fearful and anxious animals, cooperative care training, with or without sedation, is needed.

Keeping the Momentum

The Control Unleashed® Pattern 1-2-3 Game can be an effective method to keep a dog engaged and moving forward while an injection is administered.

10.13 References

1. Riemer, S., Heritier, C., Windschnurer, I., Pratsch, L., Arhant, C., & Affenzeller, N. (2021). A review on mitigating fear and aggression in dogs and cats in a veterinary setting. *Animals*, 11(1), 158.

2. Balcombe, J. P., Barnard, N. D., & Sandusky, C. (2004). Laboratory routines cause animal stress. *Journal of the American Association for Laboratory Animal Science*, 43(6), 42–51.

3. Belew, A. M., Barlett, T., & Brown, S. A. (1999). Evaluation of the white-coat effect in cats. *Journal of Veterinary Internal Medicine*, 13(2), 134–142.

4. Bragg, R. F., Bennett, J. S., Cummings, A., & Quimby, J. M. (2015). Evaluation of the effects of hospital visit stress on physiologic variables in dogs. *Journal of the American Veterinary Medical Association*, 246(2), 212–215.

5. Herron, M. E., & Shreyer, T. (2014). The pet-friendly veterinary practice: a guide for practitioners. *Veterinary Clinics: Small Animal Practice*, 44(3), 451–481.

6. Bigras-Fontaine, C., Bazin, I., & Desmarchelier, M. (2022). Clinical relevance of rectal temperature in cats showing marked signs of stress during routine veterinary visits. *Proceedings of the American College of Veterinary Behaviorists Veterinary Behavior Symposium*, 11.

7. Hall, E. J., & Carter, A. (2017). Establishing a reference range for normal canine tympanic membrane temperature measured with a veterinary aural thermometer. *Veterinary Nursing Journal*, 32(12), 369–373.

8. Smith, R., Mastrocco, A., Prittie, J., & Weltman, J. (2023). Comparison of aural and rectal temperature in dogs presenting to an emergency room. *Veterinary Medicine: Research and Reports*, 125–131.

9. Mandese, W. W., Griffin, F. C., Reynolds, P. S., Blew, A. C., Deriberprey, A. S., & Estrada, A. H. (2021). Stress in client-owned dogs related to clinical exam location: a randomised crossover trial. *Journal of Small Animal Practice*, 62(2), 82–88.

10. Mariti, C., Ricci, E., Zilocchi, M., & Gazzano, A. (2013). Owners as a secure base for their dogs. *Behaviour*, 150(11), 1275–1294.

11. Stellato, A. C., Dewey, C. E., Widowski, T. M., & Niel, L. (2020). Evaluation of associations between owner presence and indicators of fear in dogs during routine veterinary examinations. *Journal of the American Veterinary Medical Association*, 257(10), 1031–1040.

12. Yin, S. A. (2009). *Low Stress Handling, Restraint, and Behavior Modification of Dogs and Cats.* CattleDog Publishing.

13. Csoltova, E., Martineau, M., Boissy, A., & Gilbert, C. (2017). Behavioral and physiological reactions in dogs to a veterinary examination: Owner-dog interactions improve canine well-being. *Physiology & Behavior*, 177, 270–281.

14. Kuhne, F., Hößler, J. C., & Struwe, R. (2014). Behavioral and cardiac responses by dogs to physical human–dog contact. *Journal of Veterinary Behavior*, 9(3), 93–97.

15. Jones, E. (2023). Cooperative care for companion dogs: emotional health and wellness. *Companion Animal*, 28(7), 1–6.

16. Jones, E. (2023). Preparing Fearful Dogs for Vaccinations with Cooperative Care. *Animal Behaviour and Welfare Cases*, abwcases20230011.

17. Sydänheimo, A., Freeman, M., & Hunt, K. (2023). Cooperative care does not scare-Use of cooperative care training in routine husbandry in dogs. *Animal Behaviour and Welfare Cases*, abwcases20230010

18. Horowitz, A. (2021). Considering the "dog" in dog–human interaction. *Frontiers in Veterinary Science*, 8, 642821.

19. Littlewood, K. E., Heslop, M. V., & Cobb, M. L. (2023). The agency domain and behavioral interactions: assessing positive animal welfare using the Five Domains Model. *Frontiers in Veterinary Science*, 10. https://doi.org/10.3389/fvets.2023.1284869

20. Squair, C., Proudfoot, K., Montelpare, W., & Overall, K. L. (2023). Effects of changing veterinary handling techniques on canine behavior and physiology part 1: Physiological measurements. *Animals*, 13(7), 1253.

21. Heath, S. (2018). Understanding feline emotions: . . . and their role in problem behaviours. *Journal of Feline Medicine and Surgery*, 20(5), 437–444.

22. Tooley, C., & Heath, S. E. (2023). Emotional arousal impacts physical health in dogs: A review of factors influencing arousal, with exemplary case and framework. *Animals*, 13(3), 465.

23. Flanagan, T., Wahl, M. J., Schmitt, M. M., & Wahl, J. A. (2007). Size doesn't matter: needle gauge and injection pain. *General Dentistry*, 55(3), 216–217. PMID: 17511363.

24. Patout, M., Lamia, B., Lhuillier, E., Molano, L.-C., Viacroze, C., Benhamou, D., Muir, J.-F., & Cuvelier, A. (2015). A randomized controlled trial on the effect of needle gauge on the pain and anxiety experienced during radial arterial puncture. *PLoS ONE*, 10(9), e0139432.

25. Crisi, P. E., De Santis, F., Giordano, M. V., Cerasoli, I., Colucci, F., Di Tommaso, M., & Luciani, A. (2021). Evaluation of eutectic lidocaine/prilocaine cream for jugular blood sampling in cats. *Journal of Feline Medicine and Surgery*, 23(2), 185–189.

26. Flecknell, P. A., Liles, J. H., & Williamson, H. A. (1990). The use of lignocaine-prilocaine local anaesthetic cream for pain-free venepuncture in laboratory animals. *Laboratory Animals*, 24(2), 142–146.

27. Henfrey, J. I., Thoday, K. L., & Head, K. W. (1991). A comparison of three local anaesthetic techniques for skin biopsy in dogs. *Veterinary Dermatology*, 2(1), 21–27.

28. Leask, E. (2021). Efficacy of EMLA™ cream for reducing pain associated with venepuncture in felines. *Veterinary Evidence*, 6(3).

29. van Oostrom, H., & Knowles, T. G. (2018). The clinical efficacy of EMLA cream for intravenous catheter placement in client-owned dogs. *Veterinary anaesthesia and analgesia*, 45(5), 604–608.

30. Wagner, K. A., Gibbon, K. J., Strom, T. L., Kurian, J. R., & Trepanier, L. A. (2006). Adverse effects of EMLA (lidocaine/prilocaine) cream

and efficacy for the placement of jugular catheters in hospitalized cats. *Journal of Feline Medicine and Surgery*, 8(2), 141–144.

31. Hefler, L., Grimm, C., Leodolter, S., & Tempfer, C. (2004). To butterfly or to needle: The pilot phase [5]. *Annals of Internal Medicine*, 140(11), 935–936. doi:10.7326/0003–4819–140–11–20040601000027.

32. Shin, D., Nam, A., Song, K. H., & Seo, K. W. (2019). Influence of needle gauge and venepuncture difficulty on thromboelastography in healthy cats. *Journal of Feline Medicine and Surgery*, 21(8), 708–713.

33. Jensen AL, Wenck A, Koch J, et al: Comparison of results of hematological and clinical chemical analyses of blood samples obtained from the cephalic and external jugular veins in dogs. *Res Vet Sci*. 1994;56(1): 24–9.

34. Gilor S, Gilor C: Common laboratory artifacts caused by inappropriate sample collection and transport: how to get the most out of a sample. *Topics in Companion Animal Medicine*. 2011;26(2): 109–118.

35. Savvas, I., Raptopoulos, D., & Rallis, T. (2016). A "light meal" three hours preoperatively decreases the incidence of gastro-esophageal reflux in dogs. *Journal of the American Animal Hospital Association*, 52(6), 357–363.

36. Tsompanidou, P., Robben, J. H., Savvas, I., Anagnostou, T., Prassinos, N. N., & Kazakos, G. M. (2021). The Effect of the preoperative fasting regimen on the incidence of gastro-oesophageal reflux in 90 Dogs. *Animals*, 12(1), 64.

37. Ramsey, D., Fleck, T., Berg, T., Nederveld, S., DeLong, D., Tena, J. K., Aleo, M., & McCall, R. (2014). Cerenia prevents perioperative nausea and vomiting and improves recovery in dogs undergoing routine surgery. *International Journal of Applied Research in Veterinary Medicine*, 12(3).

38. Elliott, K. F., Rand, J. S., Fleeman, L. M., et al. (2011). Use of a meal challenge test to estimate peak postprandial triglyceride concentrations in dogs. *American Journal of Veterinary Research*, 72(2), 161–168.

Contributing Authors
Anneliese Heinrich MSc, DVM
Christine D. Calder DVM, DACVB

CHAPTER 11

Feline Low Stress Handling®

11.1 Introduction

Cats have a unique sensory system distinct from humans, featuring a well-developed sense of smell, ultrasonic hearing, and low-light vision that prioritizes movement detection before clarity and focus.[1–3] These sensory capabilities make them excellent hunters and significantly influence their behavior in human environments.[1–6] Additionally, cats have a relatively short socialization period (two to nine weeks), during which they exhibit a decreasing interest in social interactions with other cats or humans, coupled with a heightened sense of environmental exploration, preparing them for an independent life and making them selectively social.[1,2,4]

Understanding these aspects of feline behavior and physiology is necessary for interacting with them in a way that respects their natural instincts and minimizes stress, especially in clinical or caregiving settings. As both predator and prey species, cats often exhibit protective responses during human interactions, including handling and restraint.[5,6–11] Therefore, they should be handled with the minimal amount of restraint necessary in any situation.[5,11] Their common response to fear, such as freezing or undergoing a behavioral shutdown, should not be mistaken for compliance but recognized as signs of distress and poor welfare.[5] This understanding necessitates a gentle and empathetic approach to handling, and conducting interactions in a manner that respects their unique nature and promotes their wellbeing.[5]

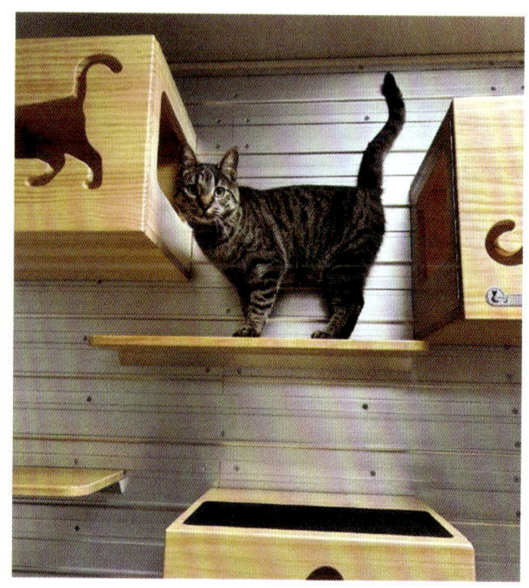

Fig. 11.1 A: Little has changed during the domestication process of cats. Understanding normal feline behavior and their needs is critical when working with cats. (Photo courtesy of Louisiana State University Small Animal Teaching Hospital Community Practice- Nancy Welborn)

Historically, common handling methods such as full body restraint, stretching, and scruffing (grabbing the loose skin at the back of a cat's neck) were used, primarily for quick control.[5–11] However, these techniques often result in protective emotions displayed as behavioral shutdown or defensive aggression (hissing, swatting, growling, biting, and scratching) in cats.[5–14] In 2011, a major shift in feline welfare occurred with the publication of the AAFP/ISFM

Table 11.1.1: Goals of Feline Friendly Low Stress Handling® Techniques

Reduced Fear, Anxiety, Frustration, and Pain	By using Low Stress Handling® techniques, the primary goal is to minimize protective emotions and pain that cats may experience during veterinary visits.
Reinforced Veterinarian-Client-Cat Bond	Trust and confidence are essential in any veterinarian-client relationship. These techniques help build a stronger bond by demonstrating empathy and gaining trust from the client.
Improved Efficiency, Productivity, and Job Satisfaction for the Veterinary Team	When cats are less stressed, they are easier and safer to handle. This efficiency leads to greater productivity and job satisfaction among veterinary staff, as they can perform their tasks more effectively and with less risk of injury.
Increased Client Compliance	Happy clients are more likely to follow veterinary advice and return for regular check-ups. When they see that their cats are being handled with care and respect, they are more likely to trust the veterinary team's recommendations and have improved client satisfaction.
Timely Reporting and Early Detection of Medical and Behavioral Concerns	An engaged cat is easier to examine, which can lead to earlier detection of potential health and behavioral issues. Additionally, caregivers are more likely to bring their cat in more frequently if they are less stressed about the process themselves. This also improves financial outcomes due to the increased number of feline patients, higher average transaction fees, an increase in annual spending and pet food sales.
Fewer Injuries to Clients and the Veterinary Team	Cats with protective emotions can scratch or bite, posing a risk to both caregivers and veterinary staff. The use of Low Stress Handling® techniques reduces these risks.
Reduced Anxiety for the Client	Knowing that their cat is being treated with care and compassion can significantly alleviate a client's anxiety about veterinary visits.

Adapted from Rodan, I, et al. "AAFP and ISFM feline-friendly handling guidelines." *Journal of Feline Medicine and Surgery* 13.5 (2011): 364–375 and Rodan I, et al. 2022 AAFP/ISFM Cat Friendly Veterinary Interaction Guidelines: Approach and Handling Techniques. *Journal of Feline Medicine and Surgery*. 2022;24(11):1093–1132.

Feline Friendly Guidelines, which included contributions from experts like Dr. Sophia Yin.[11] These guidelines advocated moving away from traditional, forceful handling methods towards Low Stress Handling® techniques. These included various towel wraps (e.g., burrito, half burrito, scarf wrap), restraint holds, and specific equipment (e.g., muzzles, gloves, nets, and cat bags).[11] They emphasized recognizing cats' stress signals and modifying the environment to reduce stress during interactions, and discussed using chemical restraint judiciously when necessary.[11]

As numerous studies have advanced, our knowledge in this field, a new shift in feline-friendly handling has emerged in 2022. The AAFP/ISFM released an update to the 2011 guidelines further emphasizing the importance of giving cats choices and control over their interactions with humans, other animals, and their environment to minimize protective emotions.[5,6] The updated guidelines now explicitly advise against practices that were once considered Low Stress Handling®, such as tight towel wraps, gloves, muzzles, cat wraps, and cat bags, due to their negative impact on feline welfare.[5,6] These methods, previously thought to be low stress, are now understood to increase the risk for pain, discomfort, and fear in cats.[5–10,15–19] Consistent use of such methods can lead to the development of protective emotions, behavioral withdrawal, and potentially defensive behaviors in subsequent interactions.[5–10,12–14] This evolution in guidelines emphasizes the importance of continuous learning and adaptation in feline interactions to consistently guarantee the most humane and effective treatment of cats.

11.2 The Misconception of Handling the "Difficult" Cat

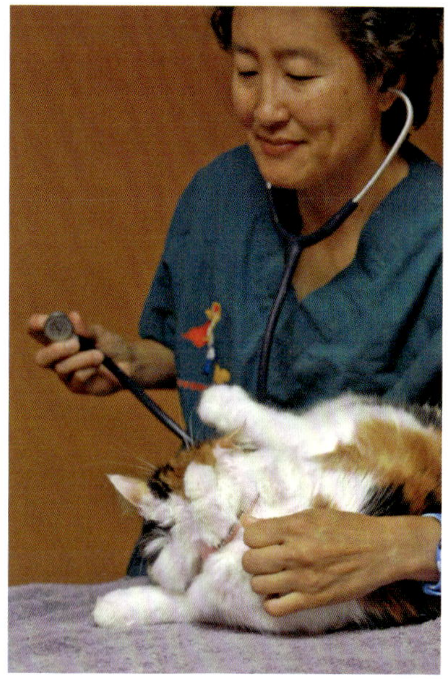

Fig. 11.2 A: Even when scruffed, cats can potentially rotate, escape, scratch, and bite, as indicated in this picture.

Often, cats are unjustly labeled as "feisty," "angry," "difficult," or even "evil."[15,20] A common dilemma faced by those caring for these misunderstood felines is how to effectively manage a seemingly uncooperative cat without resorting to equipment and safety tools such as cat bags, wraps, muzzles, full-body restraint, scruffing, or gloves. The solution to this dilemma is not found in these tools or harsh handling. Rather, it lies in the need for empathy and a deeper understanding of feline behavior.[5,6] By recognizing that such behavior often stems from protective emotions such as fear or discomfort, caregivers and team members can adopt a more compassionate approach.

Instead of resorting to forceful techniques, the solution involves considering the cat's emotional state and often the judicious use of pre-visit medications and sedation.[5,6,11] This alternative approach places a strong emphasis on ensuring the safety, emotional well-being, and overall welfare of the cat.[11] It also recognizes that a stressed, fearful, or anxious cat is less likely to cooperate during examinations and procedures.[5,11] By addressing the cat's stress through appropriate medical interventions, caregivers can cultivate a more compassionate and manageable experience for both themselves and the cat.[5,11] This approach results in better outcomes for all involved, promoting a more positive and welfare-friendly interaction.

Safety

Cats experiencing protective emotions require special care. Continuously holding, restraining, or wrestling these cats not only escalates their behavior due to fear conditioning but also increases the risk of injury to both the cat and the human involved.[5,21] This approach can strain the human-animal bond and negatively affect the emotional well-being of both the handler and the cat.[5]

Learned Helplessness

Learned helplessness is a term used to describe a situation in which cats have learned that they lack agency or control in an aversive situation. When cats exhibit signs of ***learned helplessness***, they become behaviorally inhibited and essentially give up, even if they perceive that their life is in danger.

New Guidelines

According to the 2022 Cat Friendly Veterinary Environment Guidelines, additional equipment such as cat bags, gauntlets or gloves, muzzles of any kind, Elizabethan collars, anesthetic induction boxes/vessels, pillowcases, mesh cat "nabbers," air muzzles, or any other device placed over the cat's head, cat tongs, or rabies pole are not considered cat friendly.[5,6]

In such situations, it is important to assess the necessity of the procedure. If it is not an urgent matter, consider alternative approaches like sending the cat home for carrier training, similar to how dogs are trained for muzzle use, or scheduling a return visit with pre-visit medications or sedation. In case of an emergency, instead of using a tight towel wrap or neck wrap, opt for a loosely wrapped, warm towel infused with pheromones.[5,19] Specific Low Stress Handling® restraint holds like the Ring hold, U-hold, and C-hold can also be used depending upon the situation.[22]

Pain

As a prey species, cats instinctually hide pain.[23,24] This tendency is pronounced during fear and anxiety, potentially masking or obscuring pain signs.[5,6,23] Pain, fear, and anxiety are part of the same emotional response system in cats, resulting in similar body language for both conditions.[5,6] Therefore, it is important to be aware and considerate of pain when handling cats.[5,6,24] Always use minimal handling and provide sufficient breaks to give the cat an opportunity to relax.

11.3 The Need for Choice

As discussed in other chapters, choice and a sense of control over their environment and interactions are fundamental needs for cats.[5,6,25–28] Heavy restraint, cat bags, wraps, and similar tools can strip them of this agency, potentially heightening protective emotions and triggering defensive responses.[5,6,7–10,27] Therefore, it becomes essential to provide cats with the option to choose their examination or procedure location while using minimal restraint, allowing them to move away if desired.[5,6] This approach promotes a sense of safety and reduces the likelihood of protective emotions and defensive behavior.[5,6] Effective strategies for encouraging engagement and facilitating choice include cues, lures, distractions, and cooperative care training.[5,6,22,25–28]

Cues

Cues, such as "touch" and "step-up," can be used with cats, similar to dogs, to effectively guide them to preferred locations for examinations. Utilizing platforms and non-slip mats as designated areas for body targeting can facilitate the cat's movement in a low stress manner.

Lures

Lures, such as food or toys, can be highly effective in encouraging cats to approach voluntarily and prepare for handling. For example, using wand toys or creating a trail of treats can coax cats to step onto a scale independently, eliminating the need for physical lifting. This approach not only reduces stress for the cat but also enhances safety for both the animal and the handler.

Scruffing and Clipnosis®

The common belief that scruffing is an acceptable way to handle cats is largely based on the observation that mother cats, or queens, carry their young by the scruff. However, this practice can increase defensiveness in cats, leading to potential injuries for both the cat and the handler, either immediately or over time.[7–10] Safer alternatives to scruffing include allowing the cat to take breaks, using loose towel wraps, and, if necessary, sedation.[5,6,11]

Clipnosis® involves applying steady, firm pressure to a cat's scruff using tools such as Gentle Calming Clips™ from OurPet's® or similar devices like binder clips.[8,20,29–32] While this may induce a trance-like state in cats, appearances can be deceiving. Current research indicates that what might seem like a calming effect is more likely a state of behavioral inhibition or learned helplessness.[8,20,29–34] This suggests that the cat is not truly calm or relaxed, but rather feels unable to escape or respond, potentially compromising the cat's welfare.8,20,29–34 Scruffing and clipnosis® are practices that do not align with the principles of Low Stress Handling®.[5,6,11]

Distractions

The use of distractions, such as lickable mats or toys, can greatly enhance a cat's comfort during examinations and procedures.[5,6,11,22] By documenting individual preferences, team members can tailor future visits to meet each cat's specific needs, creating a consistently low stress environment.

Cooperative Care and Intervention Visits

Cooperative care training and intervention visits are other highly effective strategies.[25–28,35] A similar process in dogs, cats can be taught to position themselves, communicate consent, and learn foundational behaviors such as stationing, lying down, sitting, and targeting.[25–28,35] This preparation is essential for successful behavior modification, especially during routine veterinary procedures, handling, and restraint positioning. By implementing these strategies, not only does it improve the well-being of cats, but also ensures safer and more effective handling practices.

11.4 Low Stress Handling® Environment

When working with cats, all team members should have a thorough understanding of feline behavior, their needs, and the best ways to interact with them.[5,6] Efforts should be made to minimize wait times and environmental stressors.[5,6,11] It is advisable that only

Table 11.4.1: Green Cats: Ok To Proceed

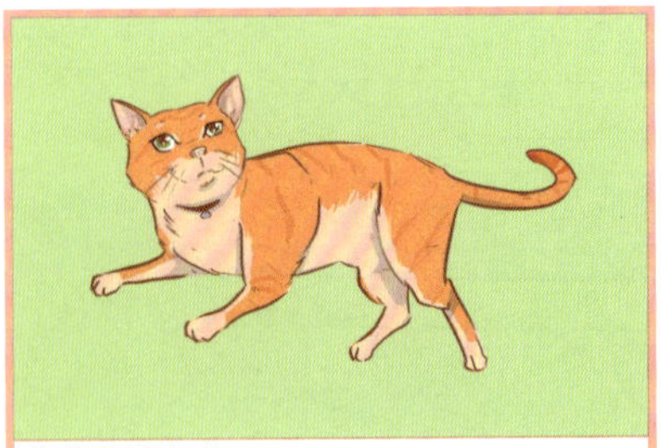

Relaxed, comfortable, and eating

Low Stress Handling® Plan

- Proceed but monitor the cat's behavior and body language throughout the procedure.
- Ensure that the cat is still willing to engage in activities like eating, playing, and interacting.
- Stop if signs of escalating emotional arousal are observed, such as fidgeting, avoidance, staring, or the cat becoming slow-moving or frozen.

experienced team members interact with cats and proper training should be provided to ensure that interactions and handling are conducted appropriately.

Acclimation

Acclimation time is essential for cats; therefore, the room should be prepared ahead of time. Frequent disruptions can increase protective emotions in cats.[5,6,12] To minimize this, gather all necessary items, including equipment for venipuncture, examination tools, and any required vaccinations or injections, before starting the procedure. Additionally, team members should observe the cat and greet them as outlined in previous chapters before handling.

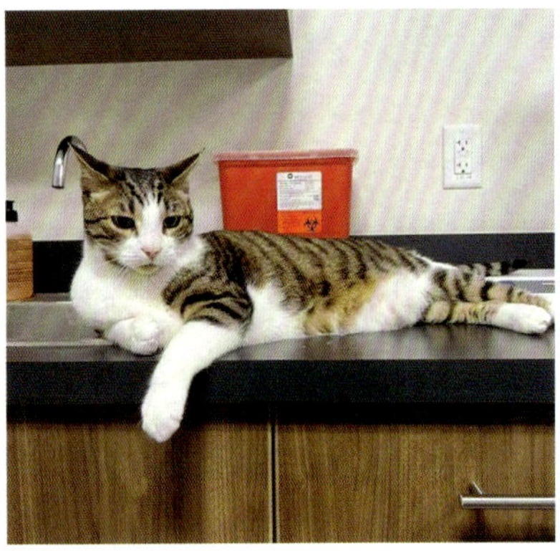

Fig. 11.4 A: Cats should be given time to acclimate to their environment and examined where they are comfortable. (Photo courtesy of Louisiana State University School of Veterinary Medicine Community Practice)

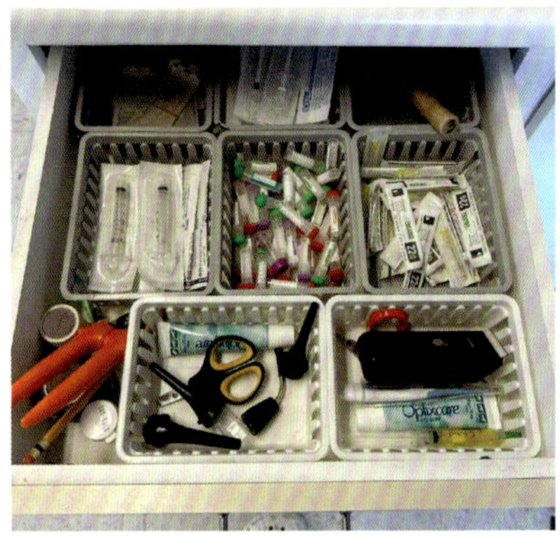

Fig. 11.4 B: Examination rooms should be well stocked with all necessary supplies. (Photo courtesy of Eliot Veterinary Hospital)

Observations

Upon arrival and during transitions (e.g., entering the examination room), support the underside of the carrier with both hands rather than carrying it like a suitcase. In the examination room, the carrier should be placed on the floor before opening its door. This allows the cat time to survey and adjust to their new surroundings while providing them with an opportunity to exit the carrier safely and at their own pace. If necessary, a trail of treats can be used to gently encourage the cat to exit.

As the cat emerges from the carrier and begins to explore the room, carefully observe their gait, posture, haircoat, body condition, and overall behavior. Simultaneously, gather information about the cat's history. Allow the cat to approach and seek attention on their own terms. While doing so, it is best to avoid direct eye contact. Instead, engage in slow blinking and gently toss treats behind the cat to encourage them to turn away, before turning back and approaching for more.

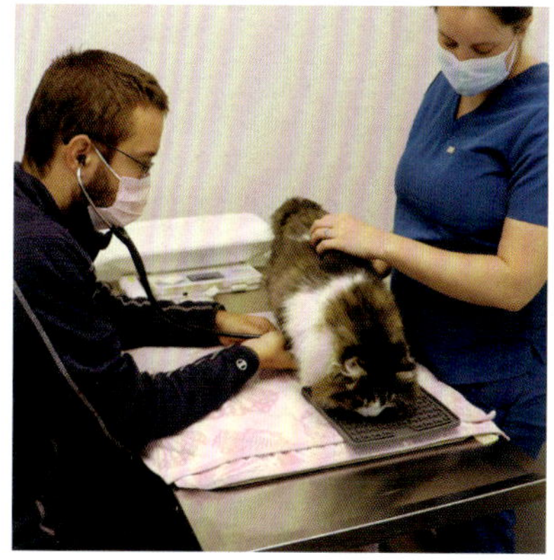

Fig. 11.4 C: Food, such as cat food smeared on a lickable mat (as shown in this photo courtesy of Portland Veterinary Emergency and Specialty Center), can serve as a valuable distraction to encourage a cat to remain standing during a procedure or examination.

Blood Pressure Measurement

When necessary, prioritize obtaining a blood pressure measurement before engaging in any other handling procedures, such as examinations, venipuncture, or diagnostic imaging.[5,] This approach helps reduce the risk of situational hypertension in cats.[5,36–38]

Ideal Environment

Blood pressure measurement should take place in a setting where the cat feels relaxed and comfortable, preferably in a position of their choice.[5] An ideal environment would be a quiet, dimly lit room.[5] Allow the cat approximately 20–30 minutes to acclimate to the surroundings before initiating the measurement process.[5] Whenever possible, cats should remain with their caregivers.

Table 11.4.2 Questions to consider for an accurate blood pressure measurement

- Is the cat willing to eat?
- Can the caregiver remain in the room?
- Should the cat remain in their carrier, covered with a pheromone-infused blanket?
- Would the cat be more comfortable in a cage with a pheromone-infused blanket?
- Would the cat be more comfortable loose in the room?
- Would the cat be more comfortable with a litterbox and water dish?
- Would pre-visit medications be beneficial?

Minimizing Stress

To prepare for the measurement, moisten the fur with a cotton ball or apply ultrasound gel. If necessary, use quiet clippers for fur trimming.[5,38] During the readings, use headphones to minimize the cat's stress from the noise.[39] Avoid applying pressure on joints or tightly holding the feet, since this can influence the readings and potentially cause discomfort.[5]

High Definition Oscillometry (HDO)

While the doppler method is commonly used for blood pressure measurement, other techniques such as High Definition Oscillometry (HDO), are also worth considering. HDO facilitates real-time scanning of pulse waves and requires less direct interaction with the cat, making it a potentially less stressful alternative.[5,41]

Blood Pressure Cuff Placement

For cats with osteoarthritis, the coccygeal (tail) placement of the cuff may be more appropriate, while radial placement of the cuff could be better for overweight cats.[5,38,40]

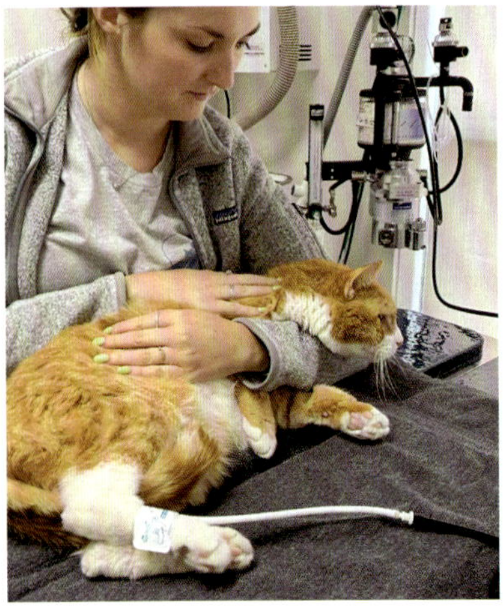

Fig. 11.4 D: Demonstrates minimal restraint while obtaining a blood pressure reading. Always allow the cat to choose a comfortable position and avoid holding the joints or feet tightly. (Photo courtesy of Eliot Veterinary Hospital)

11.5 Examinations

For examinations, find a location where the cat feels most comfortable. Options include inside their carrier, on a counter, inside a sink, or on the caregiver's lap. If an examination table is used, provide a non-slip mat for safety and comfort. Cats that prefer elevated surfaces should be gently encouraged to jump up, rather than being forced or abruptly moved. Handlers and team members must plan their approach for each cat, tailoring their handling strategies in advance to suit individual needs and preferences.

Distance Examination

The approach to examining cats, while sharing similarities to dog examinations, places a strong emphasis on minimizing stress and understanding feline behavior. The initial steps of the examination involve observing the cat's behavior and physical indicators from a distance, without making direct contact. This includes monitoring the cat's gait for any irregularities, ensuring muscle symmetry, observing the size of the pupils, assessing the respiratory rate, and checking for signs of orthopedic, dermatological, or neurological diseases. This non-invasive observation allows for an assessment of the cat's overall health without causing undue stress.

Weight and Temperature

Record the cat's weight when they are comfortably positioned on the scale. If the cat is stressed, weigh them inside their carrier and subtract the carrier's weight for accuracy. Avoid measuring temperature, before the examination to reduce stress.[37] For healthy cats, obtaining a temperature might not be necessary. Axillary or infrared thermometers may be an alternative if a temperature is needed.[42–46] Observe and record the respiratory rate before handling, noting that it often increases in a veterinary setting due to stress. In situations where respiratory disease is a concern, caregivers can record the cat's resting respiratory rate at home for comparison during visits. A digital stethoscope can be used to measure heart rate and listen to heart sounds wirelessly using a Bluetooth® enabled device.[47]

Positioning for Physical Examination

When positioning cats for a physical examination, use minimal handling. Cats should always be given the choice to sit, stand, lie down, or move freely, ensuring their comfort and choice.[5] A loosely draped, warm, pheromone-infused towel can offer a sense of security, without the need for tight wraps that restrict movement.[5,6] In this context, employing cues, lures, and cooperative care training is essential. For cats that exhibit fear, anxiety, or frustration, scheduling intervention visits can be highly beneficial.

The Hands-on Examination

The physical examination of a cat should be tailored to the unique preferences and needs of each individual animal. Minimal handling and restraint are essential, and the examination should start with the least invasive procedures from the cat's perspective, gradually moving towards more invasive ones.[5,11,22]

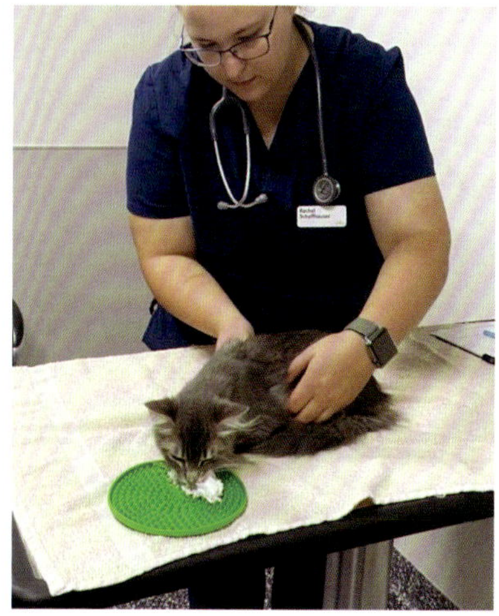

Fig. 11.5 A: Handling for examination should be done in a manner that is comfortable for the cat. (Photo courtesy of Louisiana State University School of Veterinary Medicine Community Practice)

Observations

Throughout the examination, observe the cat's body language and make necessary adjustments based upon feedback at each step of the process. This helps identify aspects of the examination that the cat may find uncomfortable or aversive such as abdominal palpation, head and neck examination, or certain types of equipment.[5] Offering frequent breaks during the examination can help minimize stress, especially if the cat appears uncomfortable during any part of the examination.[5] Dividing the examination into shorter segments can help reduce emotional arousal and facilitate cooperation.[5]

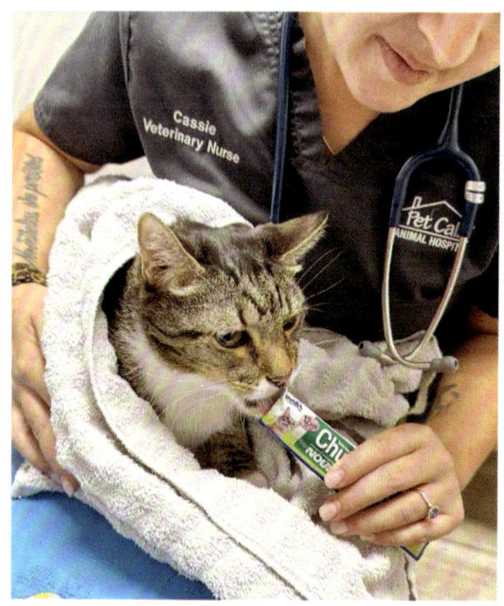

Fig. 11.5 B: A warm, pheromone infused towel and food distraction help provide comfort and feeling of security for many cats. (Photo courtesy of Adrian Novoa, FFCP (photographer) and Cassandra Vazquez, BS FFCP)

Ensuring Comfort and Security

During an examination a cat should always feel safe, supported, and secure.[5,22] This can be achieved by gently sliding hands along the cat's body for positional adjustments, rather than releasing and re-grasping, which could cause the cat to startle.[5,22] A single examiner using minimal restraint is often sufficient, and this person should be flexible, adjusting the examination order to suit the cat's comfort level and needs.

Examination Procedure

The examination should typically begin with auscultation of the heart and lungs, because for many cats, this is the least invasive step.[5] After auscultation, the examination can proceed to palpate the abdomen on the head and mouth.[5] Documenting the

Weigh Before Examining

Many cats show a preference for remaining on the scale during their examination. Consequently, it is advantageous to weigh cats before beginning the examination.[5] This way, if the examination cannot be completed for any reason, the weight will have already been recorded.[5] A current weight is necessary for sedation or if medications are prescribed.

individualized handling plan in the medical record for future visits is recommended.

Special Considerations

For assessing musculoskeletal diseases, combining physical examination findings with caregiver observations is often necessary.[5,48–50] Questionnaires and video of the cat's movement in the home environment can provide more accurate information than in-clinic observations.[5] If pain is a concern, administer analgesics.[5]

Two-Second Rule

When handling cats, always follow the two-second rule; if the cat struggles for two seconds, pause, reposition, and try again.[22] If, after two additional attempts, the cat continues to resist, stop, and determine if the procedure is urgent.[22] If yes, sedation is necessary. If no, reschedule and prescribe a pre-visit medication.

11.6 Neck, Chest, Front, and Hind End Holds

Sometimes restraint is needed but this does not mean scruffing or full body restraint. Many cats can be comfortably positioned using techniques similar to those used with dogs, such as the C-hold, U-hold, Chest hold, or Ring hold.[22] When using these holds, secure the hind end with the other hand or arm to minimize forward, backward, and lateral movements.[22]

11.7 Body Holds

As previously discussed, recent research has shown that scruffing and full-body stretching are aversive to cats and do not align with Low Stress Handling® principles. For procedures such as venipuncture, intravenous (IV) catheter placement, cystocentesis, and blood pressure measurement, the preferred positions for the cat are standing, sternal, or semi-lateral recumbent.[5] The use of lateral (placing the cat on their side) or dorsal recumbency (placing the cat on their back) should be limited to specific cases and only when the cat has been pre-medicated or sedated. Utilizing a trough or towel can enhance their comfort in these positions. Additionally,

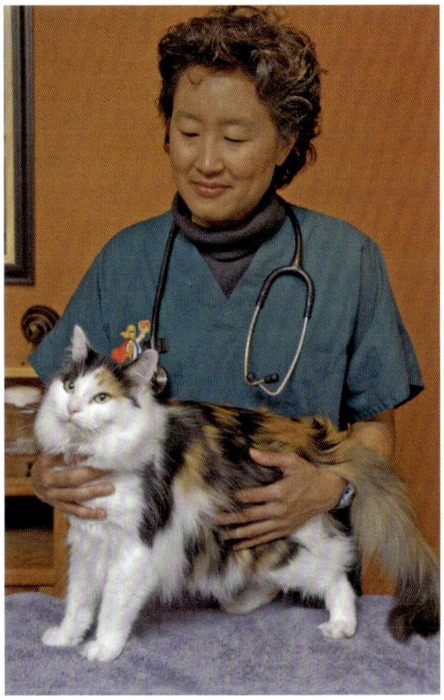

Fig. 11.6 A: This image demonstrates a U-hold loosely around the neck to reduce forward movement, with a hand placed on the lateral aspect of the hip to minimize lateral and backward movements while standing.

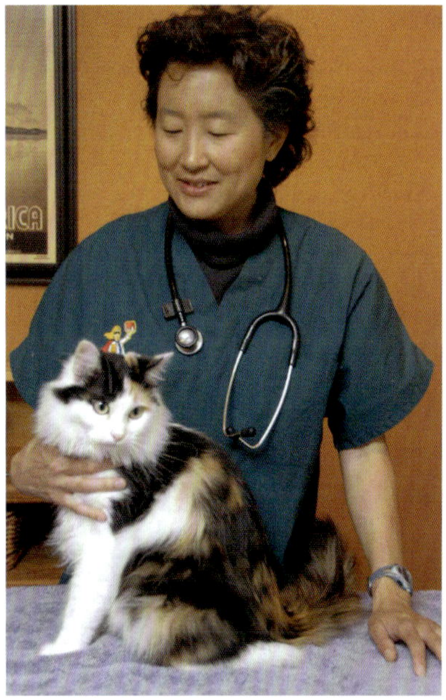

Fig. 11.6 B: This figure shows a loose C-hold to reduce forward movement, with the handler using their body to further support the cat and reduce lateral movements.

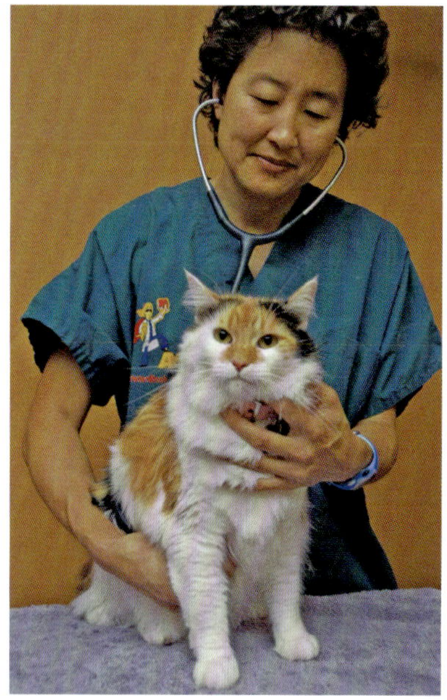

Fig. 11.6 C: This image illustrates a loose chest and upper leg hold to reduce forward and lateral movements, with the hand in front used for massaging the cat's chest, neck, and head.

intervention visits and cooperative care training are effective methods to acclimate cats to these positions, especially if they are necessary for future procedures or examinations.

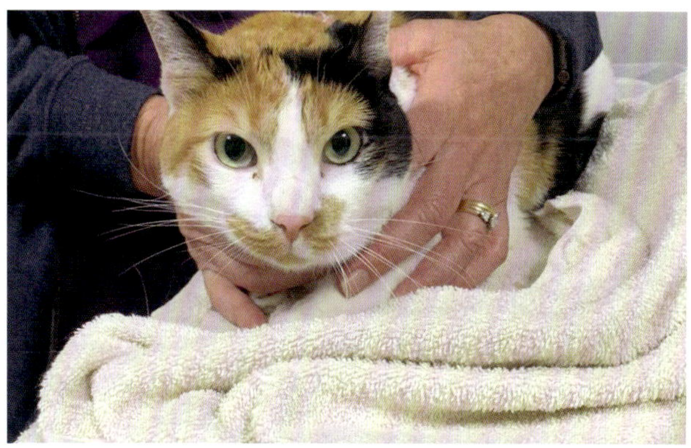

Fig. 11.6 D: This image illustrates the use of a ring hold. (Photo courtesy of Louisiana State University School of Veterinary Medicine Community Practice)

Table 11.7.1: Yellow Cats: Proceed With Caution

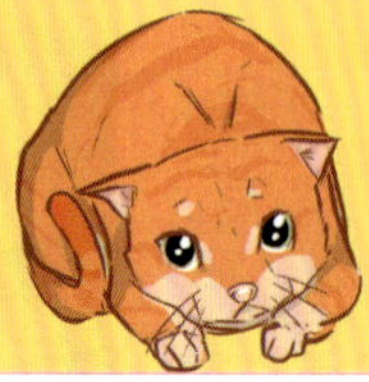

In this category, cats may display different signs of increasing arousal:

Increased Activity (Fidget and Flight)

- Cats displaying increased activity may exhibit behaviors such as fidgeting or looking for ways to flee.
- An example of this is scanning the room, including the ceiling and tops of cabinets, in search of an escape route or a place to hide.

OR

Decreased Activity (Freeze)

- Decreased activity can manifest as a freeze response.
- Examples of this behavior include slow, cautious movements, attempts to hide in the sink, behind items on the counter, or in their carrier.
- A cat might become immobilized and curl up tightly while remaining sternal, with feet tucked and tail curled around their body and head down.
- Some cats may even feign sleep during this state.
- An elevated respiratory rate is also a common indicator of stress in this scenario.

Both increased and decreased activity are serious welfare concerns and intervention is needed.

Low Stress Handling® Plan

This animal is stressed and needs to be monitored closely.

- If the cat continues to eat, play, and interact freely: **Proceed with Current Approach**
- If signs of stress escalate (e.g., stops eating, shows fidgeting, or freezes): **Immediate Action Required**

Avoid letting the cat struggle for more than 2 seconds before repositioning.

- Limit repositioning to no more than 2–3 times.
- Make carrier training a priority to ease future handling.
- Consider referral for cooperative care training and behavior modification.
- Needs:
  - Pre-visit medications +/- sedation.
  - Recognize that a serious welfare concern exist, and intervention is needed.

Standing

Many procedures, including physical examinations, abdominal ultrasounds, cystocentesis, injections, and subcutaneous (SQ) fluid administration, can be less stressful when performed with the cat in a standing position. The use of food lures and distractions helps maintain the cat's comfort and encourages cooperation during these procedures.

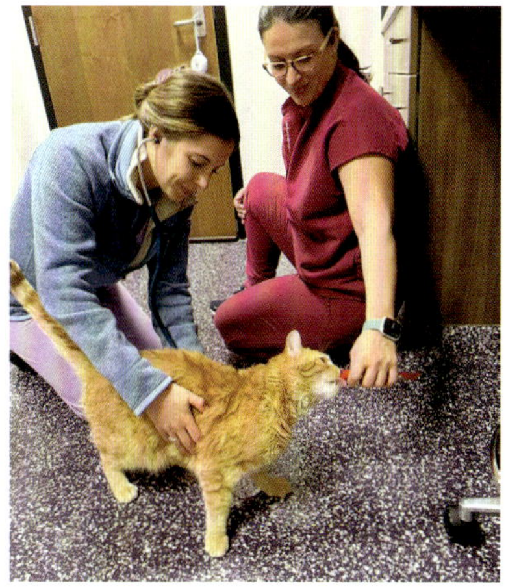

Fig. 11.7 A: Most cats are comfortable in a standing position for physical examinations. Food distractions are always helpful. (Photo of Louisiana State University Community Practice)

Cystocentesis

Cystocentesis is best performed with the cat in a standing or semi-lateral position, rather than in dorsal recumbency. Using ultrasound-guided cystocentesis improves the efficiency and success rate of the procedure while reducing pressure on the bladder.[5] This approach is particularly beneficial for minimizing discomfort in cats with painful abdomens or those suffering from osteoarthritis in their joints.[5] Additionally, ultrasound guidance helps in identifying bladder abnormalities, such as stones or masses.[5] Employing a portable ultrasound machine allows for the procedure to be conducted directly in the examination room, which avoids the stress of moving the cat to a different location.[5]

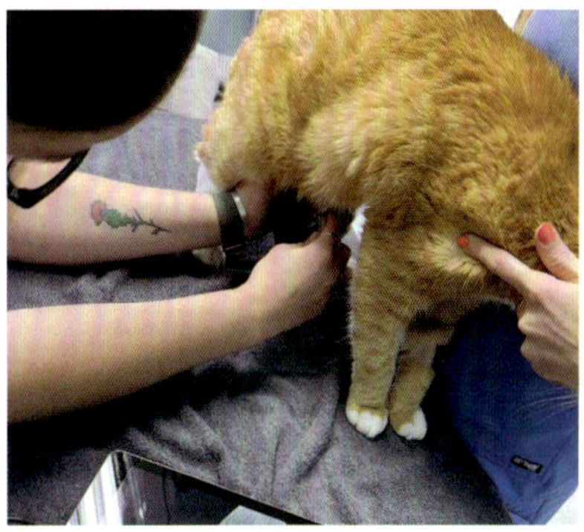

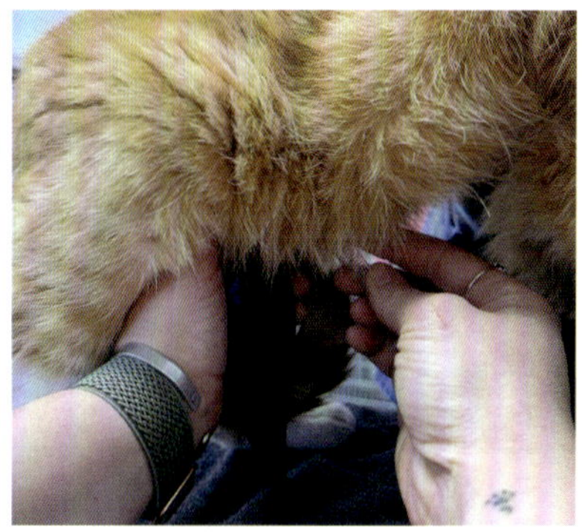

Figs. 11.7 B, C: These images demonstrate the use of minimal restraint to obtain a urine sample via cystocentesis in a standing position. (Photos courtesy of Eliot Veterinary Hospital)

Semi-Lateral Recumbency

When positioning a cat in semi-lateral recumbency avoid rough handling. Most cats will comfortably accept being rolled onto their side without resistance. In this position, the handler should support the cat's head and use their body to stabilize the cat, preventing any unwanted forward, lateral, or backward movements.[22] Place one hand gently between the hind legs and against the abdomen to support the natural alignment of the pelvis and upper hind leg.[22] Avoid holding the cat's feet in place, grasping the joints tightly, or hyper-extending the limbs, head, or neck to prevent discomfort.[5] If the cat displays signs of tension, be prepared to switch to a different handling approach. Distractions such as food, gentle petting, or massaging

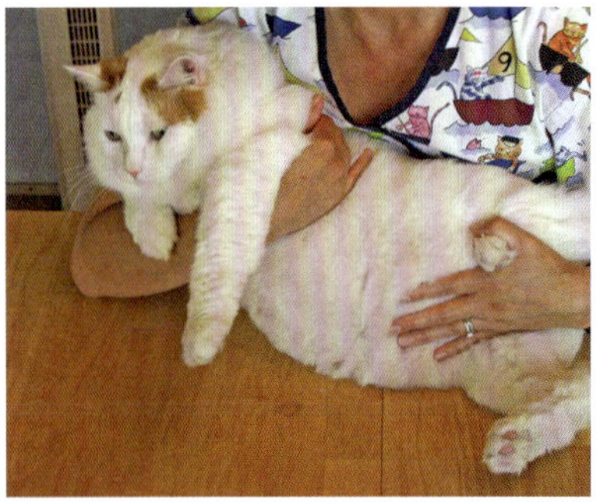

Fig. 11.7 D: This figure shows an example of semi-lateral recumbency. Notice the proper placement of the hand between the hind legs and against the abdomen.

Avoid Head Tapping

Refrain from using head tapping as a distraction technique for cats. This action can be aversive and uncomfortable for many cats.

the temporal area, are effective for keeping the cat relaxed. Never tap on their head or body as a distraction.

For certain procedures like blood pressure measurements and medial saphenous venipuncture, allow the cat to keep the front half of their body in a semi-lateral position. This position is the preferred position for many cats and removes the need for head restraint. The handler can support the front end by placing their arm under the cat's armpit, employing a C-hold around the neck, or loosely draping the front limbs with a towel.[22]

Diagnostic Imaging

Sedation is always necessary for advanced imaging such as Computed Tomography Scans (CT) and Magnetic Resonance Imaging (MRI). Often, pre-visit medications and sometimes sedation is needed for survey and diagnostic radiographs. This is because the positioning required for these procedures, including lateral recumbency and dorsal recumbency, is often uncomfortable and stressful for cats. This approach eliminates the need for gloves and muzzles, which do not align with Low Stress Handling® principles. The use of heavy sandbags and tie-downs as positioning aids is not recommended, even for sedated cats, as they can be uncomfortable, particularly for cats with osteoarthritis.[5]

11.8 Eyes, Ears, and Oral Examination

Examining the eyes and ears of cats can be a stressful experience. Therefore, pre-visit medications may be necessary to ease their discomfort. Cooperative care training and behavior modification techniques prioritize giving the cat a choice, which helps enhance cooperation and reduce protective emotions. This approach helps improve a cat's comfort level during these procedures, aligning with the principles of Low Stress Handling®.

Eye and Ear Examination

Start the eye examination by observing the cat from a distance, allowing them to become accustomed to the room or settle in their preferred spot, such as a lap or carrier. When it is time for a closer inspection, approach the cat at an angle rather than head-on, and avoid direct eye contact. You can gently massage the facial glands as you carefully lift the eyelids to examine the eye structures.[5] This low stress approach is equally important when applying fluorescein stains, eye drops, or ointments, ensuring the cat remains relaxed and comfortable throughout the procedure.

Begin the ear examination by first observing the cat's ear carriage from a distance. Similar to the eye examination process, look for any indications of pruritus (itchiness) or abnormal discharge. Before examining the external ear canal, gently massage over the

Painful Ears

When the ear is pruritic, painful or requires cleaning, both sedation and analgesics will be necessary.

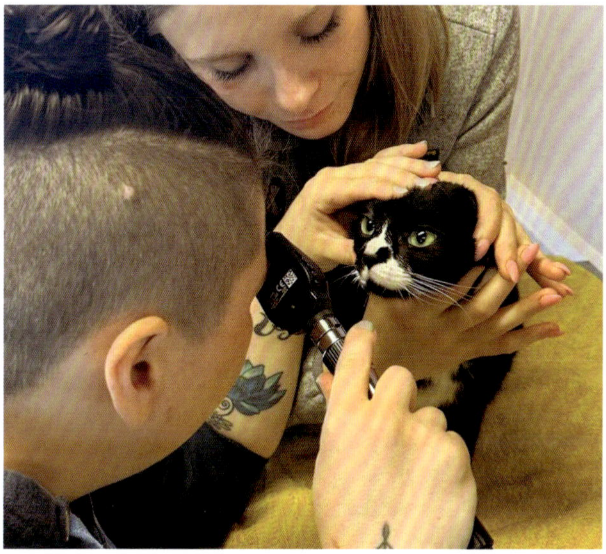

Fig. 11.8 A: This image demonstrates the use of a ring hold to stabilize the head and neck during a direct ophthalmoscopic examination. (Photo courtesy of Eliot Veterinary Hospital)

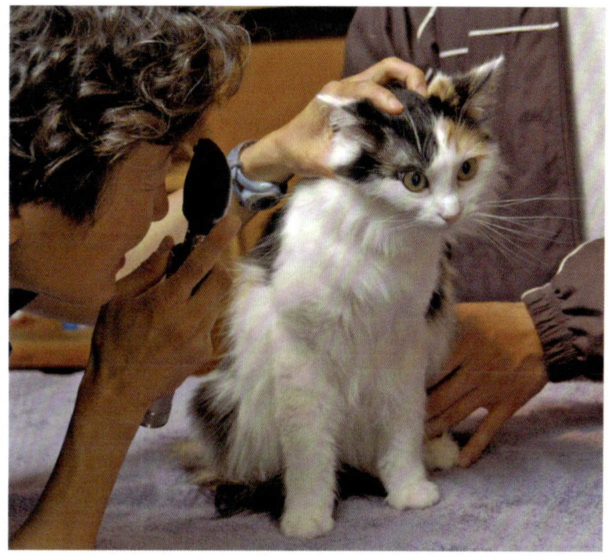

Fig. 11.8 B: This figure illustrates the approach for an eye examination. Approach the cat from an angle, avoid direct eye contact, and use minimal restraint. Massaging over the facial glands while gently lifting the eyelids to facilitate relaxation.

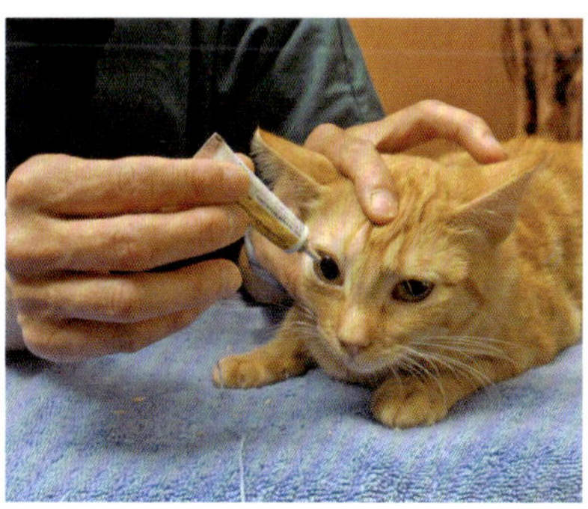

Fig. 11.8 C: This image shows how to gently open the eyelids using the index finger and thumb to massage the facial glands, facilitating the application of ointment.

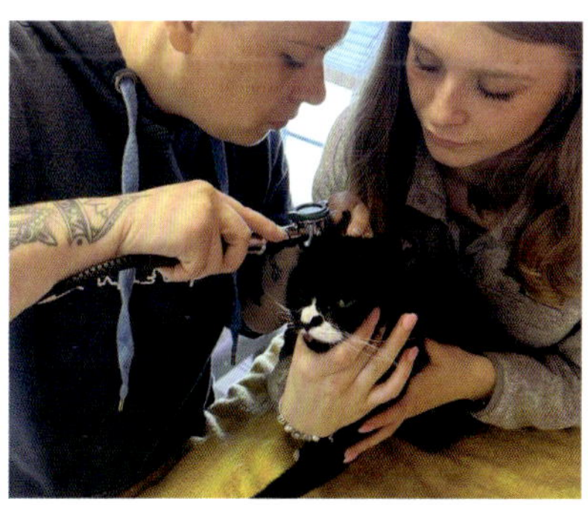

Fig. 11.8 D: In this image, a U-hold is used to stabilize the front end of the cat during an otoscopic examination, allowing the cat to remain seated comfortably. (Photo courtesy of Eliot Veterinary Hospital)

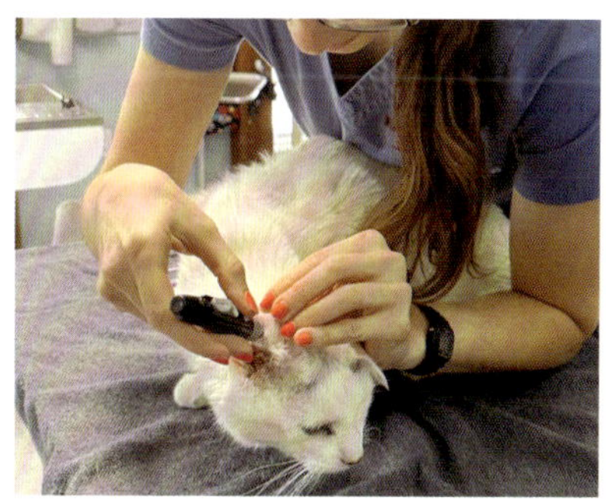

Fig. 11.8 E: This image shows the use of minimal restraint during the collection of a blood glucose sample. (Photo courtesy of Eliot Veterinary Hospital)

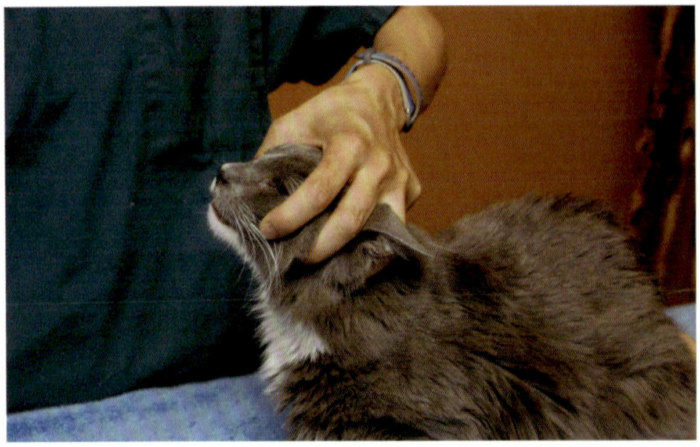

Fig. 11.8 F: Place the thumb and forefinger on the proximal aspect of the zygomatic arch (cheekbone) and gently guide the mouth slightly upward, which typically causes the mouth to open.

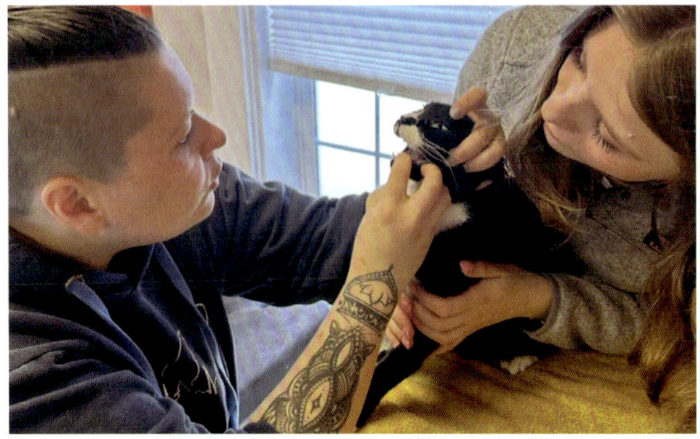

Fig. 11.8 G: This image shows how to open the mouth. Place the index finger between the mandibular canines. Avoid pulling on the jaw. If painful, sedation is needed. (Photo courtesy of Eliot Veterinary Hospital)

facial glands while holding the base of the pinna (ear flap) to ease the cat into the examination.[5] If an otoscopic examination is necessary, carefully insert the otoscope cone, gently extending the ear canal for a better view of the tympanic membrane. Be mindful of the cat's comfort throughout the procedure and consider sedation if the ear appears to be pruritic or painful.

Oral Exam

Similar to dogs, oral examinations in cats should start with an initial assessment from a distance to observe any obvious issues. Approach the cat's mouth cautiously, engaging in slow, gentle petting of the face and cheeks first.[5] This step helps to assess the cat's comfort level and detect any signs of pain. To examine the buccal surfaces of the teeth, gingiva, and cheek linings, carefully lift or lower the lips, taking care not to pull on the cat's fur.[5] Observe the cat's reaction closely; if they show any signs of discomfort or resistance, such as pulling away or hissing, pause the examination and give the cat a break.[5] In cases where the cat consistently objects or if there are signs of oral pain, sedation will be needed.

11.9 Subcutaneous Fluids and Injections

Administering subcutaneous fluids and injections is necessary for many cats throughout their lives. In emergency situations requiring quick restraint, a towel wrap may be needed, although sedation is often the preferred choice for its efficiency and reduced stress on the cat. If a towel is used, ensure it is loosely (not tightly) wrapped around the cat, with either the head (if the cat is comfortable) or feet gently secured, avoiding tight constriction.[22] To reduce stress during injections, pairing the procedure with food distractions can be effective.[5,22] Offer the cat a favorite treat or meal, holding it in a way that keeps the cat's attention focused away from the injection site. Additionally, allowing the cat to choose a comfortable position during the procedure can significantly reduce stress and resistance during the procedure.[5,22]

Cerenia® Injections

Subcutaneous injections of Cerenia® (maropitant citrate, commonly used for nausea) may cause a stinging sensation. To minimize discomfort, consider injecting directly into a pocket created by recently administered subcutaneous fluids. This method can help dilute the medication and reduce the stinging sensation.

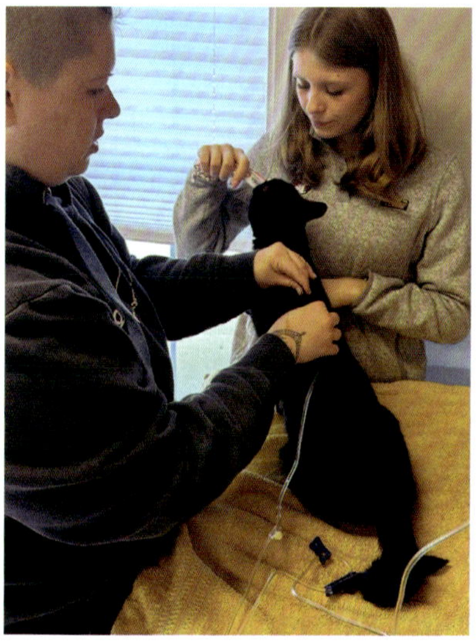

Fig. 11.9 A: Using food distractions can encourage cats to remain stationary and develop a positive association with this procedure. (Photo courtesy of Eliot Veterinary Hospital)

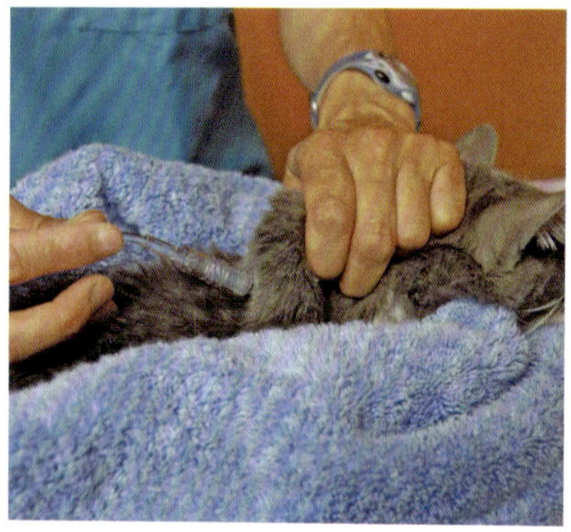

Fig. 11.9 B: This figure illustrates the use of a rolled up towel. Spraying the towel in advance with a synthetic facial pheromone and warming it can improve comfort levels. Keep the towel open at the top and avoid scruffing the cat (the scruff in this picture is tenting before placement of the needle). The towel should be at a height where a cat can comfortably rest their chin.

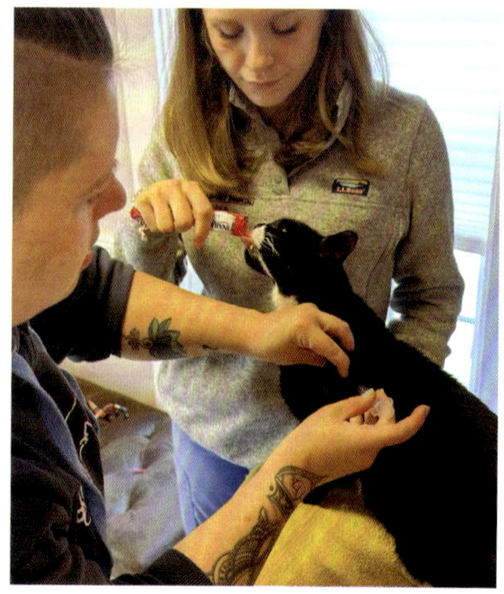

Fig. 11.9 C: Minimal restraint and food distractions are effective for subcutaneous injections. (Photo courtesy of Eliot Veterinary Hospital)

11.10 Venipuncture

During venipuncture, allow the cat a choice in terms of location and position, with the medial saphenous vein often being the least stressful option. Using a small gauge needle and butterfly catheter allows for flexibility during unexpected movements and help maintain a safe distance.[51,52] For kittens or when only a small blood volume is needed, using a specific type or size of an insulin syringe is advisable.

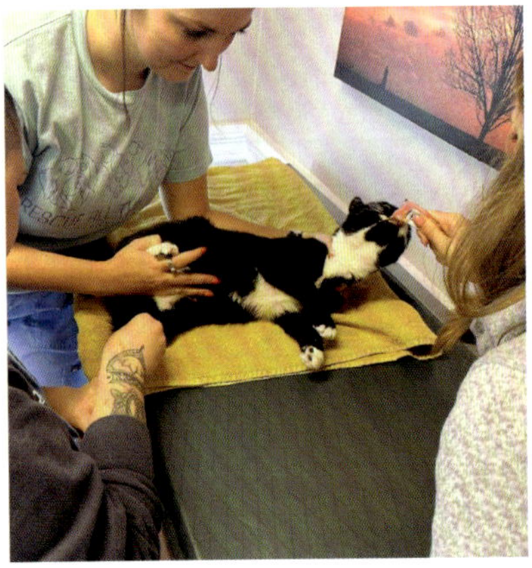

Fig. 11.10 A: Medial saphenous venipuncture tends to be the least stressful venipuncture position for many cats especially when a food distraction is added. (Photo courtesy of Eliot Veterinary Hospital)

If fur clipping is necessary, use quiet clippers and apply a topical local anesthetic about 30 minutes before the procedure.[5,6,53–59] Avoid products with a strong alcohol base, as their potent scent can be unpleasant and aversive to cats. In cases where fur clipping is not required, an alternative such as water or diluted chlorhexidine can be used.[5,6] For safety and effectiveness, ensure the chlorhexidine is appropriately diluted. Prepare for the procedure by presoaking cotton balls in this solution and storing them in an airtight container, making them readily available for use. Instead of using nozzle or squirt bottles, which can be aversive due to their association with deterrents for behaviors like counter surfing and biting, apply the solution gently using the presoaked cotton balls.

Saphenous Venipuncture

For cats with cervical or forelimb osteoarthritis, as well as those that are fearful or anxious, the medial saphenous vein is the ideal site for venipuncture. This vein is less socially invasive and allows for minimal discomfort for the cat. Semi-lateral recumbency is the recommended position for accessing this vein. Avoid forcing the cat into full lateral recumbency, which can cause stress or discomfort. When stabilizing the hind limb for sampling, handle the limb gently. Avoid grasping it tightly or bending the ankle joint excessively. Instead, hold the limb in a natural, relaxed position, and avoid pumping the foot, as this action could cause discomfort or pain.[5]

Venipuncture in a Kitten

Medial or saphenous venipuncture using an insulin syringe is an effective technique for collecting small blood samples, especially in kittens or for specific tests such as retroviral testing. To improve comfort, a towel can be lightly draped to gently secure the feet. The towel should be arranged in a manner that provides a comforting yet effective restraint, avoiding any excessive tightening that might cause distress. Continuously monitor the cat's comfort level and adjust the handling as necessary.

Cephalic Venipuncture and Catheterization

During cephalic venipuncture and catheterization, place a hand behind the elbow to advance and secure the forelimb. Avoid pumping the foot.[5] The cat should be allowed to choose its preferred handling position and location, which involves offering choices between different comfortable spots or positions.[5,22] Tight restraints around the cat's body and elbow should be avoided in favor of a secure but gentle hold.[22] For cats that prefer their head covered, a loose towel or blanket can be provided.[5]

Jugular Venipuncture

Jugular venipuncture in cats should only be attempted when the cat is relaxed and calm. Using minimal restraint, secure the cat's head by placing both thumbs behind the base of the skull and the mandible with both middle fingers, ensuring the hold is firm yet gentle.[22] Gently massage over the facial glands, avoiding firm pressure.[5,22] Carefully tilt the cat's head upwards, taking care to avoid contact with the sensitive whiskers. As an alternative method, the handler can fold in their fingers on each hand to ensure the jugular vein is not obstructed.[22]

Avoid hyperextending the cat's neck and stretching or draping the forelimbs over the edge of the table, as these actions can cause discomfort or stress.[5,22] If necessary, a towel can be loosely wrapped around the cat to allow movement of the forelimbs while still ensuring handler safety.[5] If the cat shows signs of excessive stress, sedation may be required to safely complete the procedure.

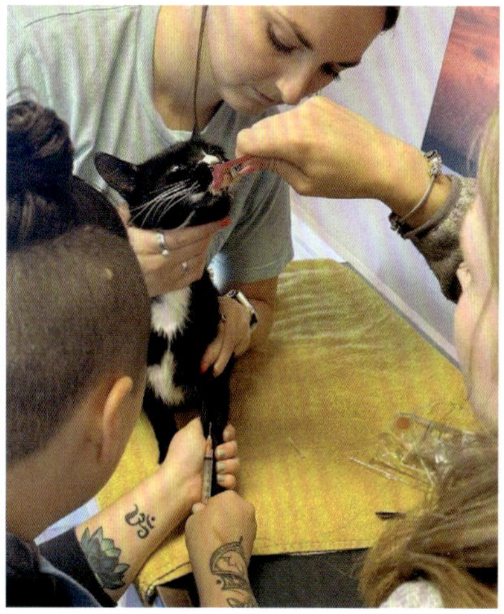

Fig. 11.10 B: Cephalic venipuncture using minimal handling and food distraction. (Photos courtesy of Eliot Veterinary Hospital)

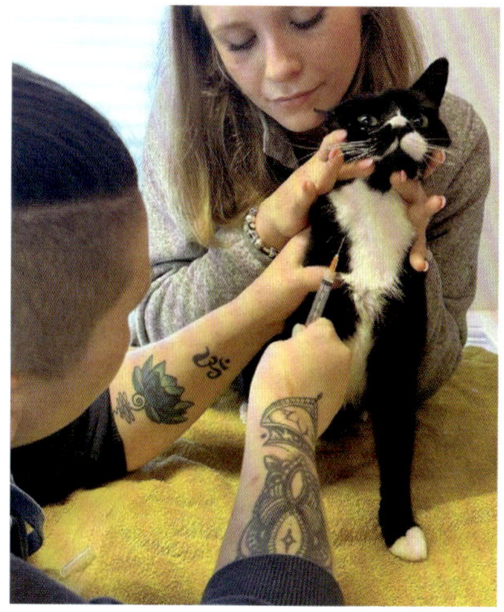

Fig. 11.10 C: This image illustrates the correct way to stabilize the cat's head for jugular venipuncture. The thumbs are placed at the base of the skull, and the mandible is supported with each middle finger, allowing the handler to massage the facial glands with their free fingers. (Photo courtesy of Eliot Veterinary Hospital)

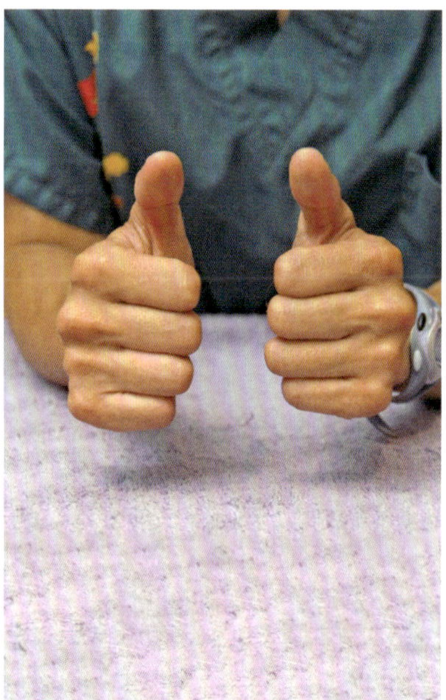

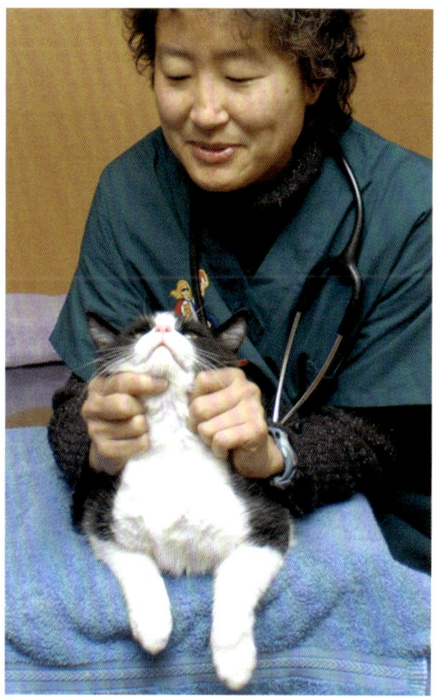

Figs. 11.10 D, E: These images illustrate alternative hand positioning for jugular venipuncture, where the handler's fingers are folded underneath the mandible to avoid obstructing the jugular vein.

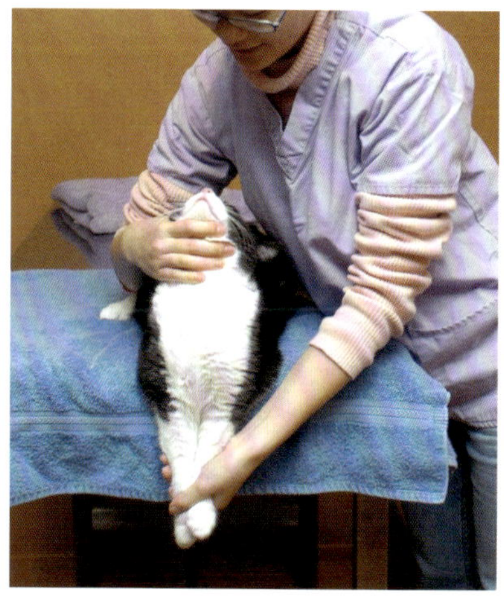

Fig. 11.10 F INCORRECT: Do not stretch cat's forelimbs over the edge of the table or hyperextend their neck. Such restraint can be painful and does not reduce lateral, forward, or backward movement. Due to a feeling of insecurity, the cat is more likely to scratch or bite.

11.11 Feline

For all cats, especially those that are fearful, carrier training is essential. Cats should be brought to the hospital in their carrier, be it soft- or hard-sided.[5,6,20,22,60] The Ninja Sedation technique can be effectively applied using the cat's carrier to facilitate the sedation process.[5,20,22] Carriers that are easy to disassemble allow for the administration of an intramuscular (IM) injection while the cat remains inside.[5,22] This approach is preferable over the use of induction chambers, as it is less stressful for the cat, decreases human exposure to anesthetic gases, and it provides accessibility to monitor and manage the cat's vital signs. Moreover, it lowers the risk of adverse effects such as hypotension, bradycardia, and stress-induced catecholamine release leading to rapid decompensation.[11]

Table 11.11.1: Red Cats: Do Not Proceed!

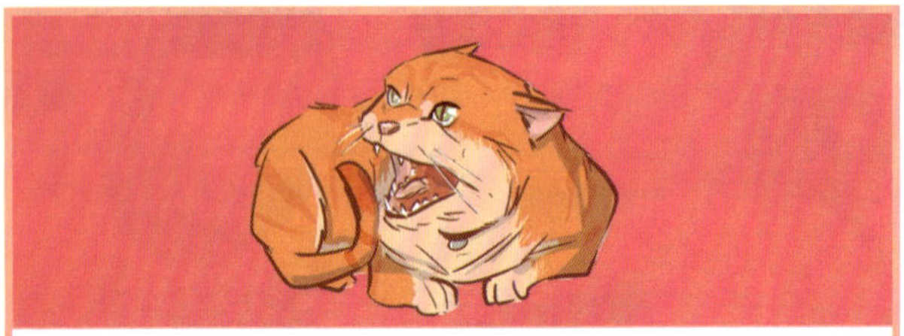

As in the yellow category, these cats may exhibit a range of behaviors indicating stress or discomfort, including:

Flight: The cat may attempt to escape or actively look for ways to flee from the situation.
Freeze: The cat might become immobile, showing signs of a freeze response, often as a defensive mechanism.
Fidget: There could be signs of restlessness or fidgeting, indicating discomfort or anxiety.
Fight: The cat will show defensive behaviors (growling, hissing, swatting, biting, and scratching) as a form of self-defense.

Low Stress Handling® Plan

- For cats exhibiting these behaviors, pre-visit medications alone are often not sufficient to alleviate their stress or anxiety effectively. In such cases, it is recommended to add intravenous or intramuscular sedation in addition to pre-visit medications.
- Refer the cat for intervention visits, cooperative care training, and behavior modification.

Individualized Handling Plan for Intramuscular Sedation in a Cat

Seraphina, a sleek Siamese cat known for her skittish nature, often struggled during veterinary visits. Her previous experiences were filled with protective emotions and defensive behaviors, making routine examinations challenging. To ease these visits for both Seraphina and her caregiver, the veterinary team developed an individualized handling plan to provide her with the necessary care while minimizing distress.

The plan started at home with Seraphina's caregivers transforming her view of the carrier from a predictor of frightening experiences to a safe, comfortable, and inviting space. They used synthetic pheromones to attract her and encourage exploration, placed treats inside, and included a soft blanket to entice her to rest there. By feeding all of Seraphina's meals inside the carrier, they hoped she would build positive associations with the carrier and choose to spend more time in it.

Once the carrier training was progressing, preparations for a rescheduled sedation visit were set in motion. Seraphina was prescribed a pre-visit medication to lessen her anxiety and facilitate an intramuscular sedation injection. This medication was administered two hours before her visit, mixed into a treat on a lickable mat.

Upon arriving at the veterinary hospital for her sedation, the team maintained a calm and relaxed approach to minimize stress. Instead of removing Seraphina from her carrier, a team member partially disassembled it just enough to insert a thick, warm towel infused with pheromones. With Seraphina securely wrapped in the towel inside the carrier, another team member quickly administered the intramuscular sedation through the same opening, before reassembling the carrier.

After the injection, the team allowed Seraphina to relax in her carrier in a quiet examination room as the sedative took effect. When it was time for her examination and rabies vaccination, she was peacefully sedated. The entire procedure, including a full physical examination and vaccinations, proceeded smoothly. Thanks to the effectiveness of the individualized handling plan, the team's preparation, and her caregiver's dedication, this time Seraphina and her caregiver left the veterinary hospital happy and anxiety-free.

The Procedure

To administer the sedative, open the carrier and slide in a warm, pheromone-infused towel or blanket to cover the cat, applying light restraint for the intramuscular injection.[5] After administering the injection, reassemble the carrier and allow the cat some time for the sedative to take effect.

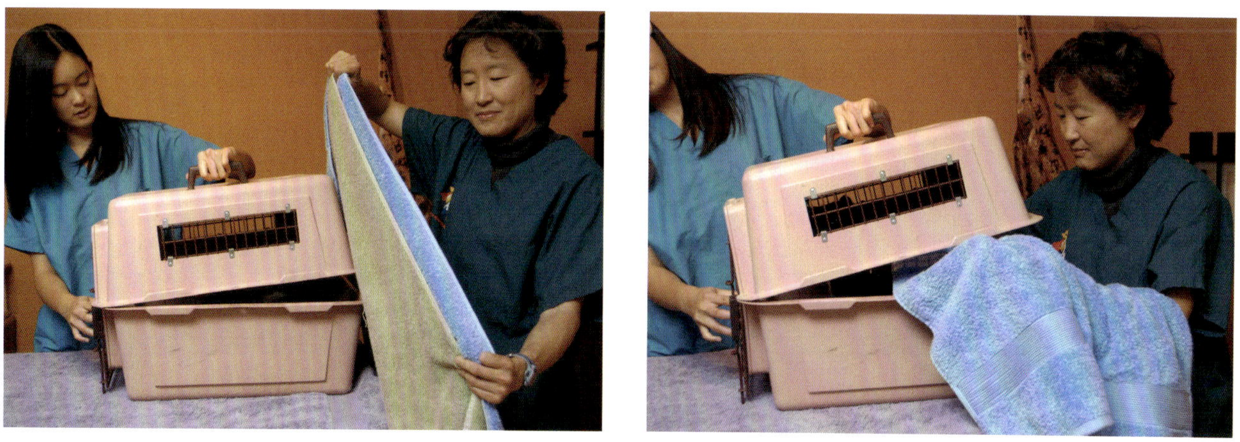

Fig. 11.11 A, B: Disassemble the carrier and lift the top slightly. Keep the front door in place to prevent the cat from darting out. One or two thick towels or blankets can be used, depending on how likely the cat is to bite or scratch.

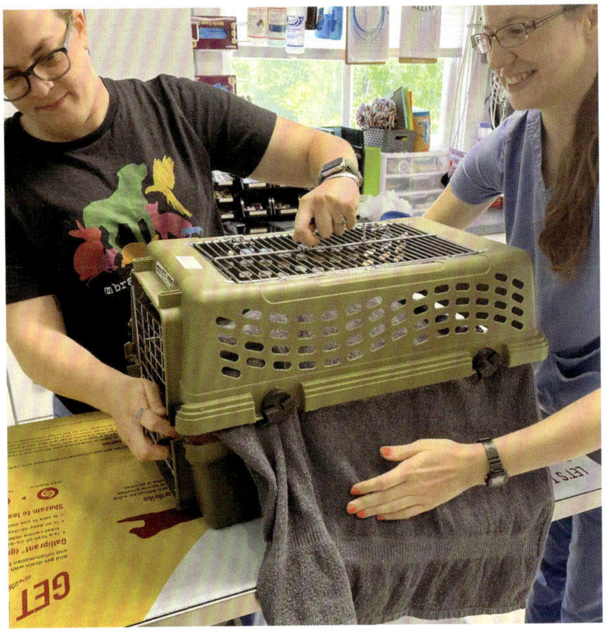

Figs. 11.11 C: Slide the towel in and cover the cat. (Photo courtesy of Eliot Veterinary Hospital)

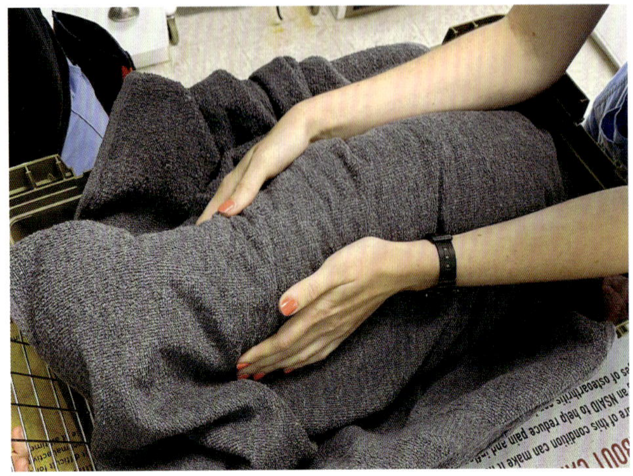

Fig. 11.11 D: This image demonstrates removing the carrier top while ensuring the door remains in place. Tuck the towel around the sides of the cat before administering the injection. Alternatively, the lid can be kept on, reaching into the carrier from the back to restrain the cat with a towel before administering the injection and then closing the carrier. (Photo courtesy of Eliot Veterinary Hospital)

11.12 Conclusion

Low Stress Handling® significantly improves welfare and safety for all. Cats should be given an opportunity to choose their preferred positioning and locations for all procedures. Always use minimal restraint and be mindful of the potential for underlying pain. Administer analgesics and sedation when necessary.

11.13 References

1. Beaver, B. V. (2003). *Feline Behavior E-Book*. Elsevier Health Sciences.
2. Houpt, Katherine A. (2018) *Domestic animal behavior for veterinarians and animal scientists*. John Wiley & Sons.
3. Overall, K. L., Rodan, I., Beaver, B. V., Carney, H., Crowell-Davis, S., Hird, N., Kudrak, S., & Wexler-Mitchel, E. (2005). Feline behavior guidelines from the American Association of Feline Practitioners. *Journal of the American Veterinary Medical Association*, 227(1), 70–84.
4. Turner, D. C. (2021). Unanswered questions and hypotheses about domestic cat behavior, ecology, and the cat–human relationship. *Animals*, 11(10), 2823. https://doi.org/10.3390/ani11102823

5. Rodan, I., Dowgray, N., Carney, H. C., Carozza, E., Ellis, S. L. H., Heath, S., Niel, L., St Denis, K., & Taylor, S. (2022). AAFP/ISFM Cat friendly veterinary interaction guidelines: Approach and handling techniques. *Journal of Feline Medicine and Surgery*, 24(11), 1093–1132.

6. Taylor, S., St Denis, K., Collins, S., Dowgray, N., Ellis, S. L. H., Heath, S., Rodan, I., & Ryan, L. (2022). ISFM/AAFP Cat friendly veterinary environment guidelines. *Journal of Feline Medicine and Surgery*, 24(11), 1133–1163.

7. Moody, C. M., Dewey, C. E., & Niel, L. (2020). Cross-sectional survey of cat handling practices in veterinary clinics throughout Canada and the United States. *Journal of the American Veterinary Medical Association, 256*(9), 1020–1033. https://doi.org/10.2460/javma.256.9.1020

8. Moody, C. M., Mason, G. J., Dewey, C. E., & Niel, L. (2020). Getting a grip: Cats respond negatively to scruffing and clips. *Veterinary Record, 186*(12), 385.

9. Moody, C. M., Mason, G. J., Dewey, C. E., Landsberg, G. M., & Niel, L. (2019). Testing two behavioural paradigms for measuring post-handling cat aversion behaviour. *Applied Animal Behaviour Science, 210*, 73–80.

10. Moody, C. M., Picketts, V. A., Mason, G. J., Dewey, C. E., & Niel, L. (2018). Can you handle it? Validating negative responses to restraint in cats. *Applied Animal Behaviour Science, 204*, 94–100.

11. Rodan, I., Sundahl, E., Carney, H., et al. (2011). AAFP and ISFM feline-friendly handling guidelines. *Journal of Feline Medicine and Surgery*, 13(5), 364–375. https://doi.org/10.1016/j.jfms.2011.03.012

12. Heath, S. (2018). Understanding feline emotions: . . . and their role in problem behaviours. *Journal of Feline Medicine and Surgery*, 20(5), 437–444.

13. Heath, S. (2020). Environment and feline health: at home and in the clinic. *Veterinary Clinics: Small Animal Practice, 50*(4), 663–693.

14. Heath, S. (2022). Feline behavioural medicine–an important veterinary discipline. *Advances in Small Animal Care, 3*(1), 13–22.

15. Adibi, & Lampl, I. (2021). Sensory adaptation in the whisker-mediated tactile system: Physiology, theory, and function. *Frontiers in Neuroscience*, 15, 770011–770011. https://doi.org/10.3389/fnins.2021.770011

16. Ikeda, R., & Gu, J. G. (2016). Electrophysiological property and chemical sensitivity of primary afferent neurons that innervate rat whisker hair follicles. *Molecular Pain, 12*, 1744806916685570.

17. Zhu, & Connors, B. W. (1999). Intrinsic firing patterns and

whisker- evoked synaptic responses of neurons in the rat barrel cortex. *Journal of Neurophysiology, 81*(3), 1171–1183. https://doi.org/10.1152/jn.1999.81.3.1171

18. Shenoda, Y., Ward, M. P., McKeegan, D., & Fawcett, A. (2020). "The cone of shame": welfare implications of elizabethan collar use on dogs and cats as reported by their owners. *Animals, 10*(2), 333.

19. Decock, L.J.G., Menuge, F., Cozzi, A., Teruel, E., Codecasa, E., Monneret, P., De Keuster, T., & Moons, C.P.H. (2023, June). Reducing feline stress in the veterinary practice: investigating the evidence. Paper presented at the 4th Annual Meeting of the European Veterinary Congress of Behavioral Medicine and Animal Welfare, Palma de Mallorca, Spain.

20. Herron, M. E., & Shreyer, T. (2014). The pet-friendly veterinary practice: a guide for practitioners. *Veterinary Clinics: Small Animal Practice, 44*(3), 451–481.

21. Brown, J. F., Taylor, S. S., & Wilson, A. M. (2021). Comparison of cat-related human injury rates in ISFM cat friendly accredited clinics and non-accredited clinics. *J Feline Med Surg, 23*, 855–856.

22. Yin, S. A. (2009). *Low Stress Handling, Restraint and Behavior Modification of Dogs & Cats:* CattleDog Publishing.

23. Gruen, M. E., Lascelles, B. D. X., Colleran, E., Gottlieb, A., Johnson, J., Lotsikas, P., Marcellin-Little, D., & Wright, B. (2022). AAHA pain management guidelines for dogs and cats. *Journal of the American Animal Hospital Association, 58*(2), 55–76.

24. Mills, D. S., Demontigny-Bédard, I., Gruen, M., Klinck, M. P., McPeake, K. J., Barcelos, A. M., Hewison, L., Van Haevermaet, H., Denenberg, S., Hauser, H., et al. (2020). Pain and problem behavior in cats and dogs. *Animals*, 10(2), 318. https://doi.org/10.3390/ani10020318

25. Jones, E. (2023). Cooperative care for companion dogs: emotional health and wellness. *Companion Animal*, 28(7), 1–6.

26. Jones, E. (2023). Preparing fearful dogs for vaccinations with cooperative care. *Animal Behaviour and Welfare Cases*, (2023), abwcases20230011.

27. Littlewood, K. E., Heslop, M. V., & Cobb, M. L. (2023). The agency domain and behavioral interactions: assessing positive animal welfare using the Five Domains Model. *Frontiers in Veterinary Science*, 10. https://doi.org/10.3389/fvets.2023.1284869

28. Sydänheimo, A., Freeman, M., & Hunt, K. (2023). Cooperative care does not scare–use of cooperative care training in routine husbandry in dogs. *Animal Behaviour and Welfare Cases*, abwcases20230010

29. Andrews, C. J., Cosner, Z., & Thomas, D. G. (2022). The efficacy of pinch-induced behavioral inhibition (clip restraint) in domestic cats (Felis Catus) declines with age. *Journal of Veterinary Behavior,* 49, 15–19.

30. Lefebvre, L., & Sabourin, M. (1977). Response differences in animal hypnosis: a hypothesis. *The Psychological Record*, 27, 77.

31. Nuti, V., Cantile, C., Gazzano, A., et al. (2016). Pinch-induced behavioural inhibition (clipthesia) as a restraint method for cats during veterinary examinations: preliminary results on cat susceptibility and welfare. *Animal Welfare,* 25, 115–123.

32. Pozza, M. E., Stella, J. L., Chappuis-Gagnon, A. C., Wagner, S. O., & Buffington, C. T. (2008). Pinch-induced behavioral inhibition ('clipnosis') in domestic cats. *Journal of Feline Medicine and Surgery*, 10(1), 82–87.

33. Riemer, S., Heritier, C., Windschnurer, I., Pratsch, L., Arhant, C., & Affenzeller, N. (2021). A review on mitigating fear and aggression in dogs and cats in a veterinary setting. *Animals*, 11(1), 158.

34. Taylor, A. F. (2020). Literature review on the handling and restraint of cats in practice and its effect on patient welfare. *Veterinary Nursing Journal*, 35(6), 162–166.

35. Howell, A., & Feyrecilde, M. (2018). *Cooperative Veterinary Care* (1st ed.). Wiley-Blackwell.

36. Belew, A. M., Barlett, T., & Brown, S. A. (1999). Evaluation of the white-coat effect in cats. *Journal of Veterinary Internal Medicine,* 13(2), 134–142.

37. Hanås, S., Holst, B. S., Ljungvall, I., Tidholm, A., Olsson, U., Häggström, J., & Höglund, K. (2021). Influence of clinical setting and cat characteristics on indirectly measured blood pressure and pulse rate in healthy Birman, Norwegian Forest, and Domestic Shorthair Cats. *Journal of Veterinary Internal Medicine*, 35(2), 801–811.

38. Whittemore, J. C., Nystrom, M. R., & Mawby, D. I. (2017). Effects of various factors on Doppler ultrasonographic measurements of radial and coccygeal arterial blood pressure in privately owned, conscious cats. *Journal of the American Veterinary Medical Association,* 250, 763–769.

39. Uematsu, S., Summers, S., Keys, D., & Quimby, J. (2023). Effect of audible static on blood pressure measurement by Doppler ultrasonic sphygmomanometry in cats. *Journal of Feline Medicine and Surgery,* 25(9), 1098612X231197084.

40. De Rosa, S. M., Drobatz, K. J., & Reineke, E. L. (2021). Evaluation of coccygeal and radial artery Doppler blood pressure measurements in sick cats with and without abnormalities in tissue perfusion. *Journal of*

Veterinary Emergency and Critical Care (San Antonio, Tex. : 2000), 31(6), 749–757.

41. Cerejo, S. A., Teixeira-Neto, F. J., Garofalo, N. A., Rodrigues, J. C., Celeita-Rodríguez, N., & Lagos-Carvajal, A. P. (2017). Comparison of two species-specific oscillometric blood pressure monitors with direct blood pressure measurement in anesthetized cats. *Journal of Veterinary Emergency and Critical Care (San Antonio, Tex. : 2000)*, 27(4), 409–418.

42. Beyer, O., Lueck, A., & Brundage, C. (2023). Comparison of axillary versus rectal temperature timing in canine and feline patients. *Veterinary Sciences,* 10(7), 475. https://doi.org/10.3390/vetsci10070475

43. Giannetto, C., Di Pietro, S., Falcone, A., Pennisi, M., Giudice, E., Piccione, G., & Acri, G. (2021). Thermographic ocular temperature correlated with rectal temperature in cats. *Journal of Thermal Biology*, 102, 103104.

44. Hall, E. J., Fleming, A., & Carter, A. J. (2019). Investigating the use of non-contact infrared thermometers in cats and dogs. *The Veterinary Nurse*, 10(2), 109–115.

45. Nutt, K. R., Levy, J. K., & Tucker, S. J. (2016). Comparison of non-contact infrared thermometry and rectal thermometry in cats. *Journal of Feline Medicine and Surgery*, 18(10), 798–803.

46. Smith, V. A., Lamb, V., & McBrearty, A. R. (2015). Comparison of axillary, tympanic membrane and rectal temperature measurement in cats. *Journal of Feline Medicine and Surgery,* 17, 1028–1034.

47. Oktivasari, P., Haryanto, F., Salman, A. H., Riandini, R., & Suprijadi, S. (2020). A real-time heart rate signal detection using an electronic stethoscope with labview. *Journal of Biomedical Physics & Engineering*, 10(3), 375–382. https://doi.org/10.31661/jbpe.v0i0.1183

48. Dowgray N, Pinchbeck G, Eyre K, et al. Aging in cats: owner observations and clinical finding in 206 mature cats at enrolment to the Cat Prospective Aging and Welfare Study. *Front Vet Sci* 2022; 9.

49. Benito, J., Gruen, M. E., Thomson, A., et al. (2012). Owner-assessed indices of quality of life in cats and the relationship to the presence of degenerative joint disease. *Journal of Feline Medicine and Surgery*, 14, 863–870.

50. Bennett, D., Ariffin, S. M. Z., & Johnston, P. (2012). Osteoarthritis in the cat: 1. How common is it and how easy to recognize? *Journal of Feline Medicine and Surgery*, 14, 65–75.

51. Hefler, L., Grimm, C., Leodolter, S., & Tempfer, C. (2004). To butterfly or to needle: the pilot phase. *Annals of Internal Medicine,* 140(11), 935–936.

52. Kirchhoff, D., Baser, R., Kwong, D., Ramanathan, L., & McCash, S. I. (2023). Comparison of a novel thin-walled 25–gauge needle push button blood collection set to a standard 23–gauge needle in a cancer patient population. *The Journal of Applied Laboratory Medicine*, 8(2), 264–271.

53. Chang, P. C., Goresky, G. V., O'Connor, G., Pyesmany, D. A., Rogers, P. C. J., Steward, D. J., & Stewart, J. A. (1994). A multicentre randomized study of single-unit dose package of EMLA patch vs EMLA 5% cream for venepuncture in children. *Canadian Journal of Anaesthesia*, 41, 59–63.

54. Chávez, C., Ubilla, M. J., Goich, M., Cañón-Jones, H., & Iturriaga, M. P. (2021). Decrease in behaviors associated with pain during catheter placement using a topical anesthetic formulation in cats. *Journal of Veterinary Behavior*, 46, 15–17.

55. Crisi, P. E., De Santis, F., Giordano, M. V., Cerasoli, I., Colucci, F., Di Tommaso, M., & Luciani, A. (2021). Evaluation of eutectic lidocaine/prilocaine cream for jugular blood sampling in cats. *Journal of Feline Medicine and Surgery*, 23(2), 185–189.

56. Hogan, M. E., Vandervaart, S., Perampaladas, K., et al. (2011). Systematic review and meta-analysis of the effect of warming local anesthetics on injection pain. *Annals of Emergency Medicine*, 58. https://doi.org/10.1016/j.annemergmed.2010.12.001

57. Oliveira, R. L. S., Soares, J. H. N., Moreira, C. M. R., Silva, C. P. P., Carrasco, L. P. S., & Souza, H. J. M. (2019). The effects of lidocaine—prilocaine cream on responses to intravenous catheter placement in cats sedated with dexmedetomidine and either methadone or nalbuphine. *Veterinary Anaesthesia and Analgesia*, 46, 492–495. Top of Form

58. van Oostrom, H., & Knowles, T. G. (2018). The clinical efficacy of EMLA cream for intravenous catheter placement in client-owned dogs. *Veterinary Anaesthesia and Analgesia*, 45(5), 604–608.

59. Wagner, K. A., Gibbon, K. J., Strom, T. L., Kurian, J. R., & Trepanier, L. A. (2006). Adverse effects of EMLA (lidocaine/prilocaine) cream and efficacy for the placement of jugular catheters in hospitalized cats. *Journal of Feline Medicine and Surgery*, 8(2), 141–144.

60. Pratsch, L., Mohr, N., Palme, R., Rost, J., Troxler, J., & Arhant, C. (2018). Carrier training cats reduces stress on transport to a veterinary practice. *Applied Animal Behaviour Science*, 206, 64–74.

Authors
Christine D. Calder DVM, DACVB
Katharine Schwarz RVT, KPA-CTP

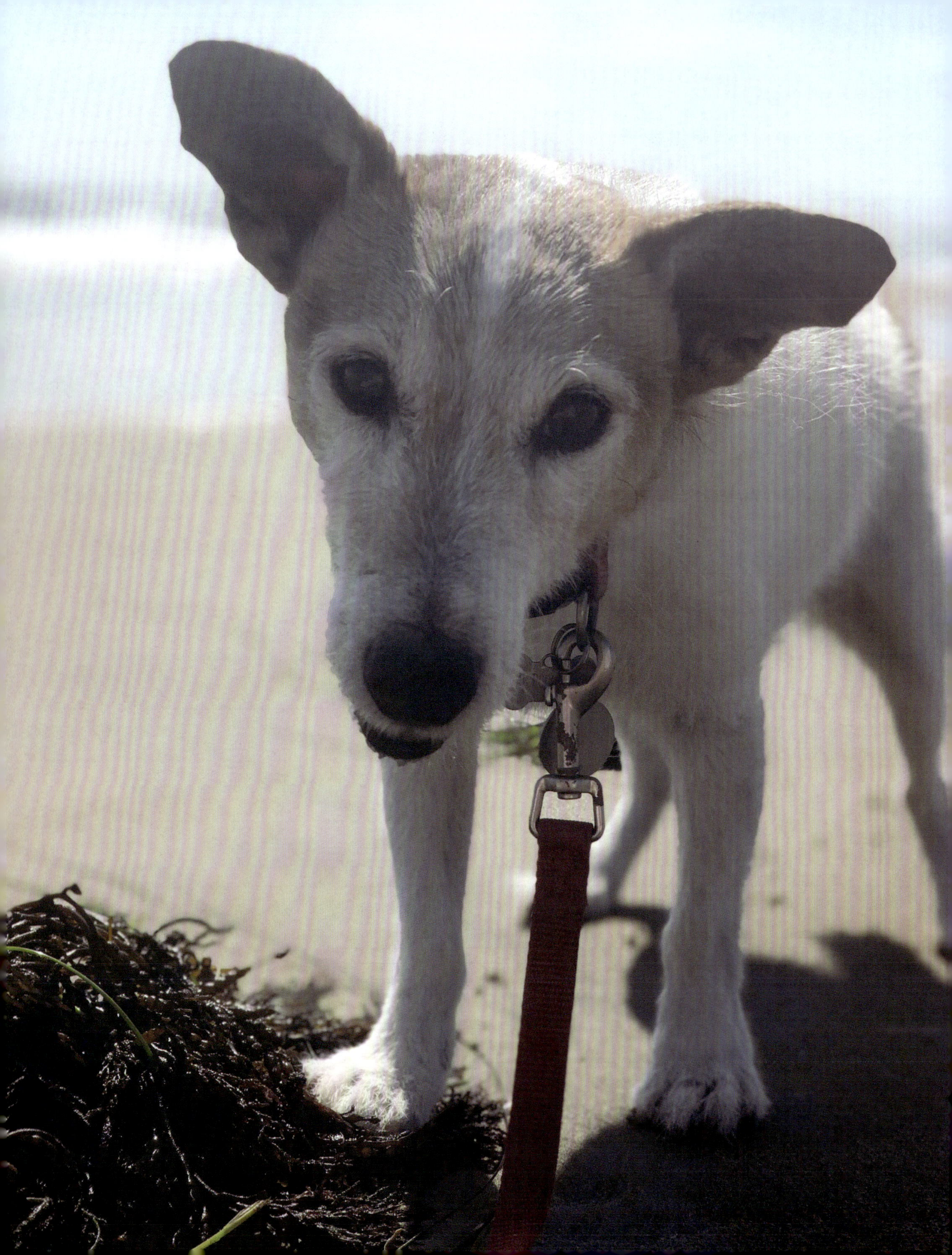

CHAPTER 12

Low Stress Handling® Algorithm and Euthanasia

12.1 Introduction

There are certain tools, restraint techniques, and strategies to only use while stabilizing an animal or in preparation for sedation. Consider other options before reaching for certain equipment, tools, or heavier restraint to get the job done. The main goals when working with animals are to provide good welfare and to reduce the risk of injury for both the handler and animal.[1] While the procedures and protocols outlined in this book should be the gold standard approach, there will be emergent situations when this may be difficult.

12.2 Low Stress Handling® Algorithm

In managing everyday cases, distinguish between the immediate wants and the long-term needs of each animal is a critical first step. Understanding and effectively managing behavior cases requires more than just medical knowledge; it involves empathetic and effective communication with caregivers. This not only ensures the well-being of the patients but also improves safety, reduces burnout, and enhances job satisfaction for the veterinary team and other animal care professionals.

Escalating Aggression in a Cat

Fluffy, a sleek black and white cat, nervously entered the examination room for his annual check-up. His wide, dilated eyes scanned the unfamiliar space, heightening his anxiety. When the crate door opened, hands quickly reached in to grab him rather than giving him a moment to acclimate, causing Fluffy to hiss with his ears flattened against his head.

He was promptly placed on the cold table, immobilized by a firm scruff. His tail lashed, and he growled, signaling his discomfort and fear. As his aggression escalated, the team opted for cat gloves and a tight towel wrap to restrain Fluffy. He swiped with extended claws as they approached, resulting in a struggle that left someone bleeding before he was securely wrapped in a towel.

Throughout the examination, Fluffy remained stiff, his ears flattened, pupils dilated, and his rapid breathing mixed with soft growls indicated his discomfort. Despite the restraint, his defensive behavior persisted, making it clear that drawing blood for his annual bloodwork was not going to be possible during this visit.

Escalating Aggression in a Dog

Blue, a cattle dog mix, entered the veterinary clinic visibly anxious, panting, pacing, and hypersalivating. Avoiding eye contact, he hid behind his caregiver when approached by the veterinary technician. After gathering a detailed history, the technician attempted to place Blue on the examination table to take his temperature, but he resisted and his distress increased. His discomfort escalated into a growl when the technician reached for his collar. Realizing the need for a different approach, a second technician entered the room, carrying a blue nylon sleeve muzzle. They made several attempts to place the muzzle but soon had to get help from Blue's caregiver. Once the muzzle was securely in place, the veterinary team decided to move Blue into a separate area, hoping he would calm down away from his caregiver.

As they moved toward the hospital's treatment area, Blue stopped every few feet to paw at his muzzle, trying desperately to remove it. In the back room, two additional team members helped hold him down. Despite his growing anxiety, they administered the necessary vaccines. The veterinarian briefly listened to his heart but was unable to conduct a full examination or perform the annual heartworm test, so Blue was returned to his caregiver. Although the team managed to restrain him in the treatment area, Blue's escalating anxiety and defensive behavior made a comprehensive physical examination and venipuncture impossible.

Creating a Plan

The cases of Fluffy and Blue are common in veterinary practice and highlight the limitations of certain tools and methods. In both instances, there is a significant risk of deteriorating behavior as protective emotions and defensive behaviors intensify.

When encountering patients like Blue and Fluffy, veterinary and animal care professionals need to approach each case with a well-thought-out plan.[2] The use of the Low Stress Handling® algorithm empowers professionals and fosters critical thinking skills, enabling them to determine the most appropriate and individualized approach for each animal in their care. This method involves a careful assessment of the animal's emotional state and the urgency of the required procedure.

Non-Urgent Procedures

For non-urgent procedures, adhering to Low Stress Handling® principles typically involves rescheduling, in addition to pre-visit medication and cooperative care training. Activities like muzzle training for dogs and carrier training for cats and small dogs are important when preparing animals for a low stress sedation process. Potentially distressing tools such as tight towel wraps, gloves, and muzzles for cats, as well as heavy restraint and forced muzzling for dogs, are not necessary to ensure safety and efficiency during the sedation process.

Urgent Procedures

In urgent cases where immediate action is required, prioritizing sedation significantly reduces the need for more forceful methods such as forced muzzling, tight towel wraps, or heavy restraint. Even in these scenarios, Low Stress Handling® techniques should be used whenever to ensuring that the process is as humane for the animal as possible.

Let us revisit the scenarios of both Fluffy and Blue, but instead of forceful techniques, Low Stress Handling® methods were used instead.

Cat

Each level includes tools and techniques from the level above, with additional considerations

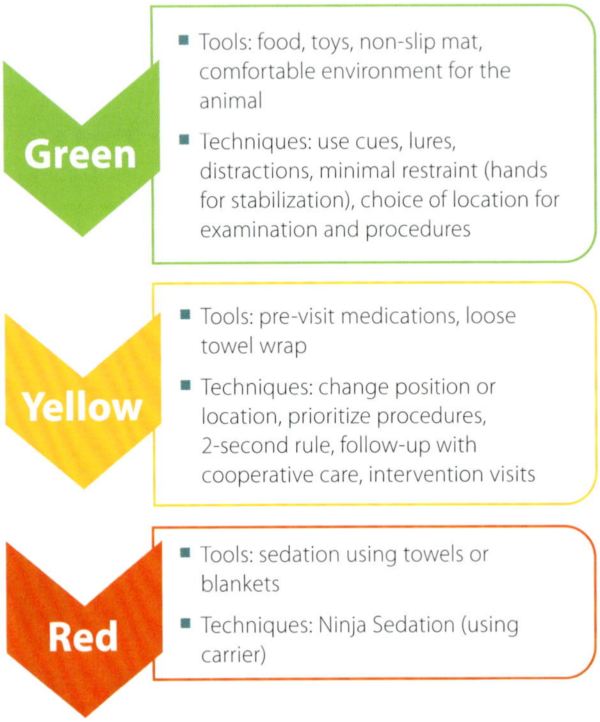

Fig. 12.2 A: Applying Low Stress Handling© principles can be challenging at times. This algorithm shows the step-by-step pathways and choices to consider when developing an individualized handling plan for cats. (Image courtesy of Desiree Broach).

Fluffy: Sedation

After adhering to the two-second rule and two attempts to restrain Fluffy, the veterinarian, Dr. Anderson, decided to stop Fluffy's appointment due to his escalating signs of stress. Prioritizing Fluffy's well-being Dr. Anderson initiated a discussion with Fluffy's caregiver, about using sedation and Low Stess Handling® methods during future visits.

Dr. Anderson: "Mrs. Tate, given Fluffy's escalating distress, prioritizing his well-being is our top priority. We recommend rescheduling his examination for later this week. At his next visit, we'll use sedation to help him relax and remain comfortable throughout the procedure. Meantime, I can prescribe pre-visit medication for you to administer at home to help relax Fluffy before his next visit. Are you familiar with Dr. Yin's Low Stress Handling® principles?"

Mrs. Tate: "I've heard of it, but I don't know the details. Why is sedation necessary?"

Dr. Anderson: "The Low Stress Handling® principles are designed to minimize fear, anxiety, and stress in animals during veterinary visits. Sedation helps him relax so that we can safely and effectively complete a thorough examination without causing distress."

Mrs. Tate: "I'm concerned about the risks associated with sedation. Can't we try without it initially and see how Fluffy responds?"

Dr. Anderson: "I appreciate your concern. From my perspective, starting with sedation early on prevents Fluffy from reaching a heightened state of anxiety or fear. Once Fluffy becomes highly stressed, it will be harder for him to relax. This could make future veterinary visits even more stressful for him. If we can provide a calm and relaxing experience from the start, then he is more likely to associate the veterinary hospital with engaging emotions instead of protective ones. Also, sedation helps us do a more comprehensive examination and get the diagnostic samples needed to evaluate Fluffy's overall health. We can than provide any treatment that he may need."

Mrs. Tate: "But are there risks associated with sedation itself?"

Dr. Anderson: "There are always risks associated with any medical procedure, including sedation. However, when administered by trained professionals following proper protocols, these risks are minimal. In this case, I believe the risk of complications from sedation is lower than the long-term impact of his protective emotions during each visit. Our goal is to create an environment where Fluffy feels safe so we can provide the best possible care."

Mrs. Tate: "I only want what's best for Fluffy. Thank you for explaining thoroughly. Okay, let's go ahead with your recommendation."

Dr. Anderson then emphasized the necessity of carrier training for Fluffy's upcoming visit and suggested leaving the carrier out with treats periodically placed inside the carrier to encourage positive associations.

Two weeks later, Fluffy was brought back for his postponed appointment by Mrs. Tate, who carried him securely in his carrier. Dr. Anderson and a team member met them in an examination room and carefully took apart the carrier, inserting a blanket between the two halves. As the team member skillfully secured Fluffy in the blanket, Dr. Anderson quickly administered a sedative injection into Fluffy's epaxial muscles. The carrier was then carefully reassembled, giving Fluffy the time for the sedation to take effect.

After Fluffy was sedated, Mrs. Tate chose to remain in the room while Dr. Anderson carried out a thorough examination, including venipuncture and cystocentesis. A reversal agent was given and Fluffy was carefully placed back in his carrier to wake up. Throughout the process, Fluffy remained peacefully unaware, and Mrs. Tate was pleased with smoothly everything went.

Dog

Each level includes tools and techniques from the level above, with additional considerations

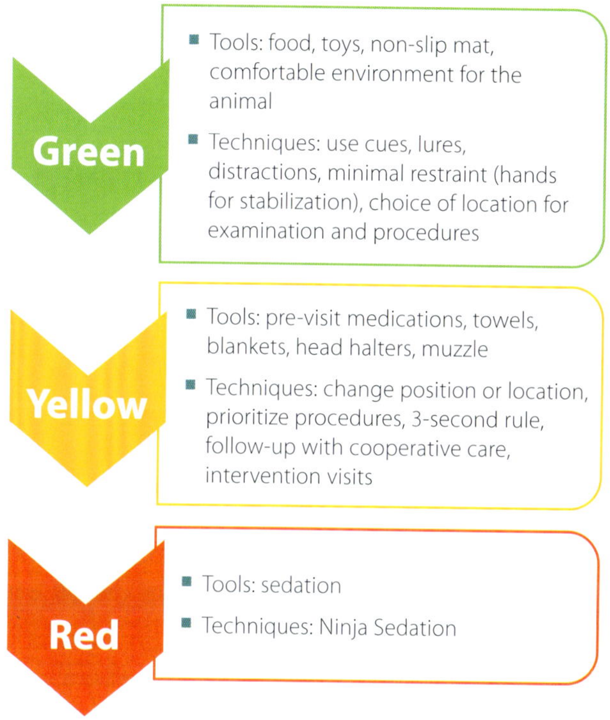

Fig. 12.2 B: This algorithm shows the step-by-step pathways and choices to consider when developing an individualized handling plan for dogs. (Image courtesy of Desiree Broach)

Blue: Sedation

In the scenario with Blue, the veterinarian stopped the procedure upon realizing a change in approach was necessary. Sedation was recommended.

In preparation, Blue was sent home with a basket muzzle and Mr. Hill was taught the 1-2-3 Game by the veterinary technician to prepare for the Ninja Sedation technique. The technician demonstrated how to properly fit the muzzle on Blue, showing Mr. Hill how to hold the muzzle in his hand and use treats to encourage Blue to willingly put his nose into it. She chose not to attempt this in the exam room to avoid stress for Blue. The goal was for Blue to have only positive experiences with the muzzle from the very beginning. Additionally, she provided Mr. Hill with resources on muzzle training and cooperative care from the CattleDog Publishing® website.

While the technician demonstrated muzzle training with Mr. Hill, the veterinarian recorded the plan in Blue's medical record and prescribed a pre-visit medication to be trialed at home and then administered on the day of Blue's sedation appointment. Once Blue was comfortable with the muzzle, the appointment would be rescheduled.

A few weeks later, Blue was brought back for his postponed appointment and, the Ninja Sedation technique was used. Mr. Hill walked Blue into the veterinary hospital, counting "1, 2, 3," giving him a treat after every "3". Engaged with each other and absorbed in the game, they moved seamlessly from the car, through the parking lot, and into the hospital waiting room. As the duo entered through the front door, the veterinarian discreetly followed, stepping out behind Blue and quickly inserting a needle with an extension set attached to a preloaded syringe into the muscles along Blue's back. Blue remained unaware of the procedure, focused solely on Mr. Hill and the anticipated treat following the count of "3."

Blue was then guided into a quiet and dimly lit examination room, equipped with a soft bed on the floor and time is given for the sedation to take effect. Once Blue is sedated, the veterinarian and a team member enter the room and perform the examination, administer vaccinations, and obtain a blood sample for an annual heartworm test. Once completed, a reversal agent is given.

Both of these scenarios demonstrate the use of Low Stress Handling strategies to minimize stress when there is a need. The individualized handling plan for both Fluffy and Blue would involve intervention visits and cooperative care training.

12.3 Emergency Use of Muzzles and Elizabethan Collars

In the practice of Low Stress Handling® methods, there is debate regarding the use of tools such as muzzles, cat gloves, and cat bags.[3,4] Some argue that these tools are sometimes necessary for safety, while others consider them outdated. If used, these tools should not substitute for pre-visit medications and sedation. Instead, emphasis should be placed on monitoring emotional states and adapting handling strategies accordingly.[3,4]

Muzzles for Dogs

Muzzles serve as an essential safety tool that all dogs should be comfortable wearing from a young age. The recommended types of muzzles are basket, cage, or vinyl muzzles. These designs allow dogs to pant, drink, eat, and even vomit, ensuring their comfort and well-being. Nylon or leather sleeve muzzles are not considered in line with Low Stress Handling® principles. These type of muzzles are more restrictive, inhibiting essential behaviors like panting, and should be avoided.

Counterconditioning to a Basket Muzzle

If a dog shows fear towards a basket muzzle, a conditioning technique using a wide-mouth container, like a yogurt container, can be useful. Start by allowing the dog to lick food from the container, which naturally encourages them to insert their nose inside while reaching for the food at the bottom. As the dog grows more accustomed to putting their nose into the container, you can gradually increase the challenge. This can be done by stepping back, which prompts the dog to move forward to continue licking and eating from the container's depths. This method progressively familiarizes the dog with the feeling of having something around their muzzle in a way that is engaging and low stress.

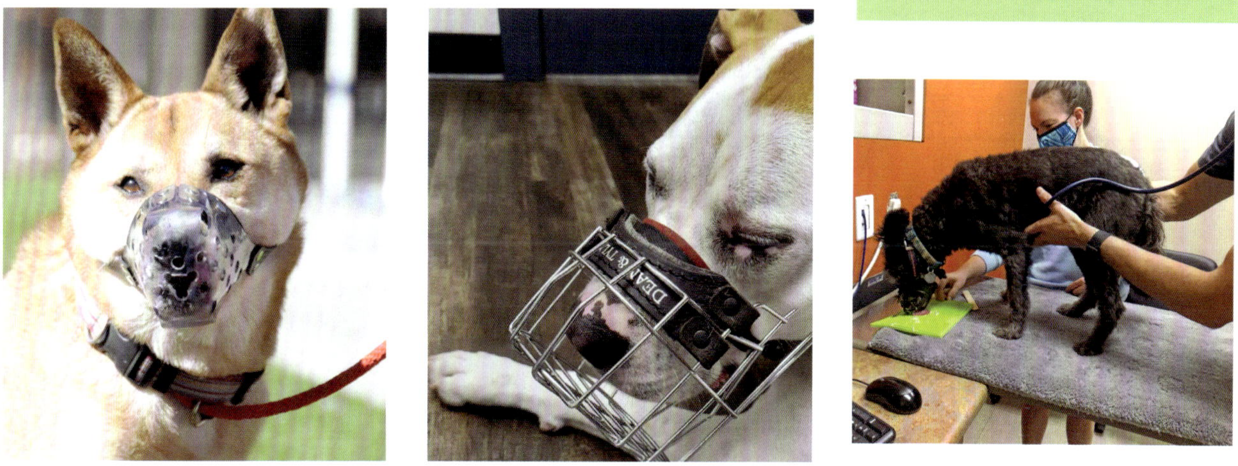

Figs. 12.3 A–C: Examples of a vinyl, wire basket, and plastic muzzle. (Photo B courtesy of Casey Paul, Photo C courtesy of Jessica Benoit)

Emergency Muzzling

In emergency situations when muzzling is necessary, entice the dog to put their nose into the muzzle with food smeared inside. As an alternative, pre-visit medication can be administered in a meatball or via an oral transmucosal (OTM) route before applying the muzzle. If the dog refuses food and muzzling is imperative, approach the dog from the side and gently scoop the muzzle onto the dog's nose from under the chin.[2] This side approach can be less intimidating and facilitates a smoother muzzling process.

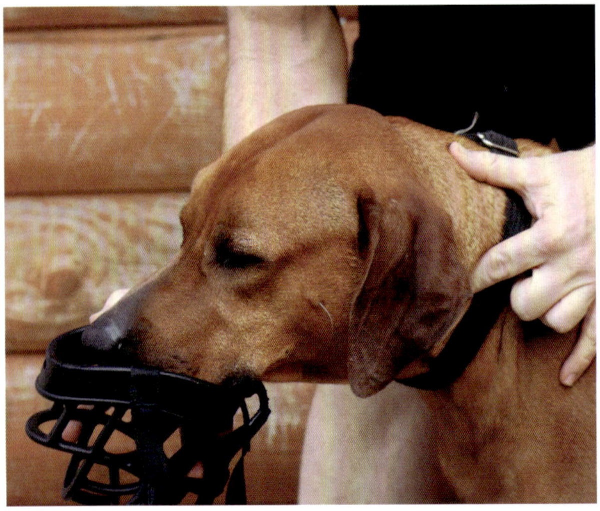

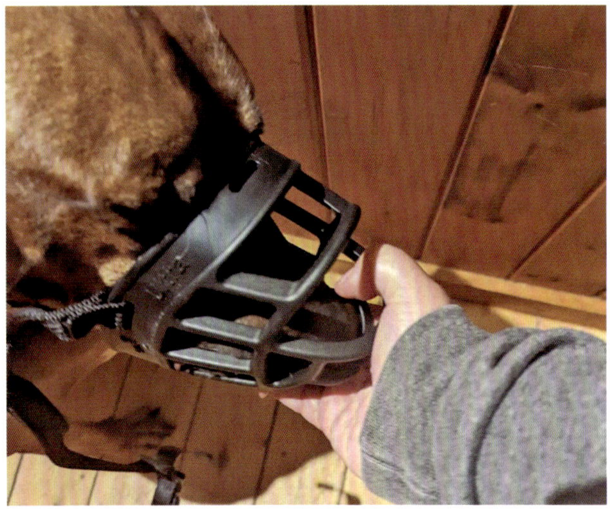

Figs. 12.3 D, E: When applying a muzzle, approach from the side, under the chin, and scoop up over the nose before clasping the straps in place. The 1–2–3 Game is a great way to build duration while wearing the muzzle.

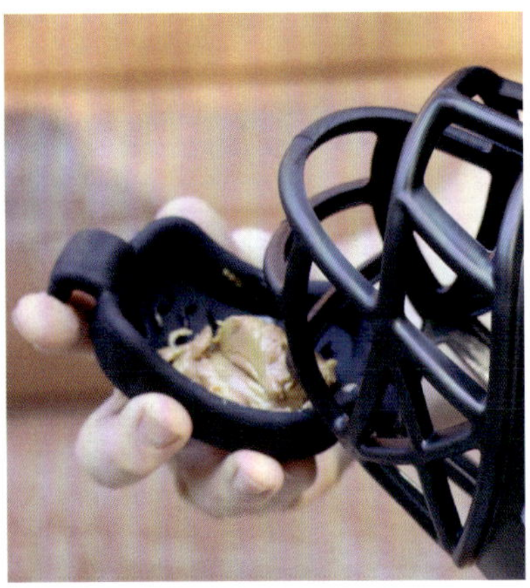

Fig. 12.3 F: Some muzzles have attachments for spreading lickable treats or frozen kibble.

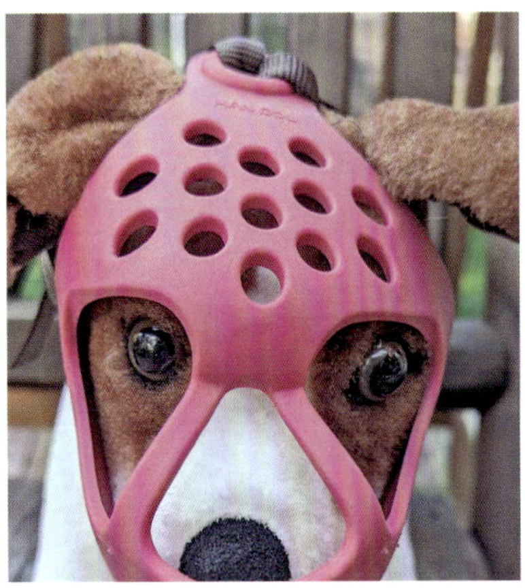

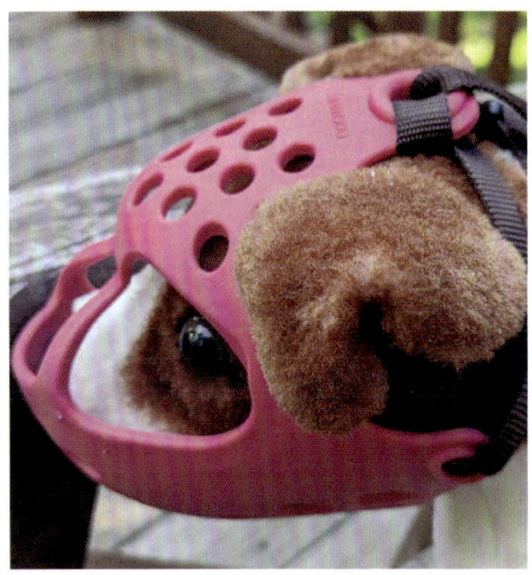

Figs. 12.3 G, H: Example of a muzzle for a brachiocephalic dog.

Nonviolent Communication Example

Nonviolent Communication (NVC), dialogue focuses on expressing feelings and needs and making requests rather than demands or judgments.[5] In this dialogue, the veterinarian (Dr. Harris) communicates with a caregiver (Sam) about the need to use a basket muzzle as part of the sedation process for a laceration repair.

Dr. Harris: "Hello Sam, I've examined your dog's laceration, and it looks like we'll need to sedate him to repair it. To do this safely, we'll need to use a basket muzzle. I understand this might be concerning, so I'd like to explain our approach."

Sam: "A muzzle? I'm worried that might scare him. He's never had to wear one before."

Dr. Harris: "I completely understand your concern, and it's our priority to make this as low stress as possible for your dog. One method we use is to encourage him to put his nose into the muzzle by using food. This can create a positive association with the muzzle for him. Have you noticed any treats or foods he particularly likes?"

Sam: "Yes, he loves peanut butter. But what if he still doesn't take to the muzzle?"

Dr. Harris: "If he's still resistant, we'll approach him gently from the side and scoop the muzzle onto his nose from under his chin. This side approach is less intimidating for dogs and helps in a smoother muzzling process. Our team is experienced in this, and we'll be as gentle as possible."

Sam: "I appreciate that, Dr. Harris. I just want to make sure he's not too stressed out by all this."

Dr. Harris: "Absolutely, Sam. We want the same. Keeping your dog calm and safe is our top priority. We'll take it step by step and keep you updated throughout the process. Do you have any other concerns or questions?"

Sam: "No, that covers it. Thank you for explaining everything and for being so considerate of his feelings."

Dr. Harris: "Of course, Sam. We're here to ensure the best care for your dog. Let's go ahead with the most comfortable approach for him."

Muzzles for Cats

According to the 2022 AAFP/ISFM Cat Friendly Veterinary Interaction Guidelines, muzzling cats is not recommended and is no longer part of Low Stress Handling®.[3,4] Instead, other alternatives should be utilized, such as a loosely wrapped, pheromone infused towel over the cat's head or body, or administering medications or sedation.[3,4] Muzzles are discouraged as they can retain pheromones from other cats, apply undue pressure on sensitive whiskers, and hinder the ability to assess a cat's facial expressions for signs of distress.[3,4,6–8] Additionally, muzzles are not bite-proof and may provide a false sense of security.

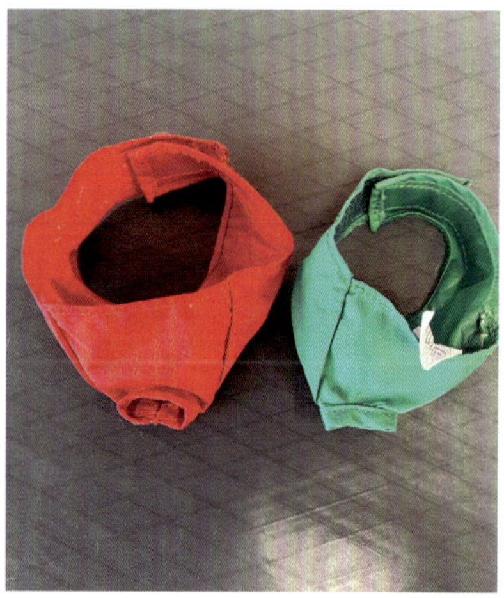

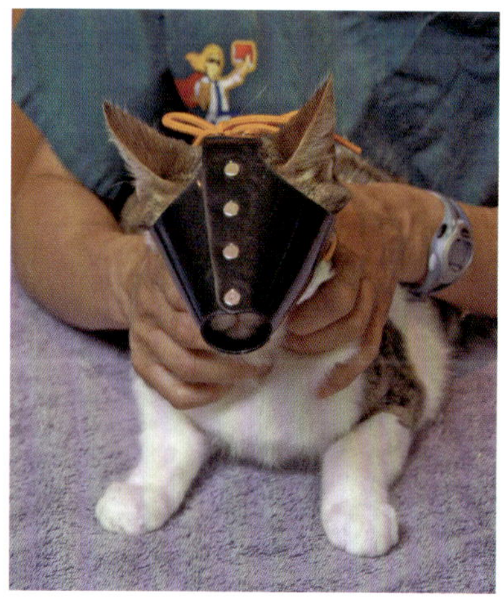

Figs. 12.3 I, J: Leather cone and nylon muzzles, which can uncomfortably press on whiskers, are not considered Low Stress Handling®. (Photo I courtesy of Eliot Veterinary Hospital)

Handling a Cat During Venipuncture

In this dialogue, the veterinarian (Dr. Lee) and a veterinary team member (Melissa) are discussing the best approach for handling a cat during venipuncture. The veterinarian is aware of the latest guidelines recommending against muzzling cats, while Melissa, the team member, initially suggests using a muzzle.

Melissa: "Dr. Lee, I think we should use a muzzle for this cat's venipuncture. It seems like the safest option to prevent any bites."

Dr. Lee: "I understand your concern for safety, Melissa. However, I recently read the 2022 AAFP/ISFM Cat Friendly Veterinary Interaction Guidelines, and they advise against muzzling cats. Muzzling isn't considered part of Low Stress Handling® anymore. It's more about understanding and addressing the cat's needs and behavior."

Melissa: "That's interesting, Dr. Lee. I wasn't aware of that. But I'm concerned about getting bitten. How do we handle the cat safely?"

Dr. Lee: "I share your concern about safety, and that's why these guidelines suggest alternatives. We could use a pheromone-infused towel to gently cover the cat's head or body, which can help calm them. Also, considering pre-visit medications or sedation might be a more effective approach. These methods reduce stress for the cat and make the process safer for us too."

Melissa: "I see your point about reducing stress for the cat. But I haven't used those methods before. How do we ensure they work effectively?"

Dr. Lee: "I can guide you through it. Let's start by gently wrapping the cat in a pheromone-infused towel. This method helps minimize their stress and movement. If we notice that the cat is still too stressed, we can then consider sedation. Our goal is to ensure the procedure is as low stress as possible for the cat, which in turn makes it safer for us."

Melissa: "Okay, I'm willing to try these methods. I guess it's all about adapting to the cat's needs and ensuring everyone's safety."

Dr. Lee: "Exactly, Melissa. It's about finding the balance between the cat's well-being and our safety. Let's work together on this, and I'm here to support you through the process."

Elizabethan Collars and Air Muzzles

Elizabethan collars and air muzzles should be reserved for urgent situations such as in brachycephalic dogs when quick intravenous access or sedation is needed. These tools are not recommended

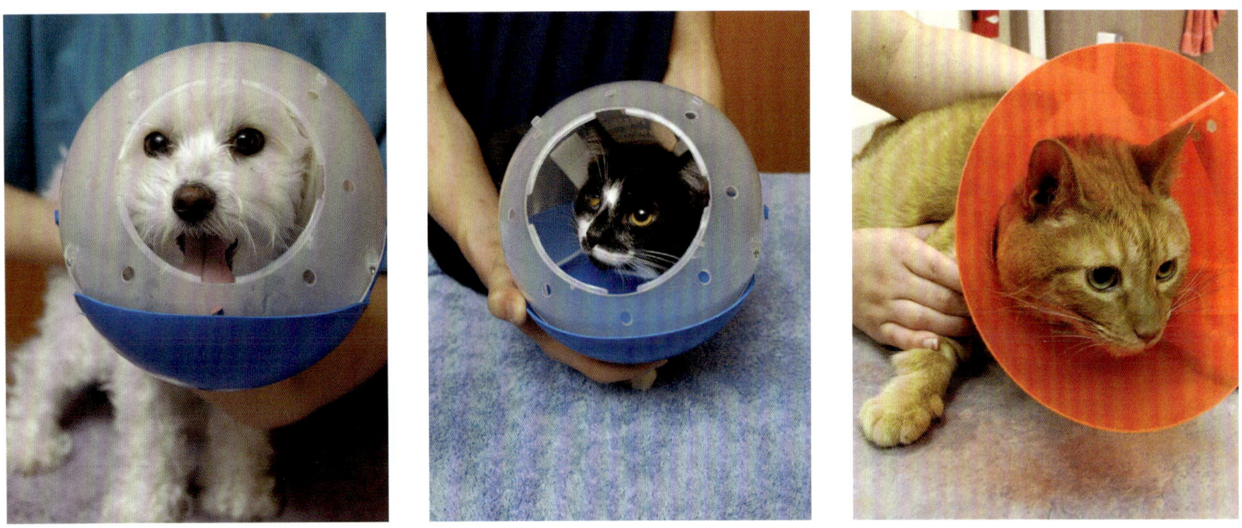

Figs. 12.3 K-M: Elizabethan collars or air muzzles should be reserved for urgent, lifesaving procedures and considered on a case-by-case basis.

for routine procedures, long-term treatments, or post-surgical care unless the animal has been previously acclimated to them through cooperative care training.[9] Air muzzles need to be used with extreme caution on cats. The weight of the muzzle puts pressure on a cat's delicate neck bones, and the contact of the whiskers with the inside of the muzzle can overstimulate their sensitive sensory system.[6–8]

Towel Scarf Wrap

A comparative study in a veterinary environment examined two methods of restraining cats: one method without using a towel and another that involved a towel scarf wrap. The research did not identify any consistent differences in overall stress levels between the two methods. However, the observation of increased tail lashing in cats restrained with the towel scarf wrap suggests that this method may be more stressful for cats.[10]

12.4 Emergency Use of Towels and Blankets

In certain situations, the use of towels and blankets can be an essential aid in handling and restraining animals. However, these items should not be used as a replacement for pre-visit medications or sedation. For increased safety, use a thicker towel or blanket to extract animals from kennels, to provide emergency restraint, or to serve as a temporary measure for dogs when an appropriate muzzle is not available.

Towel and blanket use for cats

Tight towel wraps or towel scarf wraps are no longer considered Low Stress Handling® due to their restrictive nature. Such methods can remove an animal's sense of control and choice, contributing to increased stress.[10] In emergency situations or shelter settings where medications or sedation are not readily available, the preferred alternative is to loosely-wrapped, warm blankets or towels, infused with pheromones.[11,12]

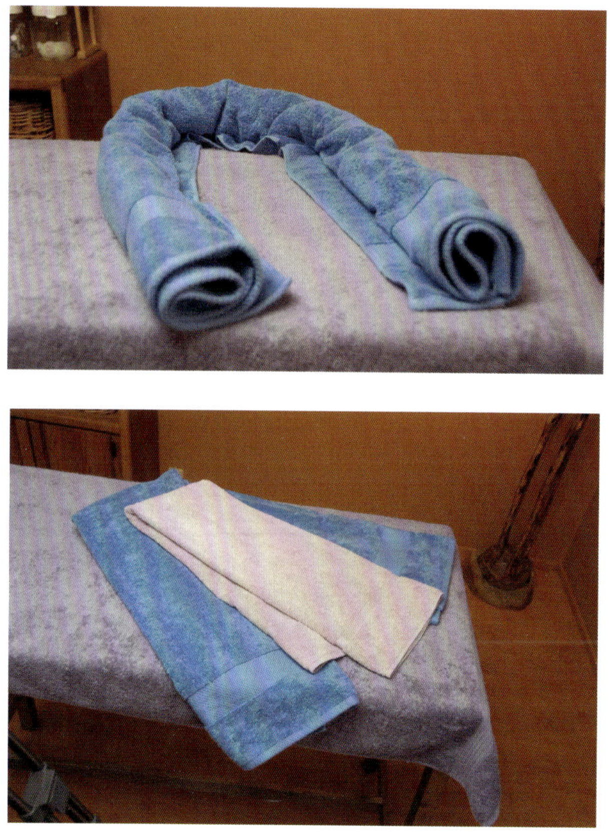

Figs. 12.4 A, B: To make a towel wrap, start with the towel rolled or folded lengthwise. Use a smaller towel for tiny dogs. The blue towel is 30 x 50 inches.

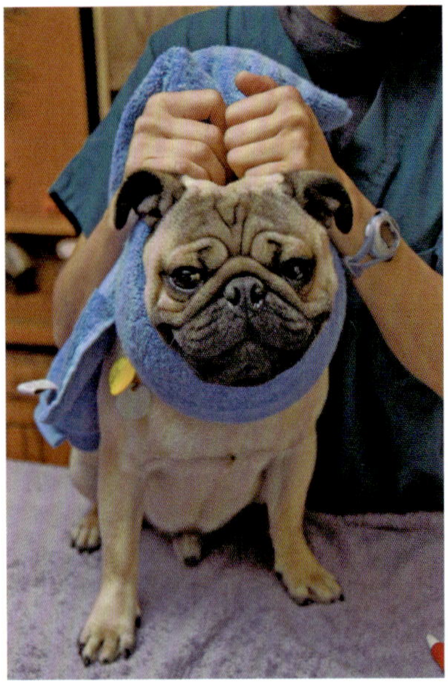

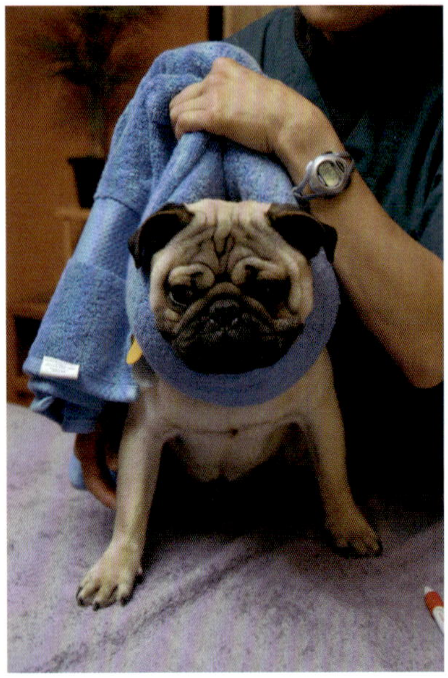

Figs. 12.4 C, D: Hold the towel at the base of the skull. Be sure to wrap it high enough so there is no space between the towel and the dog. The picture on the left shows the correct way to use a towel restraint. In the picture on the right, the towel is too loose which could be a safety hazard.

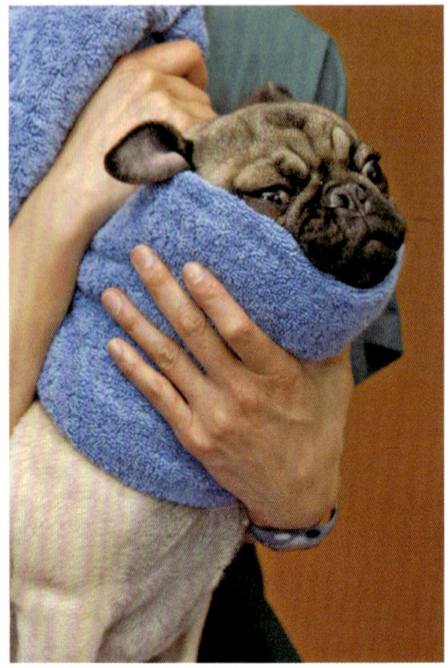

Fig. 12.4 E: For fine control of the head, use a U-hold while minimizing backward and lateral movements. Use a folded towel. Rolled towels may be too thick to allow the handler to properly feel the neck.

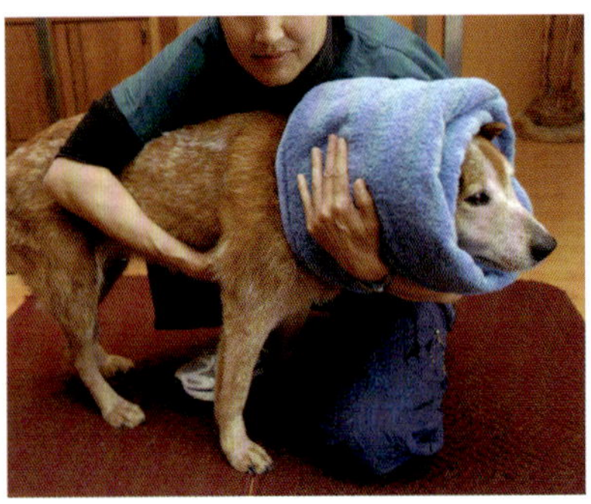

Fig. 12.4 F: A folded towel can be used to immobilize the head of some medium dogs. Some dogs will easily back out of this type of wrap. A second person behind the dog helps to minimize backward movement.

Towels and Blanket Use for Dogs

Finding suitable muzzles for brachycephalic and small dogs can be challenging. Although a custom-made muzzle is ideal, it may not be available in an emergency. In such cases, a rolled towel or blanket can be used for safe head control.[1] As with other tools, always monitor the emotional state of the animal and discontinue use if the animal becomes stressed.

Use of a Large Blanket

When managing larger dogs, particularly when only one handler is available, a large blanket can be effectively placed around the dog's head and neck for safe control. To assist in this process and to prevent the dog from backing up, position them near a door or wall. Allow the dog to choose their own position, whether lying down or standing.

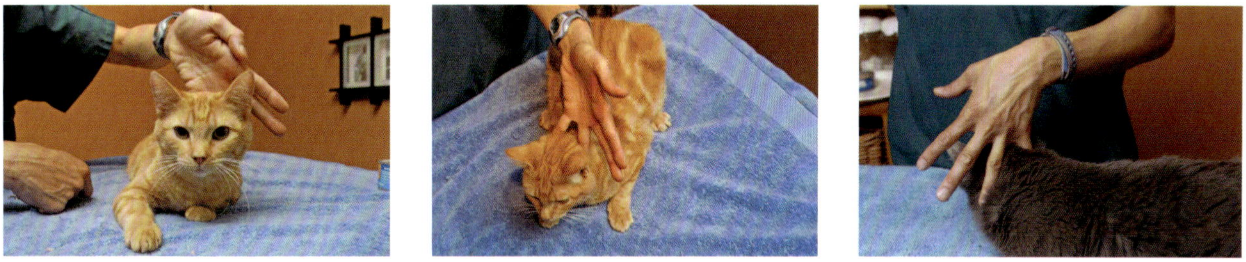

Figs. 12.5 A–C: For one-handed head restraint, place the fourth and fifth fingers behind the skull, sliding the hand down so the neck fits against the webbing between the fingers. In a relaxed cat, this technique could be used to examine the cat's eyes, ears, and mouth.

12.5 Emergency Use of Head and Body Restraint in Cats

Head restraint in cats should be reserved for urgent situations and only used for brief periods, such as looking for a towel or during sedation. Cats may find these types of holds aversive due to their restrictive nature.

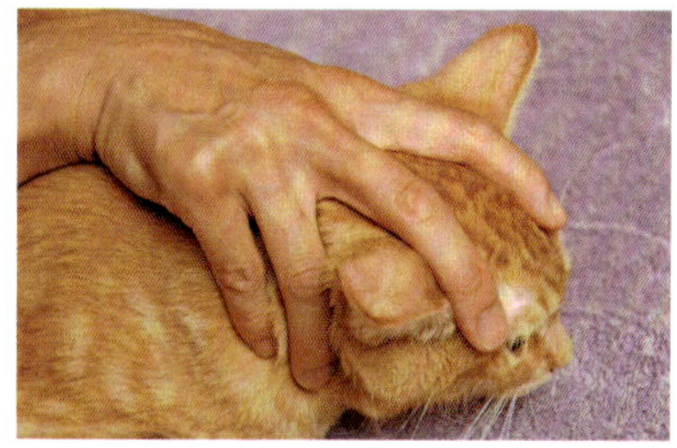

Fig. 12.5 D: An alternative is to use the outside fingers to encircle the base of the skull, with the index and middle finger gently stabilizing the head. This hold allows for head and neck massage, reducing forward movement.

Football Hold

This method is most effective with a relaxed, average-sized cat. It can be challenging for obese cats, as the handler's forearm will bear the cat's weight. When correctly executed, this hold secures the cat against the handler's body, providing gentle control over the head, front legs, and body.[1]

Initiate this hold with the cat on an elevated surface. Stand alongside the cat, wrapping one arm around their outer side, with

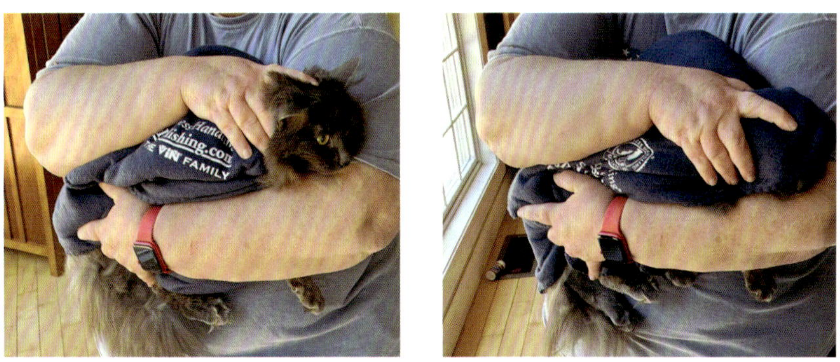

Figs. 12.5 E, F: A football hold can be stressful for some cats. A towel can be draped over the cat leaving the head exposed (E) or covering the head (F) depending on the comfort level of the cat. The football hold should not be used for painful or arthritic cats.

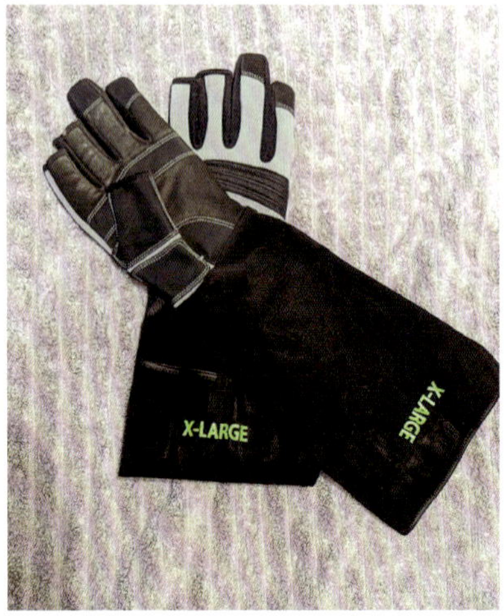

Fig. 12.6 A: Padded gloves can offer some protection against injuries from bites and scratches. However, their use is unnecessary when individualized handling plans are in place, or when pre-visit medications and sedation are appropriately used. Gloves are not recommended for routine grooming, restraining, or handling activities. They should be used only in specific situations where an animal requires sedation and when a towel or blanket alone does not provide adequate safety for handling.

the elbow near the hip and the palm along the shoulder. If the cat is restless, reconsider the approach. If the cat remains still, secure them close to your abdomen, with the other arm along the cat's spine, and the thumb and pinky over the dorsal neck and shoulder area. The middle three fingers can gently massage the head and ears.

Using Gloves for Restraint

Here is a dialogue between a veterinary team member (Alex) and a veterinarian (Dr. Smith) discussing the use of gloves for restraining cats:

Alex: "Dr. Smith, I feel concerned about using gloves for restraining cats. I've observed that gloves can sometimes escalate a cat's protective emotions and defensive behaviors. I'm worried this might not align with our commitment to Low Stress Handling®."

Dr. Smith: "I understand your concern, Alex. I feel that gloves provide a sense of safety for our team, especially when dealing with unpredictable situations. I believe they can be a necessary precaution."

Alex: "I appreciate the safety aspect, especially for our team's protection. However, I've noticed that cats often become more agitated when we use gloves. I'm worried this could be counterproductive to their emotional well-being and our safety in the long run. I'm wondering if we could explore alternatives like food distractions, or using a warm, pheromone-infused towel, which might be more in line with Low Stress Handling® principles."

Dr. Smith: "It's important to consider all options. Safety is my primary concern, but I also see the value in maintaining a low stress environment. Can you tell me more about these alternatives?"

Alex: "Certainly, Dr. Smith. For instance, we could use food distractions, familiar cues, and luring for positioning. These techniques help the cat develop engaging emotions and make them more receptive to handling. We can also practice Low Stress Handling® holds, which are designed to minimize discomfort and anxiety for the cat. Another option is to use a loosely wrapped, pheromone-infused towel, which can gently restrain the cat without causing undue stress. This approach aligns with our commitment to Low Stress Handling© and can be more effective and improve the overall welfare of our patients."

Dr. Smith: "Those sound like valid techniques, Alex. How do they compare in terms of safety and effectiveness?"

Alex: "In many cases, these methods can be just as safe, if not safer, than using gloves. They focus on reducing the cat's stress, which in turn can lower the risk of defensive behavior. This makes handling safer for us and less traumatic for the cat. Plus, pre-visit medications or sedation, when used appropriately, can greatly enhance the effectiveness and safety of these techniques, both for us and the cat."

Dr. Smith: "I see your point about the benefits of reducing stress for safety. It's important to keep both our team and the animals safe. Let's trial these methods and monitor their effectiveness. However, I would still like to keep gloves as a backup option, at least until we are confident in the alternative methods."

Alex: "That sounds reasonable, Dr. Smith. I agree that having gloves as a backup is a good idea. Meanwhile, focusing on these low stress techniques could really enhance our approach to animal care."

12.6 Emergency Use Only Tools

There are several tools available for handling and restraining animals, but not all are considered suitable under Low Stress Handling® methods.

Gloves

While gloves may seem like a practical solution for protection against bites and scratches, their use often suggests that sedation would be a more appropriate and effective approach. Gloves can unintentionally increase a cat's fear and are not effective in preventing struggles or the escalation of aggressive behavior.[3,4] In their attempts to escape, cats might target areas not covered by gloves, posing additional risks. Moreover, gloves can impair the handler's ability to make precise tactile adjustments during handling or injection procedures. Consequently, gloves are not recommended within the framework of Low Stress Handling® methods for both cats and dogs. The preferred approach should involve training dogs to become comfortable with muzzles, conditioning cats to carriers, and giving priority to sedation.

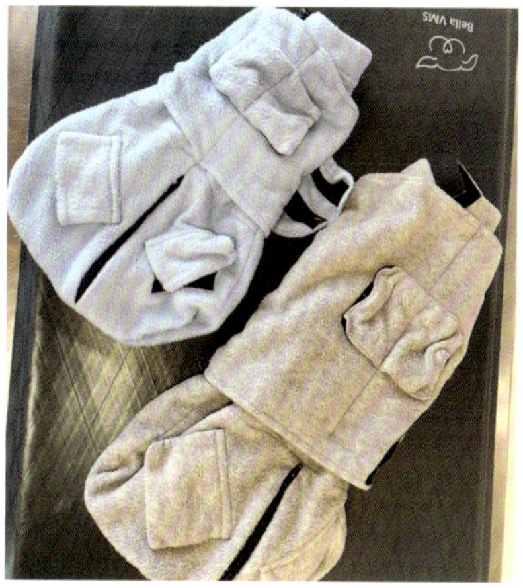

Fig. 12.6 B: Cat wraps, are not appropriate for examinations, vaccinations, venipuncture, or catheter placement. (Photo courtesy of Eliot Veterinary Hospital)

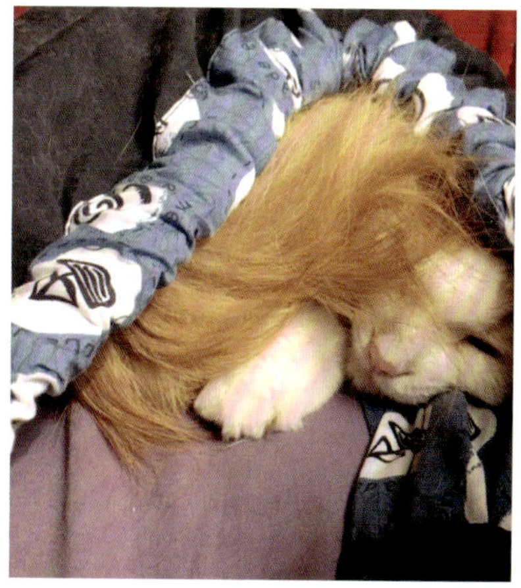

Fig. 12.6 C: This image shows a cat that freely climbs into and enjoys riding in a sling carrier.

Cat Bags, Cat Wraps, and Sling Carriers

Using a cat bag or similar device for restraining cats and some dogs can be tempting. However, unless the animal has been conditioned to these tools and enters them willingly, they should not be used. These tools

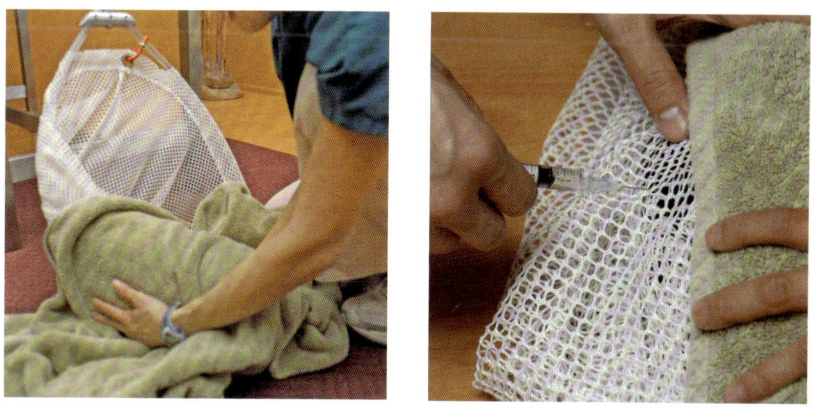

Figs. 12.6 D, E: A net should be used only in an emergency and by a skilled handler. After capture, place a towel over the cat and administer sedation through the net before transferring the cat to a secure location.

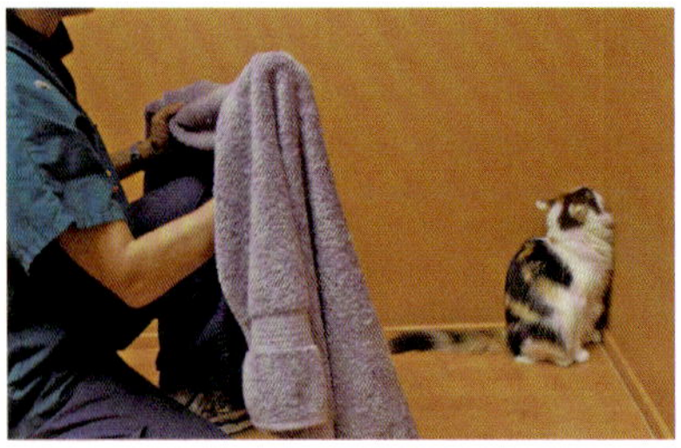

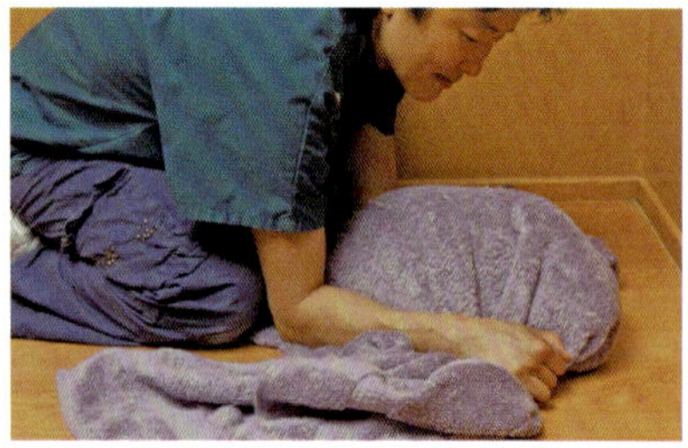

Figs. 12.6 F, G: A quick and loose blanket towel wrap is preferred for capturing escaped cats.

do not allow the animal to have choice or control over their environment.[3,4] While some animals might seem okay or relaxed, they are often emotionally shut down.

Nets

Nets are primarily for capturing escaped cats and should only be used by trained personnel.[1,12] Practicing with an inanimate object, like a ball, is advised before actual use.[1] When cats hide under objects or in tight spaces, gently coaxing them out before using a net is recommended. After capture, cover the cat with a towel and sedate before moving.[12]

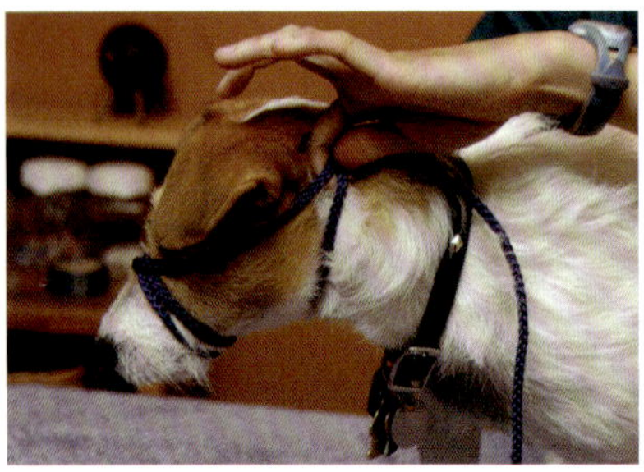

Fig. 12.7 A: A leash muzzle can cause pain and is not recognized as a Low Stress Handling® tool or technique.

Cat Nabber

The cat nabber, consisting of mesh netting attached to a metal enclosure, is sometimes used for capturing fearful or feral cats.[1,12] This device is not in line with Low Stress Handling® methods. A blanket wrap would be the preferred alternative.[3,4]

12.7 Equipment to Avoid Even in an Emergency

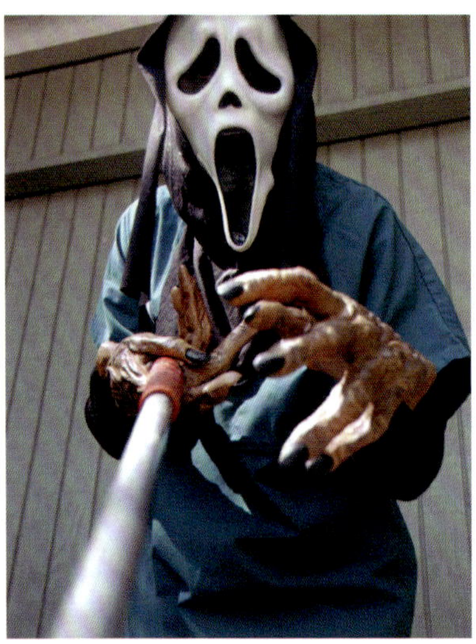

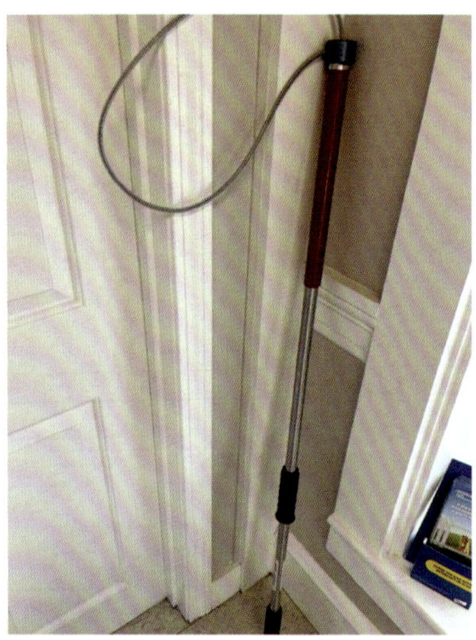

Figs. 12.7 B, C: Catch and rabies poles should be used solely for human safety when alternative handling methods are inadequate. (Photo C courtesy of Eliot Veterinary Hospital)

The following tools are not appropriate for use, even in emergencies, and should be avoided:

Leash Muzzle

Leash muzzles do not align with Low Stress Handling® methods. These can be painful, especially when used by team members who are afraid or unskilled.

A Catch or Rabies Pole

The use of a catch or rabies pole should be limited to situations where other handling techniques are insufficient to protect human safety.[12] Designed to keep a dog's head at a safe distance, these poles should not be used to lift, push, or pull a dog, and are entirely inappropriate for cats.[12] Their use can induce fear and panic and may cause serious physical harm. Only individuals with extensive experience and skill should use this device.[12]

Snappy Snare

Part pole and part slip lead, the Snappy Snare should not be used for similar reasons to catch poles.[12] The slip lead component constricts without a stopping point leading to the potential for choking.[12]

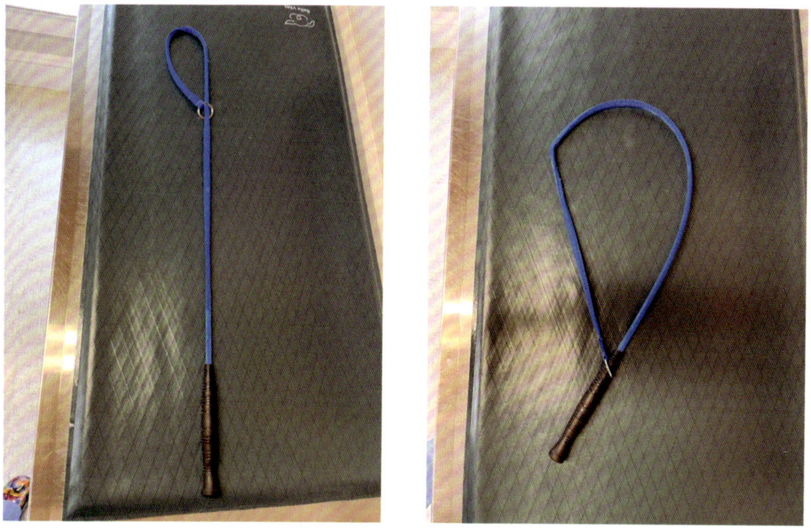

Figs. 12.7 D, E: The Snappy Snare is not a Low Stress Handling® tool and should not be used. (Photos courtesy of Eliot Veterinary Hospital)

Slip Lead for Cats

Slip leads are never appropriate for cats.[12] The risk of choking is high as the lead can tighten rapidly and be difficult to loosen. Most cats are not accustomed to neck pressure, which can lead to physical injuries and emotional trauma.

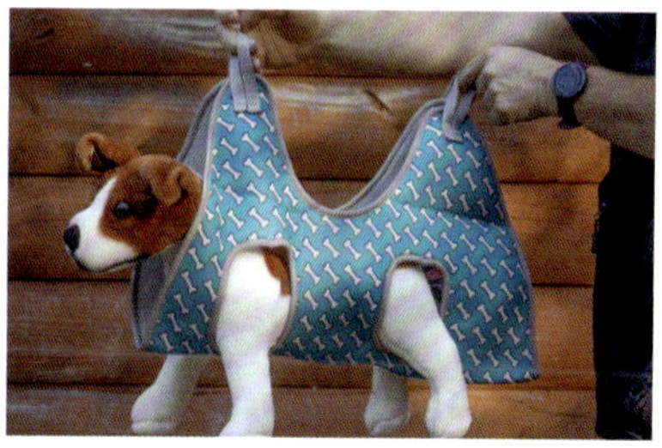

Fig. 12.7 F: Slings are never recommended to aid in nail trims or other procedures.

Hanging Slings

Both commercially available and homemade slings that suspend a dog or cat in the air are never recommended. While these tools may seem to make tasks such as nail trimming easier, they often leave dogs and cats feeling frozen and withdrawn (a state of learned helplessness), rather than cooperative. As a result, their fear, anxiety, and frustration can escalate.

Nail Trim Using a Sling vs. Cooperative Care Nail Trim

Sling Nail Trim

Rocco, a spirited French bulldog, always felt anxious about nail trimming. At the groomers, they decided to use a sling to control him better and speed up the process. However, once Rocco was secured in the sling and lifted slightly off the ground, his fear was evident. He tensed up, his eyes darted around searching for an escape, and his ears shifted slightly to the sides. With no control or way to escape, Rocco was terrified. The sling made him feel trapped, leading him to shut down emotionally and become immobilized by fear, not cooperation.

Cooperative Care Nail Trim

After learning about the benefits of cooperative care, Rocco's caregiver decided to give it a try. Rocco's introduction to this method began with mat work. Using treats relaxation was shaped from a sitting position to lying on his side.

As Rocco consistently demonstrated these relaxed postures, the desensitization and counterconditioning phase of the behavior modification began. This included gradual touches progressing to his legs, and then to handling his paws while the nail clippers were kept out of sight. As Rocco's comfort level increased, the clippers were introduced gradually, first within sight before making contact with his nails.

Transdermal Medications

Some transdermal medications, such as fluoxetine, amitriptyline, buspirone, and gabapentin, may have lower bioavailability compared to their oral counterparts.[14–19] This could result in reduced effectiveness.

At this stage, Rocco's choice to remain on the mat signaled his assent to proceed to the next step. If he lifted his head, changed position, or moved away, he communicated his dissent. Both choices were respected and reinforced, creating predictability and trust. Over time, Rocco began to associate nail trims with engaging emotions, knowing that he always had a voice in the situation.

Comparing the two methods, the differences are clear. The sling technique may have achieved the immediate goal, but overlooked Rocco's emotional well-being. The Low Stress Handling® and cooperative care approach, although more time intensive initially, laid a foundation of trust and mutual understanding. This method placed a priority on Rocco's behavioral health and overall well-being during the procedure.

12.8 Low Stress Handling® Administration of Oral Medications

Administering oral medications can be challenging, and using force may negatively impact the caregiver-animal relationship, particularly with cats. When employing a Low Stress Handling® approach, sometimes administering pre-visit medications is unavoidable.[13] If

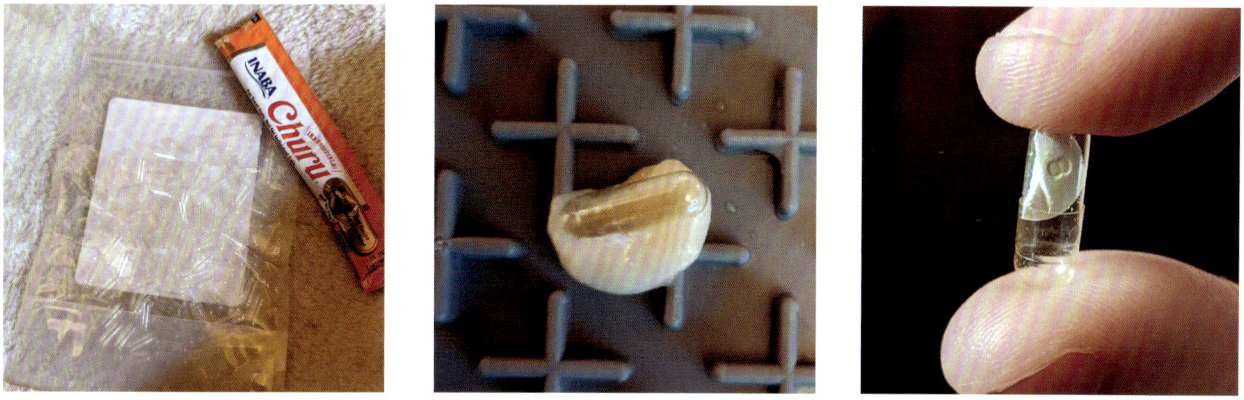

Figs. 12.8 A-C: Medications can be inserted into a commercially available gel cap for ease of administration.

an injection is not an option, alternatives such as concealing the pill in food, using a Pill Pocket™, or opting for a transdermal application may be appropriate.[13]

For pets requiring multiple medications, commercially available gel caps are useful as they allow multiple tablets to be combined into a single gel cap. For liquid medications, transfer the oral suspension into a 3-ml or 5-ml syringe and layer soft food in and around the liquid. This method encourages pets to lick the mixture from the syringe, making it more likely that they will eat it.

12.9 Emergency Restraint Techniques for Injections

Administer sedation before emotional arousal escalates for maximum efficacy, reducing the amount of medication needed and the risk of side effects. Before the sedation appointment, an individualized handling plan should be in place. Preparation includes discussing and rehearsing handling techniques with the team members and gathering all necessary supplies before the animal arrives. Such preparation not only enhances the efficiency of the process but also contributes significantly to the safety and comfort of the animal.

Medication Training

Introducing kittens to Pill Pockets™ or other methods of administering medication from an early age can make the process easier in the future. However, it is also possible to train older cats to take their medications cooperatively.

Table 12.8.1: Alternative Options for Administering Oral Medications

- Employ the three-treat technique on a mat or textured surface. Give three treats on a mat twice a day. Eventually, hide the medication in the second treat.
- Squeeze something yummy on the meds.
- Hide meds in a Pill Pocket™.
- Use cooperative care to teach dogs and cats how to take medications willingly.
- Gelatin caps can be used to combine multiple pills into one.
- Mix meds and food in a syringe.
- Give medications as a reward (marking a behavior).
- Give medications in an unexpected location (on a walk, in the yard, in their bed).
- Teach the pet to catch tossed treats.
- "Accidently" drop the medication on the floor in a yummy food disguise.

Table 12.9.1: Preparing Animals for Sedation

When preparing an animal for sedation, it is important to consider the following factors:

1. The animal's reactivity to visual stimuli, such as the presence of team members or medical equipment
2. Sensitivity to physical touch, especially during handling or examination. Signs of disorientation or pain

The Sedation Process

Before scheduling elective procedures that require sedation, dogs should first be conditioned to wear a muzzle and cats should be carrier trained.[20] In more urgent situations, a muzzle may need to be applied in-house to a dog. During the sedation process, walking dogs outside provides a useful distraction giving them time to sniff and decompress before entering the building. A different approach is needed for cats such as a loosely draped towel or thick blanket.[3,4]

12.10 Low Stress Handling® and Euthanasia

The journey towards the end of life can be incredibly challenging and emotional for both caregivers and their beloved pets. Euthanasia, while a sensitive subject, emerges as a compassionate option that offers relief from pain and emotional suffering for animals. The integration of Low Stress Handling® techniques during this delicate time guarantees that the process is conducted as gently and peacefully as possible.

Human-Animal Bond

Sharing a home with pets has countless benefits. Pets provide emotional support, and many studies have shown their positive impact on human health, reducing risks for heart disease and hypertension. Added benefits include fewer doctor visits and the alleviation of anxiety and loneliness.[21] Pets often motivate their caregivers to engage in exercise and facilitate social interactions with other people.

Guiding Caregivers Through the Decision of Euthanasia

Guiding caregivers through the emotionally difficult decision of euthanasia is a sensitive and delicate responsibility for veterinary professionals. The emotional connection between pet caregivers and their animals can be as profound as human-to-human relationships and the concept of the Human-Animal Bond (HAB) encompasses the deep connection, love, and sense of responsibility that people feel towards their pets.[21] However, given that pets generally have shorter lifespans than humans, the loss of a beloved pet can be a deeply traumatic experience.

When discussing euthanasia, effective communication skills are needed to engage in an open and honest discussion with caregivers. This includes providing a thorough explanation of all available treatment options, along with the potential benefits and limitations of each option. Through this transparent approach, veterinary professionals can help caregivers become well-informed of all options available so they can make decisions that are in the best interest of their pets.

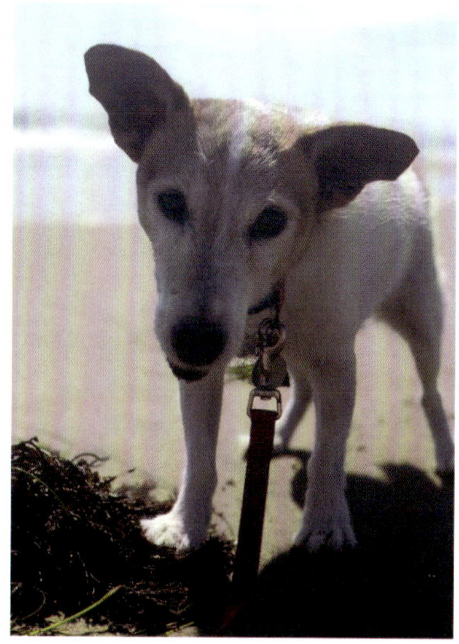

Fig. 12.10 A: The human-animal bond encompasses a deep connection, love, and sense of responsibility that people feel towards their pets, recognizing the significant ways these bonds enrich human lives. (Photo courtesy of Lauren Cole)

Proactive Discussions and Collaborative Approach

Proactively discussing a pet's quality of life during wellness visits is highly advisable, particularly for pets with chronic or terminal illnesses. Such conversations keep caregivers more informed and better prepared when faced with the difficult decision of euthanasia. When making end of life decisions, the process should be collaborative, and the concerns of everyone involved in the pet's care considered.

When effective treatments are limited or unavailable, veterinary professionals may need to provide clear and objective information to aid caregivers in the decision-making process. Veterinary professional roles can extend beyond medical advice. They are also tasked with offering emotional support and delivering detailed explanations about the euthanasia process so that it is as peaceful and comfortable as possible.

Engaged Listening and Emotional Support

Engaged listening involves fully concentrating on, understanding, responding to, and remembering what the caregiver says. This enables veterinarians to thoroughly comprehend the caregiver's concerns and emotional state while providing non-judgmental support free from the interference of personal beliefs or biases.

Cultural Sensitivity and Individual Beliefs

Different cultures and personal beliefs can significantly influence how caregivers perceive and handle the end-of-life decisions for their pets. Veterinarians should be aware of these differences and approach each case with cultural sensitivity and an understanding of individual beliefs. Demonstrate this sensitivity by asking open-ended questions, showing respect for differing viewpoints, and adapting communication styles to suit the caregiver's cultural background.

Example

Quality of Life Discussion

Dr. Carter: "Jamie, I can see how much you care for Bailey. I want you to know that I'm here to support both of you through this process. How has Bailey been doing at home recently?"

Jamie: "Dr. Carter, it's been tough. Bailey doesn't seem to have the same energy anymore. He's not eating well, and I've noticed he's in pain despite the medication. It breaks my heart to see him like this."

Dr. Carter: "It's clear you're very attentive to his needs. You've done an incredible job managing his care. Given what you've shared and his medical history, I think it's important to consider his quality of life. Has Bailey been able to enjoy any of his usual activities?"

Jamie: "Not really. He used to get so excited for walks and playtime, but now, he barely gets up to greet me when I come home. The spark in his eyes isn't there anymore."

Dr. Carter: "You've observed some significant changes, and it's natural to feel concerned about his well-being. We want Bailey to be comfortable and happy. Euthanasia is never an easy topic, but it is an option that can prevent prolonged suffering. It's a decision made from love and compassion. What are your thoughts about this?"

Jamie: "I'm struggling with the idea, but I don't want Bailey to suffer. I just don't know if it's the right time. How do I make such a decision?"

Dr. Carter: "Making this decision is one of the hardest parts of loving a pet. I can help you assess his quality of life objectively. We can look at factors like his appetite, pain levels, mobility, and overall happiness. This assessment can guide us in deciding whether it's time to say goodbye."

Jamie: "That would be helpful. I want to do what's best for Bailey, even if it's hard for me."

Dr. Carter: "Let's talk through each of these factors. Remember, the goal is to ensure Bailey's comfort and dignity. We'll consider everything you know about him, along with my professional observations, to make a compassionate decision together. How does that sound?"

Jamie: "It sounds fair. I appreciate your guidance, Dr. Carter. I just want to make sure we're not giving up too soon, but also not waiting too long."

Dr. Carter: "I understand, and that balance is important. You're not alone in this, Jamie. Let's take it one step at a time and ensure that whatever decision we make, it's with Bailey's best interest at heart."

Quality of Life Assessments

When evaluating a pet's quality of life, caregivers should closely observe their pet's physical and emotional health. Chronic pain, mobility issues, or severe physical or emotional illnesses impair the pet's quality of life.

Scales for Assessment

Caregivers are encouraged to use specialized pain scales to assess their pets' discomfort. Objectively measuring pain in animals can be difficult since they are non-verbal and the perception of pain is multifactorial and complex. Objective measurements often rely on accurately reading and interpreting body language.

Pain Scales

Several pain scales found in veterinary literature offer a variety of scoring methods that take into account both physiological and behavioral variables.[22,23] These include the Glasgow Composite Measuring Pain Scale (CMPS), University of Melbourne Pain Scale, Colorado State University Feline and Canine Acute Pain Scales, the Feline Grimace Scale, and the cat specific Botucatu University Pain Scale (UNESP-Botucatu-MCPS).[22,23]

Quality of Life

Objective tools, similar to pain scales, are available to assist in quality of life assessments.[24] One example is a scale developed by Dr. Alice Villalobos, the founder of Pawspice, a quality-of-life program for terminal pets.[25] This scale provides a thorough framework for evaluating a pet's quality of life using the HHHHHMM acronym (Hurt, Hunger, Hydration, Hygiene, Happiness, Mobility, and More Good Days than Bad). Each aspect is scored on a 0–10 scale; A total score above 35 indicates an acceptable quality of life:

1. **Hurt:** Assess pain management and oxygen needs.
   - 0: Severe pain, distress, or constant oxygen requirement.
   - 10: No pain or pain that is easily manageable without distress.
2. **Hunger:** Evaluate the pet's ability to eat and effectiveness of assisted feeding.
   - 0: Not eating; handfeeding or feeding tubes are ineffective.
   - 10: Normal eating without any assistance.
3. **Hydration:** Look at hydration levels and effectiveness of fluid management.

   - 0: Severe dehydration, unalleviated by fluids or poor tolerance.
   - 10: Well hydrated, with effective fluid management.

4. **Hygiene:** Consider the pet's cleanliness and any presence of pressure sores.
   - 0: Poor hygiene, unclean after elimination, severe pressure sores.
   - 10: Good hygiene, clean, and free of pressure sores.

5. **Happiness:** Observe the pet's interest in surroundings and signs of distress.
   - 0: No joy or interest, appears depressed or anxious.
   - 10: Expresses joy and interest, responsive to surroundings.

6. **Mobility:** Assess the pet's ability to move independently or with help.
   - 0: Unable to move, or disinterested in walks, stumbling, or severe seizures.
   - 10: Fully mobile without assistance.

7. **More good days than bad:** Consider the ratio of good days to bad days.
   - 0: More bad days, significant suffering.
   - 10: Mostly good days with minimal bad days.

Case Studies: Real Life Applications of Quality of Life Assessments

1. **Trail, the aging dog:** Trail, a 14–year-old Labrador, had been suffering from arthritis and had recently been diagnosed with bone cancer. His caregivers noted his declining interest in walks and play, decrease stamina, and obvious discomfort even with pain management. Utilizing the HH-HHHMM Scale, Trail's score was consistently below 35, indicating a diminished quality of life. This objective measurement, in addition to the veterinarian's advice, guided them towards euthanasia.

2. **Ruby's battle with chronic illness:** Ruby, a 9–year-old cat with chronic kidney disease, showed progressive weight loss and decreased activity. Her caregivers noticed her reluctance to eat and her frequent hiding over the past several weeks, which was unusual for her. After consultation and using the HHHHHMM Scale, it became clear that Ruby was experiencing more bad days than good, leading to the difficult but compassionate decision of euthanasia.

Table 12.10.1: Preparing Caregivers for Euthanasia

Preparation	Details
Procedure	Veterinarians should clearly explain the euthanasia process, including the medications used and their effects.
Providing options	Offer choices for caregivers to be present throughout the entire euthanasia process or to say good-bye beforehand, respecting individual needs.
Forms	Have caregivers complete and sign all legal forms before the procedure, including decisions about handling their pet's remains (private/group cremation, take home) and permissions for paw or nose print and/or fur clippings.
Collect payment	Collect payment in a way that avoids making caregivers wait in the reception area, such as offering to collect payment ahead of time, in the car, or in the room, allowing them to leave directly after the procedure.
Scheduling	Schedule euthanasia appointments during quieter times of the day, such as early morning or late evening.
Items from home	Encourage pet caregivers to bring special blankets, beds, toys from home, and favorite foods for the pet to enjoy before and during the procedure.

Preparing Caregivers for the Euthanasia Procedure

Caregivers often struggle with the decision to euthanize. Open communication about what to expect can alleviate some of their fears and uncertainties. Ways to help prepare the caregiver emotionally can be found in Table 12.10.1 above.

Example

Euthanasia Procedure Conversation

In a softly lit consultation room, Dr. Anderson sits with Melissa, who gently strokes Willow's fur. The atmosphere is quiet, with gentle music playing in the background.

Dr. Anderson: "Melissa, before we go any further, I want to make sure you understand what will happen today. We're here to make this as peaceful as possible for both you and your cat, Willow."

Melissa: "I want to be with her until the very end."

Dr. Anderson: "And you shall be. You can hold her throughout the process. I'm here to help you with anything you need. Before we proceed, we have some forms to take care of."

Dr. Anderson slides a form across the table to Melissa.

Dr. Anderson: "This form includes your consent for the procedure and also asks for your preferences regarding Willow's remains—whether you would like a private cremation or another option. We can also prepare a paw print and fur clippings for you to keep."

Melissa takes a moment to read through the form, her eyes moist with tears, and signs.

Dr. Anderson: "Thank you, Melissa. Now, let's take care of the payment. This way, once the procedure is completed, you can take all the time you need with Willow without worrying about anything else."

Melissa nods, and a customer service representative processes the payment in the quiet of the room.

Dr. Anderson: "Now that the formalities are out of the way, we can focus on Willow. If you have her favorite blanket or a toy, feel free to make her comfortable with them."

Melissa places a soft blanket around Willow and sets a small toy beside her.

Dr. Anderson: "Perfect. I'll apply a topical anesthetic to Willow's leg, which will numb the area before we place the butterfly catheter. It's a less stressful method, especially for cats, and allows for movement if Willow wants to adjust her position."

Dr. Anderson applies the cream and waits a moment.

Dr. Anderson: "We're ready for the sedative now. It will help Willow relax completely. This won't hurt her; it's just like falling into a deep sleep."

Melissa strokes Willow, whispering softly to her as Dr. Anderson administers the sedative. Willow's eyes gently close as she relaxes into Melissa's arms.

Dr. Anderson: "She's comfortable now. When you feel the time is right, give me a nod, and I will proceed with the final step."

After a pause, Melissa gives a small nod. Dr. Anderson administers the euthanasia medication gently and with reverence. Within moments, Willow passes peacefully.

Dr. Anderson: "She's at peace now, Melissa."

Melissa leans down, kisses Willow's head, and murmurs a heartfelt goodbye. Dr. Anderson steps out, giving Melissa the privacy to grieve.

Once Melissa has left, Dr. Anderson ensures that Willow is treated with respect and dignity, following through with the aftercare according to Melissa's wishes.

Creating a Tranquil Environment

Whether at a veterinary hospital, in a shelter or home setting, arrange the space in a way that minimizes stress for both pets and their caregivers. Keep foot traffic to a minimum, close the blinds, and lock the door to reduce exposure to potential stressors like unfamiliar people, other animals, or loud equipment. Dimmed lights can bc soothing, benefiting both the pet and the caregiver, especially if they are grieving. Pheromone diffusers and sprays can have a calming effect along with species-specific music.

Location of Euthanasia Procedure

Choosing the right location for euthanasia can significantly impact the experience for both the animal and caregiver. Table 12.10.2 below lists some of the pros and cons for each location.

Table 12.10.2: Pros and Cons of Euthanasia Locations

Location	Pros	Cons
Home	Familiar environment, privacy, reduced stress from not traveling	Emotional attachment to location, challenges in performing the procedure, more complex disposal of remains
Hospital	Immediate access to tools and medications, trained staff on hand	Can feel sterile, potential for long wait times, exposure to other pets and caregivers
Outside	Opportunity for natural setting, ample space, calming environment	Lack of control over environment, potential weather-related delays, provision of seating for caregivers necessary
Car	Some feel more secure and safe in the car. It is familiar	Challenging location to administer injections
In a lap or comfortable space	Personal touch, comfort for the animal	Challenging location to administer injections

Preparing the Room

When setting up a room for euthanasia, all necessary items should be within reach. This includes stocking the room with medications, syringes, and needles. Comfort should be a priority for both indoor and outdoor procedures. If euthanasia is to be performed on a caregiver's lap, place a non-absorbent sheet between two layers of blankets, beds, or towels to manage any spills effectively. Paper towels need to be readily available for quick cleanup. Remove all waste and the trash can to reduce odors. For outdoor procedures, bring all necessary equipment, paper towels, and trash bags to the site.

Soft music and lighting help create a soothing atmosphere. In the reception area, lighting an unscented candle and placing signs on doors serve as gentle reminders for others to keep their voices low and minimize noise. Barking, noisy dogs, or families with loud children should be placed in a distant examination room to minimize noise and stress. If the procedure includes placing an intravenous catheter, try to do this in the room if possible. For some pets, a butterfly catheter may be less stressful due to its flexibility. Apply topical anesthetic cream at least 10 minutes before catheter placement to minimize the pet's discomfort during the procedure.

Personal Effects

Collars, leashes, wheelchairs, or other mobility aids should not be removed from the animal until after the procedure has been completed. Since these items are integral parts of their daily routine, their removal can be distressing for the animal and may signal a cause for concern.

Euthanasia Procedure

Explain to the caregiver each step of the process including potential complications such as involuntary movements, vocalizations, or apnea. Pre-visit medications and sedation can help reduce fear and anxiety before arrival and throughout the process.

Some caregivers request other animals or children be present during the euthanasia. While the presence of a household companion animal may provide comfort to some pets, it could cause distress in others. The decision to have other animals present should be made with careful consideration of each pet's individual preferences and history. With children, some may want to say goodbye; however, their emotional response may be overwhelming to the pet. Parents should prepare and support their children throughout the process.

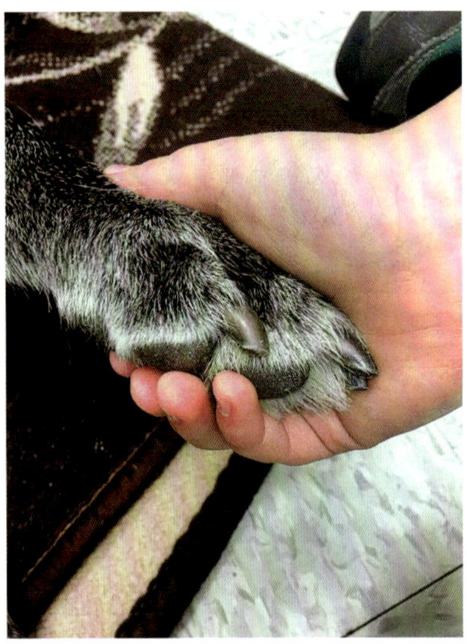

Figure 12.10 B: Handling euthanasia with care and respect acknowledges the importance of the human-animal bond. (Photo courtesy of Amelia/stock.adobe.com)

Positioning

Lure or use familiar cues to guide the animal rather than forcing them into position. Allow them to find and maintain a position that is most comfortable before administering the euthanasia solution. Avoid placing a tarp or stretcher under the animal until after the procedure is complete. For the injection, use the limb that is furthest from the caregiver and confirm the animal is fully sedated before administering the euthanasia solution.

After the Euthanasia Procedure

Handle the post-euthanasia procedures with care and respect. Remove the deceased animal discreetly and wait until the caregiver has left the area before the transfer process. This helps maintain privacy and allows the caregiver to depart without seeing their beloved pet being moved. Close all blinds and doors in the area to maintain privacy during the transfer to show respect for both the animal and the grieving caregiver.

Euthanasia in the Shelter

Euthanasia in the shelter should follow the same guidelines as pets. All animals should receive pre-euthanasia medications to minimize fear, anxiety, stress, and discomfort. Conduct the procedure in a location where the animal feels most at ease, which may include areas outside the shelter building. Never euthanize in the presence of other animals or near areas designated for disposal, such as the freezer.

Tools such as rabies or catch poles, slip leads, catch nets, and cat gloves should be avoided. Similarly, syringe poles, which can cause muscle trauma and pain, should not be used. Instead, light towel wraps, carriers, and Low Stress Handling® methods should be employed. The Ninja Sedation technique is more humane and effective. If needed, a basket muzzle is preferable to a sleeve muzzle for dogs. Cats should not be muzzled.

Medications

Pre-visit medications should be given prior to all scheduled euthanasias. Medication choices are similar to those given prior to veterinary visits. For some animals, high dosages of trazodone combined with gabapentin may be sufficient. In other cases, oral administration of different medications may be necessary. Options include phenobarbital, powdered tiletamine/zolazepam (Telazol©) mixed in a meatball, or transmucosal forms of acepromazine or dexmedetomidine.

When administering oral medications, incorporating them into the animal's favorite foods or creating medication-laden meatballs can be an effective approach. These can be used as rewards for responding to cues, making the process less stressful for the animal. Engaging the animal in activities like playing "go find it" or using Pattern Games are less confrontational methods to administer oral medications.

Intramuscular or intravenous injection of a combination like dexmedetomidine, ketamine, and butorphanol (DTK) might be needed to safely administer the euthanasia solution. In these situations, employing distractions and the Ninja Sedation techniques can be particularly beneficial.

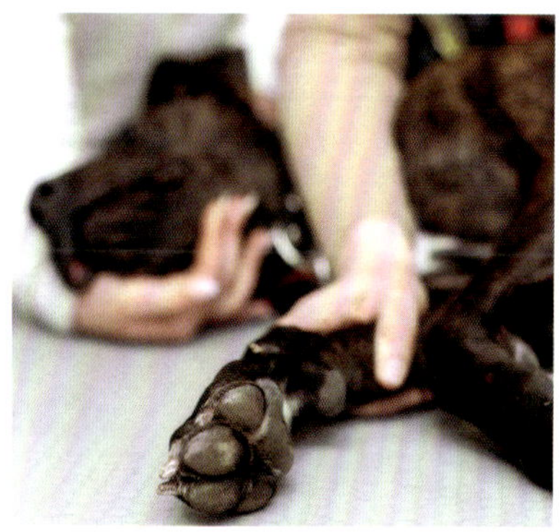

Fig. 12.10 C: Caregivers facing the loss of a pet often benefit from resources to help them manage their grief. (Photo courtesy of Ekaterina Eukota/stock.adobe.com)

Behavioral Euthanasia

Euthanizing due to behavioral concerns is an exceptionally difficult decision for everyone involved. In such cases, the quality of life of the animal and the safety of those around them are often the primary concerns. Making hasty decisions should be avoided and underlying medical causes identified and treated. Referral to a board-certified veterinary behaviorist (DACVB) can provide valuable insights and possible alternatives to euthanasia.

Many animals suffering from mental illnesses may appear physically healthy. Approach these cases without judgment and empathy for the caregiver.

Resources

Caregivers who are facing the loss of a pet, whether due to medical or behavioral reasons, often benefit from accessing resources that can help them understand and manage their grief. Local and online support groups are beneficial in this regard. These groups offer a platform for caregivers to share their experiences and emotions, make informed and objective decisions about their pet's quality of life, and find comfort and understanding among others who have faced similar situations.

There are several resources available to assist in this process. For instance, the Argus Institute at Colorado State University offers pet loss support, which can be accessed at ***https://vetmedbiosci.colostate.edu/argus/pet-loss-support/***. Another valuable resource is the University of Tennessee's Veterinary Social Work program, which addresses grief and bereavement and can be found at ***http://vetsocialwork.utk.edu/grief-and-bereavement/***.

For those dealing specifically with behavioral euthanasia, specialized resources, such as Losing Lulu (www.losinglulu.com), a website dedicated to assisting caregivers through the grieving process after a behavioral euthanasia. This site and similar resources provide individualized support, understanding, and guidance to help caregivers navigate the complex emotions associated with this type of loss.

12.11 Conclusion

The Low Stress Handling® Algorithm offers a variety of humane and effective alternatives that should be utilized before resorting to tools such as muzzles, padded gloves, or cat bags. The focus should be on the animal's well-being and safety even when medication and sedation options are limited.

Prioritizing the well-being of the animals during the euthanasia process contributes to their comfort and leads to a safer and more efficient handling experience. By choosing methods that reduce stress and fear, the process can be as respectful as possible while providing a higher level of care.

12.12 References

1. Yin, S. A. (2009). *Low Stress Handling, Restraint, and Behavior Modification of Dogs and Cats.* CattleDog Publishing.

2. Herron, M. E., & Shreyer, T. (2014). The pet-friendly veterinary practice: a guide for practitioners. *Veterinary Clinics: Small Animal Practice*, 44(3), 451–481.

3. Rodan, I., Dowgray, N., Carney, H. C., Carozza, E., Ellis, S. L. H., Heath, S., Niel, L., St Denis, K., & Taylor, S. (2022). AAFP/ISFM Cat friendly veterinary interaction guidelines: Approach and handling techniques. *Journal of Feline Medicine and Surgery*, 24(11), 1093–1132.

4. Taylor, S., St Denis, K., Collins, S., Dowgray, N., Ellis, S. L. H., Heath, S., Rodan, I., & Ryan, L. (2022). ISFM/AAFP Cat friendly veterinary environment guidelines. *Journal of Feline Medicine and Surgery*, 24(11), 1133–1163.

5. Rosenberg, M. B., & Chopra, D. (2015). *Nonviolent Communication: A Language of Life: Live Changing Tools for Healthy Relationships.* PuddleDancer Press.

6. Adibi, & Lampl, I. (2021). Sensory adaptation in the whisker-mediated tactile system: Physiology, theory, and function. *Frontiers in Neuroscience*, 15, 770011–770011. https://doi.org/10.3389/fnins.2021.770011

7. Ikeda, R., & Gu, J. G. (2016). Electrophysiological property and chemical sensitivity of primary afferent neurons that innervate rat whisker hair follicles. *Molecular Pain*, 12, 1744806916685570.

8. Zhu, & Connors, B. W. (1999). Intrinsic firing patterns and whisker-evoked synaptic response of neurons in the rat barrel cortex. *Journal of Neurophysiology*, 81(3), 1171–1183. https://doi.org/10.1152/jn.1999.81.3.1171

9. Shenoda, Y., Ward, M. P., McKeegan, D., & Fawcett, A. (2020). The cone of shame: Welfare implications of Elizabethan collar use in dogs and cats as reported by their owners. *Animals,* 10(2), 333.

10. Decock, L. J. G., Menuge, F., Cozzi, A., Teruel, E., Codecasa, E., Monneret, P., De Keuster, T., & Moons, C. P. H. (2023, June). Reducing feline stress in the veterinary practice: investigating the evidence. Paper presented at the *4th Annual Meeting of the European Veterinary Congress of Behavioral Medicine and Animal Welfare*, Palma de Mallorca, Spain.

11. Arrandale, L., & Buckley, L. (2017). Towels versus hides: which are best at reducing acute stress in the newly hospitalised domestic cat (Felis sylvestris catus)? *Veterinary Nursing Journal*, 32(10), 285–288. https://doi.org/10.1080/17415349.2017.1343536

12. The Association of Shelter Veterinarians. (2022). The guidelines for standards of care in animal shelters: Second edition. *Journal of Shelter Medicine and Community Animal Health*, 1(2), 1–76. https://doi.org/10.56771/ASVguidelines.2022

13. Taylor, S., Caney, S., Bessant, C., & Gunn-Moore, D. (2022). Online survey of owners' experiences of medicating their cats at home. *Journal of Feline Medicine and Surgery*, 24(12), 1283–1293.

14. Adrian, D., Papich, M. G., Baynes, R., Stafford, E., & Lascelles, B. D. X. (2018). The pharmacokinetics of gabapentin in cats. *Journal of Veterinary Internal Medicine*, 32(6), 1996–2002.

15. Ciribassi, J., Luescher, A., Pasloske, K. S., Robertson-Plouch, C., Zimmerman, A., & Kaloostian-Whittymore, L. (2003). Comparative bioavailability of fluoxetine after transdermal and oral administration to healthy cats. *American Journal of Veterinary Research*, 64(8), 994–998.

16. Denenberg, S., & Dubé, M. B. (2018). Tools for managing feline problem behaviours: Psychoactive medications. *Journal of Feline Medicine and Surgery*, 20(11), 1034–1045.

17. Eichstadt, L. R., Corriveau, L. A., Moore, G. E., Knipp, G. T., Cooper, B. R., & Gwin, W. E. (2017). Absorption of transdermal fluoxetine compounded in a lipoderm base compared to oral fluoxetine in client-owned cats. *Int J Pharm Compd*, 21, 242–246.

18. Mealey, K. L., Peck, K. E., Bennett, B. S., Sellon, R. K., Swinney, G. R., Melzer, K., Gokhale, S. A. & Krone, T. M. (2004). Systemic absorption of amitriptyline and buspirone after oral and transdermal administration to healthy cats. *Journal of Veterinary Internal Medicine*, 18(1), 43–46.

19. Slovak, J. E., & Costa, A. P. (2021). A pilot study of transdermal gabapentin in cats. *Journal of Veterinary Internal Medicine*, 35(4), 1981–1987.

20. Pratsch, L., Mohr, N., Palme, R., Rost, J., Troxler, J., & Arhant, C. (2018). Carrier training cats reduces stress on transport to a veterinary practice. *Applied Animal Behaviour Science*, 206, 64–74.

21. Whipple, E. E. (2021). The human-animal bond and grief and loss: Implications for social work practice. *Families in Society*, 102(4), 518–528.

22. Evangelista, M. C., Steagall, P. V. Agreement and reliability of the Feline Grimace Scale among cat owners, veterinarians, veterinary students and nurses. *Sci Rep* 11, 5262 (2021). https://doi.org/10.1038/s41598–021–84696–7

23. Hernandez-Avalos, I., Mota-Rojas, D., Mora-Medina, P., Martínez-Burnes, J., Casas Alvarado, A., Verduzco-Mendoza, A., Lezama-García, K., & Olmos-Hernandez, A. (2019). Review of different methods used for clinical recognition and assessment of pain in dogs and cats. *International Journal of Veterinary Science and Medicine,* 7(1), 43–54. https://doi.org/10.1080/23144599.2019.1680044

24. Fulmer, A. E., Laven, L. J., & Hill, K. E. (2022). Quality of life measurement in dogs and cats: A scoping preview of generic tools. *Animals : an open access journal from MDPI*, 12(3), 400. https://doi.org/10.3390/ani12030400

25. Villalobos, A. E. (2011). Quality-of-life assessment techniques for veterinarians. *Veterinary Clinics: Small Animal Practice*, 41(3), 519–529.

Author
Christine Calder DVM, DACVB

Medications for Veterinary Visits

At-Home Medications

Drug	Dosage
Acepromazine	0.5–2 mg/kg PO DOG or CAT
Alprazolam	0.02–0.1 mg/kg PO DOG; 0.0125–0.25 mg/kg PO CAT
Clonidine **(DOGS ONLY)**	0.01–0.05 mg/kg PO 90 minutes prior to departure
Dexmedetomidine OTM (Sileo®) **(DOGS ONLY)**	USE LABELED DOSE
Diazepam **(DOGS ONLY)**	0.5–2 mg/kg PO
Gabapentin	10–50 mg/kg PO DOG; 50–100 mg PO **PER CAT** **reduce dosage by 50–75% for cats with kidney disease and increased frailty scores**
Lorazepam	0.02–0.1 mg/kg PO DOG; 0.125–0.25 mg PO **PER CAT**
Maropitant (Cerenia®)	8 mg/kg PO DOG; 1 mg/kg PO CAT for motion sickness
Pregabalin	5 mg/kg PO DOG or CAT
Melatonin **(DOGS ONLY)**	1–4 mg PO **PER DOG**
Trazodone	2–12 mg/kg PO DOG; 25–50 mg PO **PER CAT**

In-Clinic Sedation

Drug	Dosage	Duration/Comments
Acepromazine	0.01–0.1 mg/kg IV, IM, SC DOG or CAT	6–8 hours
Acepromazine OTM	0.025–0.05 mg/kg DOGS or CATS	
Alfaxalone	1–2 mg/kg IV or 2.5 mg/kg IM SMALL DOG; 0.5–5 mg/kg IV, IM CAT	15–20 minutes
Buprenorphine	0.01–0.02 mg/kg IM, IV, SC, OTM DOG or CAT	
Butorphanol	0.2–0.4 mg/kg IM, IV, SC DOG or CAT	30–90 minutes
Dexmedetomidine	2–40 mcg/kg (0.002–0.04 mg/kg) IM, IV DOG or CAT	30–90 minutes
Dexmedetomidine OTM	DOGS: 40 µg/kg CATS: lower dosages 5–10 µg/kg may be all that is needed especially, when combined with alfaxalone	
Diazepam	0.1–0.5 mg/kg IV DOG or CAT	Diazepam is not ideal to use as a sole agent in cats; midazolam may be a safer choice.
Hydromorphone	0.05–0.1 mg/kg IV, IM, SC DOG or CAT	every 2–4 hours
Ketamine	2.5–10 mg/kg IV, IM DOG or CAT	30–60 minutes
Ketamine OTM	5–10 mg/kg (DOG or CAT)	Tastes bitter; hide in salty food like squeeze cheese or feed separately after the dexmedetomidine/butorphanol is given
Methadone	0.1–0.5 mg/kg IM or IV (DOG or CAT)	4–8 hours
Midazolam	0.1–0.4 mg/kg IM, IV, SC DOG or CAT	
Tiletamine-Zolazepam	2–15 mg/kg IV, IM DOG or CAT	Higher dosages IM only.
Tiletamine-Zolazepam OTM	Light to moderate sedation: 5–7.5 mg/kg (DOG or CAT)	

Combinations

Desired Effect	Drug Options	Healthy Dog	Healthy Cat	Compromised or Sick Dog	Compromised or Sick Cat
Oral Pre-visit medication	Gabapentin	20–40 mg/kg PO 2–3 hours before visit	50–150 PO mg **PER CAT** 2–3 hours before		Reduce dose by 50% if renal disease is present.
	Trazodone	3–8 mg/kg PO 2–3 hours before visit			
	Alpha 2 agonist	Sileo® label dose			
Light sedation	Opioid	Butorphanol 0.2–0.4 mg/kg IV/IM	Butorphanol 0.2–0.4 mg/kg IV/IM	Butorphanol 0.2–0.4 mg/kg IV/IM	Butorphanol 0.2–0.4 mg/kg IV/IM
	Benzodiazepine	Midazolam 0.2 mg/kg IV/IM	Midazolam 0.2 mg/kg IV/IM	Midazolam 0.2 mg/kg IV/IM	Midazolam 0.2 mg/kg IV/IM
Moderate Sedation	Opioid	Butorphanol 0.4 mg/kg IM	Buprenorphine 0.02 mg/kg OTM	Butorphanol 0.4 mg/kg IM	Buprenorphine 0.02 mg/kg OTM
	Tranquilizer	Acepromazine 0.01–0.03 mg/kg IM Maximum 2–3 mg total dose	Acepromazine 0.025–0.1 mg/kg IM Maximum 1 mg total dose		
	Benzodiazepine	Midazolam 0.2 mg/kg IV/IM	Midazolam 0.2 mg/kg IV/IM	Midazolam 0.2 mg/kg IV/IM	Midazolam 0.2 mg/kg IV/IM
	Alpha 2 agonist	Dexmedetomidine 3–7 µg/kg IM	Dexmedetomidine 3–10 µg/kg OTM		
Heavy Sedation	Opioid	Butorphanol 0.2–0.4 mg/kg IM	Butorphanol 0.2–0.4 mg/kg IM	Butorphanol 0.2–0.4 mg/kg IM	Butorphanol 0.2–0.4 mg/kg IM
	Benzodiazepine		Midazolam 0.2 mg/kg IV/IM	Midazolam 0.2 mg/kg IV/IM	Midazolam 0.2 mg/kg IV/IM
	Alpha 2 agonist	Dexmedetomidine 7–15 µg/kg IM	Dexmedetomidine 10–20 µg/kg IM		
	Neurosteroid		Alfaxalone 1–2 mg IM	Alfaxalone 1–2 mg/kg IM	Alfaxalone 1–2 mg IM
	Dissociative	Ketamine 5–10 mg/kg IM	Ketamine 1–2 mg/kg IM		Ketamine 1–2 mg/kg IM

Adapted from: Grubb, T., Sager, J., Gaynor, J. S., et al. (2020). 2020 AAHA anesthesia and monitoring guidelines for dogs and cats. *Journal of the American Animal Hospital Association*, 56(2), 59–82. 10 µg/kg = 0.01 mg/kg OTM= Oral transmucosal administration

References

1. Aarnes, T. K., Dent, B. T., Lakritz, J., KuKanich, B., Wavreille, V. A., Lerche, P., Pereira, C. H. R., & Bednarski, R. M. (2023). Pharmacokinetics and pharmacodynamics of intramuscular dexmedetomidine in dogs. *American Journal of Veterinary Research*, 84(4).

2. Abrams, J., Brennen, R., & Byosiere, S. E. (2020). Trazodone as a mediator of transitional stress in a shelter: Effects on illness, length of stay, and outcome. *Journal of Veterinary Behavior*, 36, 13–18.

3. Adrian, D., Papich, M. G., Baynes, R., Stafford, E., & Lascelles, B. D. X. (2018). The pharmacokinetics of gabapentin in cats. *Journal of Veterinary Internal Medicine*, 32(6), 1996–2002.

4. Amengual, M., Flaherty, D., Auckburally, A., Bell, A. M., Scott, E. M., & Pawson, P. (2013). An evaluation of anaesthetic induction in healthy dogs using rapid intravenous injection of propofol or alfaxalone. *Veterinary anaesthesia and analgesia*, 40(2), 115–123.

5. Arnold, A., Davis, A., Wismer, T., & Lee, J. A. (2021). Suspected hepatotoxicity secondary to trazodone therapy in a dog. *Journal of Veterinary Emergency and Critical Care*, 31(1), 112–116.

6. Barletta, M., & Raffe, M. (2016). Behavioral response and cost comparison of manual versus pharmacologic restraint protocols in healthy dogs. *The Canadian Veterinary Journal*, 57(3), 258.

7. Bergeron, R., et al. (2002). Physiology and behavior of dogs during air transport. *Canadian Journal of Veterinary Research*, 66(3), 211.

8. Biermann, K., Hungerbühler, S., Mischke, R., & Kästner, S. B. (2012). Sedative, cardiovascular, haematologic and biochemical effects of four different drug combinations administered intramuscularly in cats. *Veterinary anaesthesia and analgesia*, 39(2), 137–150.

9. Bleuer-Elsner, S., Medam, T., & Masson, S. (2021). Effects of a single oral dose of gabapentin on storm phobia in dogs: A double-blind, placebo-controlled crossover trial. *Veterinary Record*, 189(7).

10. Chen, H., Yang, H., Li, M., Peng, H., Guo, W., & Li, M. (2023). Effect of oral administration of gabapentin on the minimum alveolar concentration of isoflurane in cats. *Frontiers in Veterinary Science*, 10, 1117313.

11. Cohen, A. E., & Bennett, S. L. (2015). Oral transmucosal administration of dexmedetomidine for sedation in 4 dogs. *The Canadian Veterinary Journal*, 56(11), 1144.

12. Costa, R. S., Jones, T., Robbins, S., Stein, A., & Borns-Weil, S. (2023). Gabapentin, melatonin, and acepromazine combination prior to

hospital visits decreased stress scores in aggressive and anxious dogs in a prospective clinical trial. *Journal of the American Veterinary Medical Association*, 1(aop), 261(11), 1660–1665.

13. de Azevedo, A. F., Veronezi, T. M., Zardo, I. L., Ferronatto, J. V. B., Franck, K. R., Spiering, A. G., Nunes, L. N., & da Costa, F. V. A. (2023). Does preappointment gabapentin affect neurological examination findings? A prospective, randomized and blinded study in healthy cats. *Journal of Feline Medicine and Surgery*, 25(2),

14. Dean, R. (2017). Using dexmedetomidine to alleviate noise-induced fear and anxiety in dogs. *The Veterinary Record*, 181(25), 688.

15. Dent, B. T., et al. (2019). Pharmacokinetics and pharmacodynamic effects of oral transmucosal and intravenous administration of dexmedetomidine in dogs. *American Journal of Veterinary Research*, 80(10), 969–975.

16. Di Cesare, F., Negro, V., Ravasio, G., Villa, R., Draghi, S., & Cagnardi, P. (2023). Gabapentin: Clinical use and pharmacokinetics in dogs, cats, and horses. *Animals*, 13(12), 2045.

17. Di Franco, C., Evangelista, F., & Briganti, A. (2023). Multiple uses of dexmedetomidine in small animals: A mini review. *Frontiers in Veterinary Science*, 10, 1135124.

18. Elsner, S., Medam, T., & Masson, S. (2021). Effects of a single oral dose of gabapentin on storm phobia in dogs: A double-blind, placebo-controlled crossover trial. *Veterinary Record*, 189(7)

19. Erickson, A., Harbin, K., MacPherson, J., Rundle, K., & Overall, K. L. (2021). A review of pre-appointment medications to reduce fear and anxiety in dogs and cats at veterinary visits. *The Canadian Veterinary Journal*, 62(9), 952.

20. Gilbert-Gregory, S. E., Stull, J. W., Rice, M. R., & Herron, M. E. (2016). Effects of trazodone on behavioral signs of stress in hospitalized dogs. *Journal of the American Veterinary Medical Association*, 249(11), 1281–1291.

21. Gioeni, D., et al. (2020). Oral transmucosal or intramuscular administration of dexmedetomidine–methadone combination in dogs: Sedative and physiological effects. *Animals*, 10(11), 2057.

22. Grubb, T., Sager, J., Gaynor, J. S., et al. (2020). AAHA anesthesia and monitoring guidelines for dogs and cats. *Journal of the American Animal Hospital Association*, 56(2), 59–82.

23. Gruen, M. E., & Sherman, B. L. (2008). Use of trazodone as an adjunctive agent in the treatment of canine anxiety disorders: 56 cases (1995–2007). *Journal of the American Veterinary Medical Association*, 233(12), 1902–1907.

24. Gruen, Margaret E., Simon C. Roe, Emily H. Griffith, and Barbara L. Sherman. The Use of Trazodone to Facilitate Calm Behavior after Elective Orthopedic Surgery in Dogs: Results and Lessons Learned from A clinical Trial. *Journal of Veterinary Behavior* 22 (2017): 41–45.

25. Gurney, M., & Gower, L. (2022). Randomised clinical trial evaluating the effect of a single preappointment dose of gabapentin on signs of stress in hyperthyroid cats. *Journal of Feline Medicine and Surgery*, 24(6), e85–e89.

26. Hauser, H., Campbell, S., Korpivaara, M., Stefanovski, D., Quinlan, M., & Siracusa, C. (2020). In-hospital administration of dexmedetomidine oromucosal gel for stress reduction in dogs during veterinary visits: a randomized, double-blinded, placebo-controlled study. *Journal of Veterinary Behavior*, 39, 77–85.

27. Hopfensperger, M. J., et al. (2013). The use of oral transmucosal detomidine hydrochloride gel to facilitate handling in dogs. *Journal of Veterinary Behavior*, 8(3), 114–123.

28. Horsley, K. T., Olby, N. J., Mitchell, M. A., Aulakh, K. S., & Gines, J. A. (2021). Effect of sedation on the neurological examination of the patellar and withdrawal reflexes in healthy dogs. *Frontiers in Veterinary Science*, 8, 664150.

29. Jay, A. R., Krotscheck, U., Parsley, E., Benson, L., Kravitz, A., Mulligan, A., Silva, J., Mohammed, H., & Schwark, W. S. (2013). Pharmacokinetics, bioavailability, and hemodynamic effects of trazodone after intravenous and oral administration of a single dose to dogs. *American Journal of Veterinary Research,* 74(11), 1450–1456.

30. Johnson, B. A., Aarnes, T. K., Wanstrath, A. W., Pereira, C. H. R., Bednarski, R. M., Lerche, P., & McLoughlin, M. A. (2019). Effect of oral administration of gabapentin on the minimum alveolar concentration of isoflurane in dogs. *American Journal of Veterinary Research*, 80(11), 1007–1009.

31. Jones, C. T., & Fransson, B. A. (2019). Evaluation of the effectiveness of preoperative administration of maropitant citrate and metoclopramide hydrochloride in preventing postoperative clinical gastroesophageal reflux in dogs. *Journal of the American Veterinary Medical Association*, 255(4), 437–445.

32. Karna, S. R., Chambers, P., Singh, P., Lopez-Villalobos, N., & Kongara, K. (2022). Evaluation of analgesic interaction between morphine, maropitant and dexmedetomidine in dogs undergoing ovariohysterectomy. *New Zealand Veterinary Journal*, 70(1), 10–21.

33. Kim, S. A., Borchardt, M. R., Lee, K., Stelow, E. A., & Bain, M. J. (2022). Effects of trazodone on behavioral and physiological signs of stress in dogs during veterinary visits: a randomized double-blind

placebo-controlled crossover clinical trial. *Journal of the American Veterinary Medical Association*, 260(8), 876–883.

34. Korpivaara, M., Huhtinen, M., Aspegrén, J., & Overall, K. (2021). Dexmedetomidine oromucosal gel reduces fear and anxiety in dogs during veterinary visits: A randomised, double-blind, placebo-controlled clinical pilot study. *Veterinary Record*, 189(12)

35. Korpivaara, M., Huhtinen, M., Pohjanjousi, P., & Overall, K. (2022). Tasipimidine, a novel orally administered alpha-2 adrenoceptor agonist, alleviates canine acute anxiety associated with owner departure—A pilot study. *Journal of Veterinary Behavior*, 58, 54–61.

36. Kruszka, M., Graff, E., Medam, T., & Masson, S. (2021). Clinical evaluation of the effects of a single oral dose of gabapentin on fear-based aggressive behaviors in cats during veterinary examinations. *Journal of the American Veterinary Medical Association*, 259(11), 1285–1291.

37. Lamminen, T., Doedée, A., Hyttilä-Hopponen, M., & Kaskinoro, J. (2022). Pharmacokinetics of single and repeated oral doses of pregabalin oral solution formulation in cats. *Journal of Veterinary Pharmacology and Therapeutics*, 45(4), 385–391.

38. Lamminen, T., Korpivaara, M., Aspegrén, J., Palestrini, C., & Overall, K. L. (2023). Pregabalin alleviates anxiety and fear in cats during transportation and veterinary visits—A clinical field study. *Animals*, 13(3), 371.

39. Lueck, L. C., Cameron, S., & Zidan, N. (2022). Effects of trazodone administration on the neurologic examination in healthy dogs. *Journal of Veterinary Internal Medicine*, 36(6), 2142–2148.

40. Maney, J. K., Shepard, M. K., Braun, C., et al. (2013). A comparison of cardiopulmonary and anesthetic effects of an induction dose of alfaxalone or propofol in dogs. *Veterinary Anaesthesia and Analgesia*, 40(3), 237–244.

41. Mathews, K. A., Sinclair, M., Steele, A. M., & Grubb, T. (2018). *Analgesia and anesthesia for the ill or injured dog and cat*. John Wiley & Sons.

42. Meason, C., Salazar, R., & Gentry, C. M. (2023). Alfaxalone provides reliable sedation for intradermal allergen testing in dogs and does not significantly affect results when compared to dexmedetomidine. *Veterinary Dermatology* 34(5), 404–414.

43. Messenger, K. M., Hopfensperger, M., Knych, H. K., & Papich, M. G. (2016). Pharmacokinetics of detomidine following intravenous or oral-transmucosal administration and sedative effects of the oral-transmucosal treatment in dogs. *American Journal of Veterinary Research*, 77(4), 413–420.

44. Muir, W., Lerche, P., Wiese, A., Nelson, L., Pasloske, K., & Whittem, T. (2009). The cardiorespiratory and anesthetic effects of clinical and supraclinical doses of alfaxalone in cats. *Veterinary Anaesthesia and Analgesia,* 36(1), 42–54.

45. Murphy, L. A., Barletta, M., Graham, L. F., Reichl, L. J., Duxbury, M. M., & Quandt, J. E. (2017). Effects of acepromazine and trazodone on anesthetic induction dose of propofol and cardiovascular variables in dogs undergoing general anesthesia for orthopedic surgery. *Journal of the American Veterinary Medical Association*, 250(4), 408–416.

46. Nagore, L., Soler, C., Gil, L., Serra, I., Soler, G., & Redondo, J. I. (2013). Sedative effects of dexmedetomidine, dexmedetomidine–pethidine and dexmedetomidine–butorphanol in cats. *Journal of veterinary pharmacology and therapeutics*, 36(3), 222–228.

47. Ogata, N., & Dodman, N. H. (2011). The use of clonidine in the treatment of fear-based behavior problems in dogs: An open trial. *Journal of Veterinary Behavior*, 6(2), 130–137.

48. Pankratz, K. E., Ferris, K. K., Griffith, E. H., et al. (2018). Use of single-dose oral gabapentin to attenuate fear responses in cage-trap confined community cats: A double-blind, placebo-controlled field trial. *Journal of Feline Medicine and Surgery*, 20(6), 535–543.

49. Park, L. S., & Hoelzler, M. G. (2021). Retrospective evaluation of maropitant and perioperative factors affecting postoperative appetite in cats. *The Canadian Veterinary Journal*, 62(9), 969.

50. Petty, M. C. (2014). Use of trazodone to facilitate postsurgical confinement in dogs. *Journal of the American Veterinary Medical Association*, 245(6), 629–629.

51. Posner, L., & Burns, P. (2009). Sedative agents: tranquilizers, alpha-2 agonists and related agents. In J. Riviere & M. Papich (Eds.), *Veterinary Pharmacology and Therapeutics* (9th ed., pp. 337–380). Wiley-Blackwell.

52. Rankin, D. C. (2015). Sedatives and tranquilizers. In K. A. Grimm, L. A. Lamont, W. J. Tranquilli, et al. (Eds.), *Veterinary Anesthesia and Analgesia* (5th ed., pp. 196–206). Ames, Iowa: Wiley Blackwell.

53. Quimby, J. M., Lorbach, S. K., Saffire, A., Kennedy, A., Wittenburg, L. A., Aarnes, T. K., Creighton, K. J., et al. (2022). Serum concentrations of gabapentin in cats with chronic kidney disease. *Journal of Feline Medicine and Surgery*, 24(12), 1260–1266.

54. Simon, B. T., & Steagall, P. V. (2020). Feline procedural sedation and analgesia: When, why, and how. *Journal of Feline Medicine and Surgery*, 22(11), 1029–1045.

55. Slovak, J. E., & Costa, A. P. (2021). A pilot study of transdermal gabapentin in cats. *Journal of Veterinary Internal Medicine*, 35(4), 1981–1987.

56. Spano, V., Springer, C. M., & Albright, J. D. (2023). Effects of transdermal mirtazapine and oral gabapentin as pre-veterinary visit pharmaceuticals for shelter cats. *Journal of Veterinary Behavior* 64, 47–53.

57. Stevens, B. J., Frantz, E. M., Orlando, J. M., Griffith, E., Harden, L. B., Gruen, M. E., & Sherman, B. L. (2016). Efficacy of a single dose of trazodone hydrochloride given to cats prior to veterinary visits to reduce signs of transport-and examination-related anxiety. *Journal of the American Veterinary Medical Association*, 249(2), 202–207.

58. Stollar, O. O., Moore, G. E., Mukhopadhyay, A., Gwin, W., & Ogata, N. (2022). Effects of a single dose of orally administered gabapentin in dogs during a veterinary visit: a double-blinded, placebo-controlled study. *Journal of the American Veterinary Medical Association*, 260(9), 1031–1040.

59. Tamura, J., Ishizuka, T., Fukui, S., et al. (2015). The pharmacological effects of the anesthetic alfaxalone after intramuscular administration to dogs. *Journal of Veterinary Medical Science*, 77(3), 289–296.

60. Tucker, L. E., Sanchez, A., Valverde, A., Blois, S., Uccello, O., Rutherford, A., Monteith, G., et al. (2023). Pharmacokinetic, sedative, and physiological effects of oral compounded formulations of trazodone alone or in combination with gabapentin in male cats. *Journal of Veterinary Pharmacology and Therapeutics,* 46(5), 300–310.

61. Väisänen, M., Raekallio, M., Kuusela, E., et al. (2002). Evaluation of the perioperative stress response in dogs administered medetomidine or acepromazine as part of the preanesthetic medication. *American Journal of Veterinary Research*, 63, 969–975.

62. Van Haaften, K. A., Forsythe, L. R. E., Stelow, E. A., & Bain, M. J. (2017). Effects of a single preappointment dose of gabapentin on signs of stress in cats during transportation and veterinary examination. *Journal of the American Veterinary Medical Association*, 251(10), 1175–1181.

63. Violette, N. P., Newbold, G. M., Chen, C., Miller, E. J., & Gemensky-Metzler, A. J. (2022). Effects of gabapentin and trazodone on electroretinographic responses in clinically normal dogs. *American Journal of Veterinary Research*, 83(8).

64. Warne, L. N., Beths, T., Whittem, T., Carter, J. E., & Bauquier, S. H. (2015). A review of the pharmacology and clinical application of alfaxalone in cats. *The Veterinary Journal*, 203(2), 141–148.

Index